W. Domschke H. G. Dammann (Eds.)

Prostaglandins and Leukotrienes in Gastrointestinal Diseases

B. M. Peskar K. H. Holtermüller (Co-Eds.)

Springer-Verlag
Berlin Heidelberg New York
London Paris Tokyo

W. Domschke, Prof. Dr. med.
Med. Klinik mit Poliklinik
der Universität Erlangen-Nürnberg
Krankenhausstraße 12
D-8520 Erlangen

B. M. Peskar, Prof. Dr. med.
Arbeitsgruppe Experimentelle
Klinische Medizin
Ruhr-Universität Bochum
D-4630 Bochum 1

H. G. Dammann, Prof. Dr. med.
Krankenhaus Bethanien
Martinistraße 44-66
D-2000 Hamburg 20

K. H. Holtermüller, Prof. Dr. med.
St. Markus-Krankenhaus
Wilhelm-Epstein-Straße 2
D-6000 Frankfurt/Main 50

ISBN-13: 978-3-540-18744-8 e-ISBN-13: 978-3-642-73316-1
DOI: 10.1007/978-3-642-73316-1

Library of Congress Cataloging-in-Publication Data
Prostaglandins and leukotrienes in gastrointestinal diseases.
Includes index.
1. Gastrointestinal system – Diseases – Chemotherapy.
2. Prostaglandins – Therapeutic use – Testing.
3. Leukotrienes – Therapeutic use – Testing. I. Domschke, Wolfram. II. Dammann, Hanns Gerd. [DNLM: 1. Gastrointestinal Diseases – metabolism. 2. Leukotrienes B – metabolism. 3. Prostaglandins – metabolism.
WI 100 P966]
RC802.P75 1988 616.3'3061 88-4489

Preface

In October 1986, recognized authorities from a variety of disciplines met in Lisbon, Portugal, to review recent knowledge on eicosanoids – i.e., prostaglandins, thromboxane A_2, and leukotrienes – and their role in gastrointestinal diseases.

Briefly, in the stomach endogenous as well as exogenous prostaglandins may mediate cytoprotective actions in that they stimulate gastric mucus production, bicarbonate secretion and cellular regeneration while providing adequate mucosal blood flow. In contrast, thromboxane A_2 by vasoconstriction may act as an ulcerogenic substance. Diarrheal states may be associated with prostaglandins of types E and F as they are capable to enhance intestinal water and electrolyte secretions. In chronic inflammatory bowel disease, mucosal synthesis of leukotrienes was found to be increased more markedly than that of prostaglandins suggesting that leukotrienes may have a major part in the pathogenesis of that disease.

In this volume, which is an elaborated collection of the papers given on occasion of the above-mentioned symposium, the facts and problems associated with prostanoid substances are dealt with in four sections on

1. biochemistry, biology and pharmacology of eicosanoids,
2. physiologic and pathophysiologic aspects,
3. established therapeutic implications, and
4. treatment perspectives.

We believe that the publication of these contributions by leading workers in the given fields provides a comprehensive and up-to-date appraisal of the role of eicosanoids in gastrointestinal diseases, and it is hoped that this volume will be of value to both basic scientists and practicing clinicians.

The editors would like to express their thanks to the authors, and in particular to the Bayer Company for sponsorship of the Lisbon symposium which was a scientifically stimulating event.

January 1988

W. Domschke
H. G. Dammann
B. M. Peskar
K. H. Holtermüller

Contents

Biology and Pharmacology of Prostaglandins and Leukotrienes

Protective Effects on the Gastrointestinal Mucosa. New Aspects of the Last two Years

Contributors

BAUMGARTNER, A.
Gastrointestinal Unit, Inselspital Bern, 3010 Bern, Switzerland

BERNIER
Clinique de Gastro-Entérologie de L'Hopital Saint Lazare,
107 Rue du Faubourg Saint-Denis, 75010 Paris, France

BERTACCINI, G.
Instituto die Farmacologia, Università di Parma, 43100 Parma, Italy

BEUBLER, E.
Institut für experimentelle und klinische Pharmakologie,
Universität Graz, Universitätsplatz 4, 8010 Graz, Austria

BIANCHI PORRO, G.
L. Sacco Hospital, Via G. B. Grassi 74, 20157 Milano, Italy

BOYD, E. J. S.
Gartnavel General Hospital, 1053 Great Western Road,
Glasgow G 12 OYN, United Kingdom

BUKHAVE, K.
Department of Medical Gastroenterology, Herlev Hospital,
University of Copenhagen, 2400 Copenhagen NV, Denmark

BUSS, P.
Abteilung für Allgemeine Chirurgie, Chirurgische Universitätsklinik
Hugstetter Straße 55, 7800 Freiburg, Germany

COHEN, M. M.
Department of Surgery, University of Toronto and Mount Sinai Hospital,
440-600 University Avenue, Toronto Ontario M5G 1X5, Canada

CORUZZI, G.
Instituto die Farmacologia, Università di Parma, 43100 Parma, Italy

DAMMANN, H. G.
Krankenhaus Bethanien, Martinistraße 44-66, 2000 Hamburg, Germany

DAU, B.
Krankenhaus Bethanien, Martinistraße 44-46, 2000 Hamburg, Germany

DEMOL, P.
BAYER AG, Klinische Forschung I, 5600 Wuppertal-Elberfeld, Germany

DOMSCHKE, W.
Medizinische Klinik mit Poliklinik der Universität Erlangen-Nürnberg, Krankenhausstraße 12, 8520 Erlangen, Germany

DREYER, M.
Krankenhaus Bethanien, Martinistraße 44-46, 2000 Hamburg, Germany

EGGSTEIN, ST.
Abteilung für Allgemeine Chirurgie, Chirurgische Universitätsklinik, Hugstetter Straße 55, 7800 Freiburg, Germany

FARTHMANN, E. H.
Abteilung für Allgemeine Chirurgie, Chirurgische Universitätsklinik, Hugstetter Straße 55, 7800 Freiburg, Germany

FLEMSTRÖM, G.
Department of Physiology and Medical Biophysics, Uppsala University Biomedical Center, P.O.B. 572, 751 23 Uppsala, Sweden

FLORENT, CH.
Hopital Saint Antoine, Rue du Faubourg Saint-Antoine, 75012 Paris, France

FORD-HUTCHINSON, A. W.
Merck Frosst Canada Inc., P.O.B. 1005, Pointe Claire-Dorval, Quebec H9R 4P8, Canada

FRITSCH, W. P.
II. Medizinische Klinik, Städtisches Krankenhaus, Weinberg 1, 3200 Hildesheim, Germany

GRAHAM, D. Y.
Digestive Disease Section, VA Medical Center (111D), 2002 Holcombe Boulevard, Houston TX 77211, USA

GRANSTRÖM, E.
Department of Physiological Chemistry, Karolinska Institutet, P.O.B. 60400, 104 01 Stockholm, Sweden

HALTER, F.
Gastrointestinal Unit, Inselspital Bern, 3010 Bern, Switzerland

HOLTERMÜLLER, K. H.
1. Medizinische Klinik, St. Markus-Krankenhaus, Wilhelm-Epstein-Straße 2, 6000 Frankfurt 50, Germany

IMDAHL, A.
Abteilung für Allgemeine Chirurgie, Chirurgische Universitätsklinik, Hugstetter Straße 55, 7800 Freiburg, Germany

JOHANSSON, C.
Gi Unit, Department of Medicine, Karolinska Hospital, 104 01 Stockholm, Sweden

KOBAYASHI, Y.
Department of Geriatric Medicine, Faculty of Medicine, Kyoto University, Kyoto 606, Japan

KOELZ, H. R.
Gastrointestinal Unit, Inselspital Bern, 3010 Bern, Switzerland

LANGMAN, M. J. S.
Department of Therapeutics, Queens Medical Centre, Nottingham NG7 2UH, United Kingdom

MIYAKE, T.
Department of Geriatric Medicine, Faculty of Medicine, Kyoto University, Kyoto 606, Japan

MÜLLER, P.
Abteilung für Gastroenterologie, Medizinische Universitätsklinik Heidelberg, Bergheimer Straße 58, 6900 Heidelberg, Germany

MURAKAMI, M.
Department of Geriatric Medicine, Faculty of Medicine, Kyoto University, Kyoto 606, Japan

O'BRIEN, P.
Department of Surgery, Monash University, Alfred Hospital, Commercial Road, Prahran 3181, Melbourne, Australia

PARENTE, F.
L. Sacco Hospital, Vika G. B. Grassi 74, 20157 Milano, Italy

PESKAR, B. M.
Arbeitsgruppe Experimentelle Klinische Medizin,
Ruhr-Universität Bochum, 4630 Bochum 1, Germany

PIHAN, G.
Department of Pathology, Brigham and Women's Hospital,
75 Francis Street, Boston MA 02115

RACHMILEWITZ, D.
Department of Gastroenterology, Hadassah University
Hospital, P.O.B. 12000, Jerusalem 91120, Israel

RAMPTON, D. S.
Department of Hospital Therapeutics, Newham General
Hospital, London E13 8SL, United Kingdom

RASK-MADSEN, J.
Section of Gastroenterology, Department of Medicine B,
Bispebjerg Hospital, University of Denmark,
2400 Copenhagen NV, Denmark

REES, W. D. W.
Department of Gastroenterology, Hope Hospital, University
of Manchester, Salford M6 8HD, United Kingdom

RUPPIN, H.
Medizinische Klinik mit Poliklinik der Universität Erlangen-Nürnberg,
Krankenhausstraße 12, 8520 Erlangen, Germany

SCHIESSEL, V.
I. Chirurgische Universitätsklinik, Alser Straße, 1090 Wien, Austria

SCHUMPELICK, V.
Chirurgische Klinik, Klinikum der RWTH, Pauwelstraße,
5100 Aachen, Germany

SHARON, P.
Gastroenterology Unit, Department of Internal Medicine, Biker Cholin Hospital,
2–5 Strauss Street, P.O.B. 492, Jerusalem 91002, Israel

SHORROCK, C. J.
Department of Gastroenterology, Hope Hospital, University
of Manchester, Salford M6 8HD, United Kingdom

SIMON, B.
Krankenhaus Schwetzingen, Bodelschwingstraße 11, 6830 Schwetzingen

OLL, A. H.
/A Wadsworth Hospital Center, Building 115, Los Angeles CA 90073, USA

SONTAG, S. J.
Veterans Administration, Edward J. Hines Hospital (11C2),
Hines IL 60141, USA

SZABO, S.
Department of Pathology, Brigham and Women's Hospital,
75 Francis Street, Boston MA 02115, USA

WALTER, T. A.
Krankenhaus Bethanien, Martinistraße 44-46, 2000 Hamburg, Germany

WHITTLE, B. J. R.
Department of Mediator Pharmacology, Wellcome Research Laboratories,
Langley Court, Beckenham Kent BR3 3BS, United Kingdom

WORMSLEY, K. G.
Ninewells Hospital and Medical School, Dundee DD1 9SY, Scotland

Biology and Pharmacology of Prostaglandins and Leukotrienes

Biosynthesis and Metabolism of Prostaglandins and Thromboxanes. Quantitative Determination in Biological Material

E. GRANSTRÖM

Introduction

The eicosanoids constitute a large and still growing family of oxygenated and biologically active compounds, which are derived from certain polyunsaturated, essential fatty acids. The best known of these are the prostaglandins (PGs) and thromboxanes (TXs) of the 2-series, i.e. bisenoic compounds originating in arachidonic acid.

Biosynthesis

The biosynthesis of prostaglandins and thromboxanes proceeds via several steps shared by the two types of substances. The first step, which is also the rate-limiting one, is liberation of the precursor fatty acid from phospholipid stores, presumably mainly by phospholipase A_2 hydrolysis (see review in [1]). The free arachidonic acid is then converted into two prostaglandin endoperoxides, PGG_2 and PGH_2, by the action of endoperoxide synthetase. The first step in this conversion is introduction of molecular oxygen at C-9 and C-11, which is catalyzed by the ubiquitous enzyme, fatty acid cyclooxygenase (see review in [2]). PGG_2 and PGH_2 are highly potent and unstable compounds, which can undergo a variety of different chemical and metabolic fates. PGH_2 is in fact the immediate precursor of at least six different major compounds: the "classical" prostaglandins (PGD_2, PGE_2 and $PGF_{2\alpha}$), prostacyclin (PGI_2), thromboxane A_2 (TXA_2), and 12-hydroxy-heptadecatrienoic acid (HHT), the latter with the concomitant formation of malondialdehyde (MDA).

PGH_2 is converted enzymatically or nonenzymatically into PGD_2 and PGE_2 by isomerization, and in the presence of a reductase or reducing factors also into $PGF_{2\alpha}$. Several endoperoxide isomerases have been studied and partially purified [2]. Formation of PGD_2 is also greatly enhanced by albumin. The occurrence of an endoperoxide reductase, cartalyzing the biosynthesis of $PGF_{2\alpha}$ from PGH_2, is somewhat less certain.

Metabolism and Quantitative Determination

Attempts to elucidate the biological roles of these potent compounds rely to a great extent on accurate methods for their quantitation. Several serious difficulties are, however, encountered in this field. Firstly, because of their high potencies, PGs and

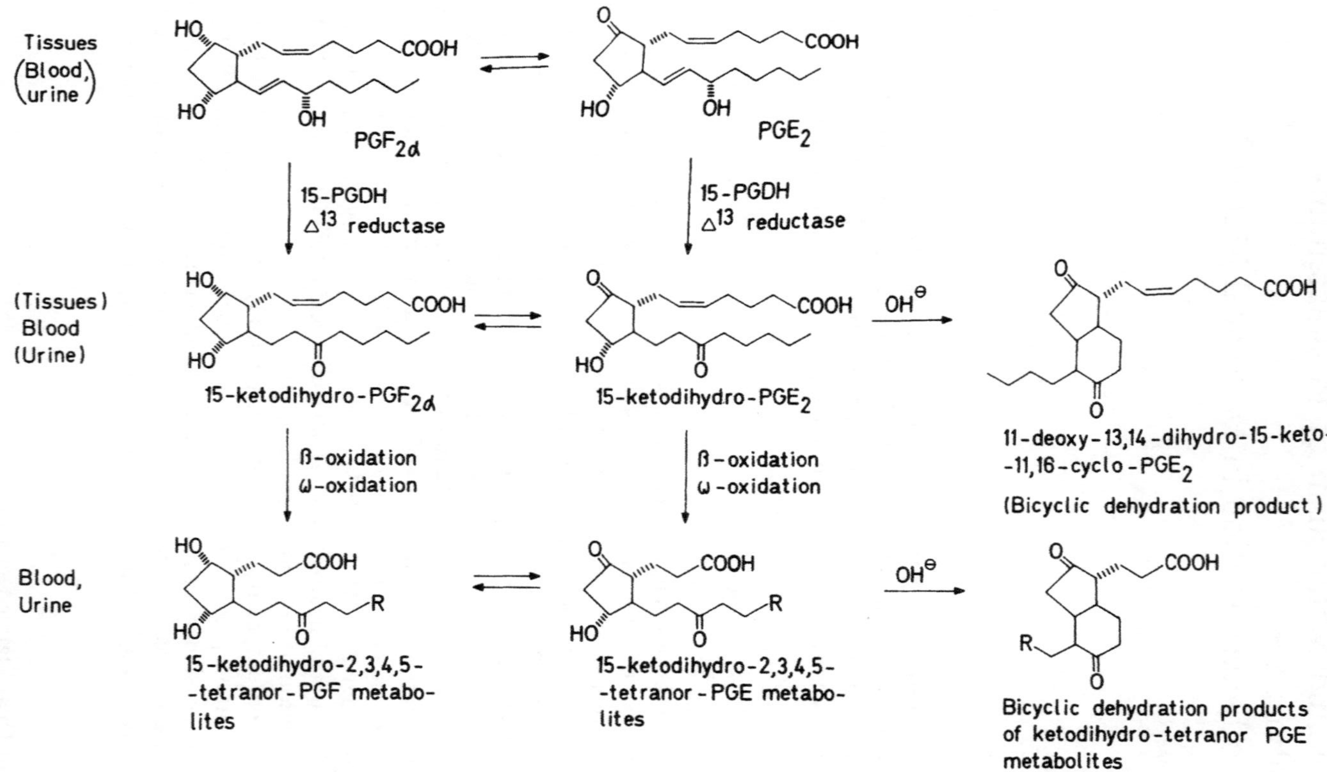

Fig. 1. Metabolism of PGE_2 and $PGF_{2\alpha}$ with structures of major metabolites and stable degradation products. Note extensive interconversion at all levels. Suggestions for most suitable compounds for monitoring in different biological material are given; less suitable materials are given within *parentheses*

TXs occur only in very low amounts in most biological material. Secondly, many tissues have a high capacity for PG and TX biosynthesis as well as further metabolism, which may be elicited ex vivo as an artifact. Thus estimation of the true in vivo amounts of a certain compound may be difficult.

To some extent, the latter difficulty may be circumvented by monitoring a different target molecule. For example, early attempts to quantitate $PGF_{2\alpha}$ biosynthesis in the body by measurement of the primary compound in peripheral plasma gave highly misleading results, whereas monitoring a major circulating metabolite, 15-keto-13,14-dihydro-$PGF_{2\alpha}$, reliably reflected the endogenous situation [3], (see Fig. 1).

Another possibility is the measurement of highly degraded metabolites, tetranor dicarboxylic compounds (Fig. 1), which appear later in the circulation after PG release and also have longer half-lives. The latter factor renders these compounds particularly suited for assay in studies based on few or even single blood samples. The highly degraded compounds are also major PGF metabolites in the urine of most studied species, and are thus suitable targets for assay in this biological fluid and serve as an index of total body PGF production [3]. $PGF_{2\alpha}$ itself, as well as other primary PGs, is also excreted in small amounts into urine but reflects mainly the renal biosynthesis.

Metabolic fates of PGE compounds are similar to those of PGFs, and assay methods for 15-keto-13,14-dihydro-PGE_2 (blood) and its tetranor dicarboxylic counterpart (urine) have been developed. However, the chemical instability of all PGEs suggests a different approach. Quantitative conversion of the unstable PGE compounds into stable degradation products prior to assay (such as the bicyclic substances depicted in Fig. 1) has proved a safer method [3].

The metabolism of PGD_2 has been elucidated comparatively recently [see review, 4]. The compound is even more unstable than PGE_2 and is rapidly dehydrated in the ring structure as well as the methyl side chain. Three major degradation products have been identified (Fig. 2) [5, 6]. The half-life of PGD_2 in aqueous medium is thus rather short, particularly in the presence of albumin. The best alternative for the scientist interested in assaying PGD_2 in vitro is either to monitor one of the degradation products, or to convert the unstable compound rapidly into a stable derivative such as the 11-methoxime prior to assay [7].

In vivo, however, the situation is quite different. One of the major metabolic fates of PGD_2 is reduction of the 11-keto group to a hydroxyl. Thus, a PGF compound is formed which is chemically quite stable [4]. In extensive metabolic studies by the Vanderbilt group, it was discovered that the 11-hydroxyl group had the β configuration in the majority of PGF products, in contrast to structurally similar metabolites derived from $PGF_{2\alpha}$ [8, 9] (Fig. 2). The major urinary metabolite in the human is 9α,11β-dihydroxy-15-keto-2,3,18,19-tetranorprost-5-ene-1,20-dioic acid, which can form a unique tricyclic structure by a combination of hemiketal formation and lactonization: this compound is thus particularly suitable for assay, since it originates exclusively in PGD_2 and cannot be confused with other sources.

Prostacyclin and Thromboxane

Two products of PGH_2 metabolism which can only be formed by enzymatic catalysis are PGI_2 and TXA_2. These highly potent compounds have some features in common:

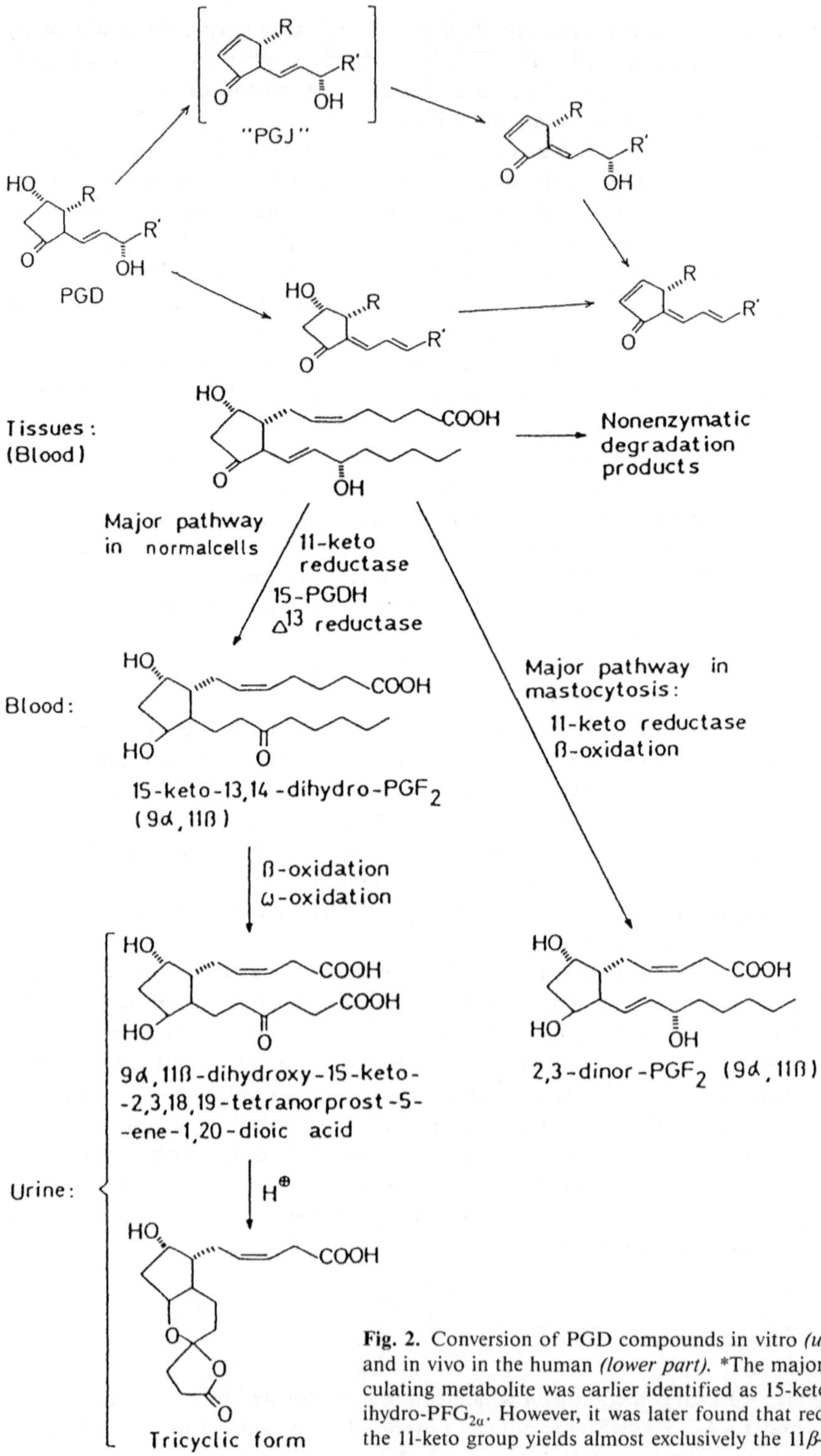

Fig. 2. Conversion of PGD compounds in vitro *(upper part)* and in vivo in the human *(lower part)*. *The major circulating metabolite was earlier identified as 15-keto-13,14-ihydro-$PFG_{2\alpha}$. However, it was later found that reduction of the 11-keto group yields almost exclusively the 11β-hydroxyl

they are chemically very unstable, and decompose by spontaneous hydrolysis into biologically inactive products, 6-keto-$PGF_{1\alpha}$ and TXB_2, respectively [see reviews, 10, 11]. Biologically, however, they are rather the opposites of one another.

Metabolism of these compounds has mainly been studied using their hydrolysis products as starting material. While PGI_2 later became available for direct metabolic studies, the corresponding situation has not yet become possible for elucidation of thromboxane metabolism, although chemical synthesis of the compound has now been accomplished [12].

Initially reported differences in the metabolism of 6-keto-$PGF_{1\alpha}$ and PGI_2 were later found to be mainly caused by differences in employed doses and were thus only apparent discrepancies. The metabolic fates of PGI_2 are rather similar to those of other PGs: dehydrogenation at C-15, reduction of the Δ^{13} double bond, β-oxidation, and ω-oxidation. Certain differences are, however, also seen: in contrast to the classical PGs, PGI_2 is not taken up by the lung; β-oxidation stops at the dinor stage; and biliary excretion of metabolites is prominent [4].

6-Keto-$PGF_{1\alpha}$ is the most commonly monitored prostacyclin metabolite in the circulation. As is the case with other PGs, however, reported levels of this compound far exceed the theoretically possible ones. The likely explanation is, again, uncontrolled formation of PGI_2 during sample collection or processing, and this necessitates the monitoring of a different metabolite. Two prominent compounds in the circulation as well as urine are 2,3-dinor-6,15-diketo-13,14-dihydro-$PGF_{1\alpha}$ and its ω-carboxylated counterpart; dinor-6-keto-$PGF_{1\alpha}$ is the major urinary compound but it less prominent in the circulation. Measurement of 6-keto-$PGF_{1\alpha}$ in the urine provides an index of the renal prostacyclin production.

Increased thromboxane biosynthesis is postulated to be associated with various cardiovascular diseases such as unstable angina [13]. Numerous attempts to study the biological roles of TXA_2 have been based on measurement of TXB_2 in plasma. However, reported levels are unrealistically high and far in excess of the true endogenous concentration. The high measured levels in blood samples are no doubt caused by the local formation of thromboxane during normal hemostatic events at the puncture site as well as by mechanically stimulated blood cells ex vivo [14].

To avoid such sources of error, a different metabolite should be assayed: either a urinary metabolite or a circulating compound that is not formed as an artifact under any circumstances. Urinary dinor-TXB_2 has been successfully monitored in a number of studies but may not be a suitable assay target for the detection of shortlasting thromboxane release. A number of other metabolites have been identified [15], and some of these occur in blood as well as urine [16, 17]. A prominent TXB_2 metabolite in several species is 11-dehydro-TXB_2, which seems to fulfill the required criteria for a suitable thromboxane parameter [16–18]. However, it should be pointed out that this compound is a metabolite of TXB_2. Whether 11-dehydro-TXB_2 is also a major metabolite of TXA_2 remains to be established.

Summary

In summary, when selecting the optimal compound for quantitative studies, several factors have to be considered: the biosynthetic capacity and profile of the studied biological system; the chemical stability of the chosen compound; the time aspect, and so on. It should be pointed out in this context that the earlier prevailing attitude in this field, viz. to develop highly specific methods for the measurement of single compounds, in order to pin-point their biological roles, is now gradually beeing replaced by the opposite one. A great deal of effort is at present being devoted to the development of profiling assay methods, where the aim is to obtain as complete a picture of formed products as possible. Even so interpretation of data is very difficult. Extensive interconversion of PGs into one another is known to take place, and established increases in the level of one compound are not necessarily caused by an overproduction. They may as well be caused by a more distal block of a metabolic step. Quantitative studies are only one tool for elucidation of the biological roles of the eicosanoids, and they should preferably be combined with studies of inhibitors, receptors, biological effects of relevant compounds, and so on.

Acknowledgement. This review was supported in part by a grant from the Swedish Medical Research Council, project no. 03X-05915.

References

1. Irvine RF (1982) How is the level of free arachidonic acid controlled im mammalian cells? Biochem J *204:* 3–6
2. Yamamoto S (1983) Enzymes in the arachdonic acid cascade. *In:* Prostaglandins and Related Substances (Pace-Asciak CR and Granström E, eds), New Comprehensive Biochemistry. Elsevier, vol *5:* pp 171–202
3. Oliw E, Granström E and Änggård E (1983) The prostaglandins and essential fatty acids. *Ibid,* pp –44
4. Granström E and Kumlin M (1987) Metabolism of prostaglandins and lipoxygenase products: Relevance for eicosanoid assay. *In:* Prostaglandins and Related Substances: A Practical Approach, (Slater TF, McDonald-Gibson RG, Nigam S and Benedetto C, eds), IRL Press, Oxford pp 5–27
5. Fitzpatrick FA and Wynalda MA (1983) Albumin-catalyzed metabolism of prostaglandin D_2. Identification of products formed in vitro. J Biol Chem *258:* 11713–11718
6. Kikawa Y, Narumiya S, Fukushima M, Wakatsuka H and Hayaishi O (1984) 9-Deoxy-Δ^9, Δ^{12}-13, 14-dihydroprostaglandin D_2, a metabolite of prostaglandin D_2formed in human plasma. Proc Natl Acad Sci USA *81:* 1317–1320
7. Maclouf J, Corvazier E and Wang Z (1986) Development of a radioimmunoassay for prostaglandin D_2 using an antiserum against 11-methoxime prostaglandin D_2. Prostaglandins *31:* 123–132
8. Liston TE and Roberts LJ II (1985) Metabolic fate of radiolabeled prostaglandin D_2 in a normal human male volunteer. J Biol Chem *260:* 13172–13180
9. Liston TE and Roberts LJ II (1985) Transformation of prostaglandin D_2 to 9α, 11β-prostaglandin F_2): A unique biologically active prostaglandin produced enzymatically in vivo in humans. Proc Natl Acad Sci USA *82:* 6030–6034
10. Pace-Asciak CR and Gryglewski R (1983) The prostacyclins. *In:* Prostaglandins and Related Substances (Pace-Asciak CR and Granström E, eds), New Comprehensive Biochemistry, Elsevier, vol *5:* pp 95–126
11. Granström E, Diczfalusy U and Hamburg M (1983) The thromboxanes. *Ibid,* pp 45–94
12. Bhagwat SS, Hamann PR, Still WC, Bunting S and Fitzpatrick FA (1985) Synthesis and structure of the platelet aggregation factor thromboxane A_2. Nature *315:* 511–513
13. Lewis HD, Davis JW, Archibald DG, Steinke WE, Smitherman TC, Doherty JE III, Schnaper HW, LeWinter MM, Linares E, Pouget JM, Sabharwal SC, Chesler E and DeMots H (1983) Protective effects of aspirin against acute myocardial infarction and death in men with unstable angina. Results of a veterans adminstration cooperative study. N Engl J Med *309:* 396–403

14. Granström E (1986) Methodology in prostaglandin and thromboxane assay. Progr Lipid Res *25:* 119–127
15. Roberts LJ II, Sweetman BJ and Oates JA (1981) Metabolism of thromboxane B_2 in man. J Biol Chem *256:* 8384–8393
16. Westlund P, Kumlin M, Nordenström A and Granström E (1986) Circulating and urinary thromboxane B_2 metabolites in the rabbit: 11-dehydro-thromboxane B_2 as parameter of thromboxane production. Prostaglandins *31:* 413–442
17. Westlund P, Granström E, Kumlin M and Nordenström A (1986) Identification of 11-dehydro-TXB_2 as a suitable parameter for monitoring thromboxane production in the human. Prostaglandins *31:* 929–960
18. Lawson JA, Patrono C, Ciabattoni G and FitzGerald GA1986) Long-lived enzymatic metabolites of thromboxane B_2 in the human circulation. Anal Biochem *155:* 198–205

Discussion Following the Report of Prof. Granström

WHITTLE

A widely used technique used for the measurement of the effects of aspirin and other nonsteroidal anti-inflammatory drugs on thromboxane formation is to administer the drugs and then to take the blood, allow it to clot in vitro, and then measure the TXB_2 levels in that serum. Do you know whether there is any metabolism of thromboxane in those samples? And whether it is a good measure of TXB_2 formation?

GRANSTRÖM

I think that the system is fairly safe to use and resistant against artifacts. It will, of course, reflect the biosynthetic capacity rather than anything endogenous. Both we and the Vanderbilt group have looked into the possible in vitro formation of metabolites in clotting as well as in nonclotting blood, and the formation of, for instance, 11-dehydro-TXB_2 is less than 1% of TXB_2 formed. So I think that is a reasonably safe approach to study the effects of these drugs.

PESKAR

Is TXA_2 metabolized the same way as TXB_2? You have shown that there is a difference for the metabolism of PGI_2 as compared to 6-keto-PGF_1.

GRANSTRÖM

Unfortunately, I think there is some risk that it is metabolized in a slightly different way. We know of some metabolic fates of TXA_2 that have to do with its enormous reactivity. It is, for instance, bound to albumin in different ways, and we do not know whether it is exclusively released again as TXB_2 or not. And there has been some controversy about the formation of, for instance, 15-keto-dihydro-TXB_2, which is very seldom seen as a metabolite of TXB_2 but may be a rather major metabolite of TXA_2 under some circumstances; so we have this additional uncertainty. 11-Dehydro-TXB_2 may rather be an indicator of TXB_2 formation, so we can only hope that TXB_2 is a reasonably major metabolite of TXA_2 in the body. Nobody knows yet, and I think it will be some time before anyone can study the metabolism of TXA_2 in vivo. I do not know how this should be done technically.

LANGMAN

Can you tell me a little about how you get to your starting point?

GRANSTRÖM

I personally do not know very much about it, but there is a lot known. Arachidonic acid exists in many different phospholipid classes, and it depends on which type of cell you are studying. Also the release mechanism may differ. I think the usually dominating mechanism is by activation of a phospholipase A_2, but there are also other ways by which it could be released.

PESKAR

If one wants to monitor prostaglandin or thromboxane formation in man, would you suggest to measure plasma levels on the urinary excretion of prostaglandin or thromboxane metabolites. What is more reliable?

GRANSTRÖM

It would depend on what you are looking for. I think, if you can be sure technically that you get complete collection of all the urine from a patient during a 24-h period, it is a rather safe index of a total body production. But I very much doubt that a small, local, short-lasting increase in prostaglandin formation, say from a small site somewhere in the body, would be reflected in the urinary levels. So, if you are looking for something specific, for example, local production of thromboxane in coronary vessels during a short attack of angina, you may have to use a different approach.

WHITTLE

When you measure the urinary metabolites of the various eicosanoids do you not have the complicating factor that you are also measuring the release not only into the systemic circulation but also from the kidneys themselves? Thus, if you have a pathogenic situation, for example, where the kidneys may be inflamed, will you not get an imbalance of the profile of products in the urine not necessarily reflecting whole-body formation?

GRANSTRÖM

This is very true. And I think this is probably the reason why people are turning to profiling assays instead, for we have seen many examples of changes in the metabolic pattern during different conditions, such as the mastocytosis example I showed some time ago. And there is also the problem of interpretation of data: If you do find increased amounts of a certain compound, it does not necessarily mean that there is an increase in the formation of it. It could also reflect a block in the further metabolism of the compound.

Involvement of the Eicosanoids, Thromboxane A_2 and Leukotriene C_4 in Gastric Mucosal Damage

B. J. R. WHITTLE

Introduction

The metabolites of arachidonic acid, the eicosanoids, formed by the cyclo-oxygenase and lipoxygenase enzymes exert potent actions on the function and integrity of the gastric mucosa. Since local ischaemia may be involved in the pathogenesis of various forms of gastric damage and ulceration, the local vasodilator actions exerted by many of the anti-ulcer prostanoids such as PGE_2 [2] may contribute to the overall process of mucosal protection. A direct action on the vascular endothelium may also contribute, and it has been demonstrated that the potent protective prostanoid, 16,16-dimethyl PGE_2, can prevent the microcirculatory stasis induced by the damaging agent ethanol [3].

Not all eicosanoids, however, exert protective effects on the gastric mucosa. Thus the cyclo-oxygenase product, thromboxane A_2 (TxA_2), derived predominantly from platelets, is a potent vasoconstrictor in many vascular beds. It is a highly labile moiety, with a half-life of less than 30 seconds under physiological conditions, and to study its pharmacological actions, it therefore must be generated locally, Thus when its precusor arachidonic acid was infused into the canine gastric arterial circulation so as to incubate with the blood-borne platelets to generate TxA_2, dose-related vasonconstriction in the gastric circulation was observed. When the canine gastric mucosa was concurrently exposed to a weak topical irritant such as the bile salt, sodium taurocholate, extensive mucosal damage rapidly ensued [14]. To extend these observations further, studies using the chemically-stable endoperoxide analogue, 11α-9α epoxy-methano-PGH_2 (U-46619) which behaves as a thromboxane mimetic [1] were conducted.

Pro-Ulcerogenic Effects of the Thromboxane Mimetic

A segment of acid-secreting fundic mucosa of the stomach of the pentobarbital-anaesthetized dog was encased *in situ* in a lucite chamber consisting of two compartments and the vasculature was pump-perfused with blood (10 ml min^{-1}) from a cannulated femoral artery [14]. The endoperoxide analogue U-46619 (Upjohn Company, Kalamazoo) was infused locally into the arterial blood line, close to stomach.

Topical instillation into the gastric chamber of acid (100 mM HCl) or an acid-taurocholate (5 mM in 100 mM HCl) mixture caused only a low incidence of

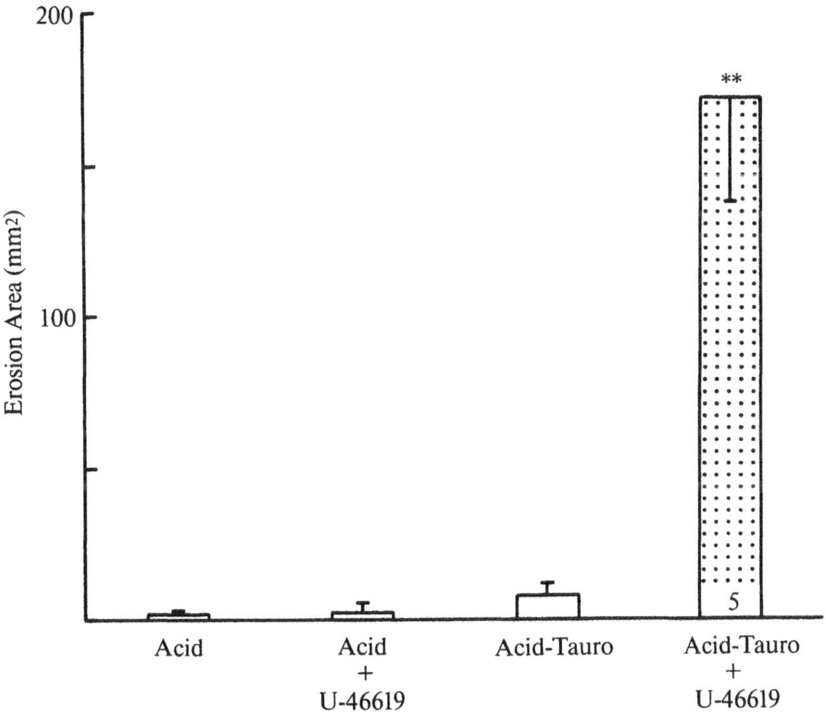

Fig. 1. Gastric mucosal damage following a 30 min period of topical application of acid (100 mM HCl), or acidified taurocholate (5 mM in 100 mM HCl) either alone or during local intra-arterial infusion of the thromboxane mimetic, U-46619 (5 ng $kg^{-1}min^{-1}$) in the dog gastric chamber preparation. Results, shown as lesion area, are the mean ± s.e.m. of 5 experiments, where statistical significant change from control is $^{**}P < 0.01$. Data are adapted from [15]

macroscopically visible gastric mucosal damage during the 30 min observation period. Likewise, intra-arterial infusion of the epoxy-methano-endoperoxide analogue (5 ng $kg^{-1}min^{-1}$) during exposure to the acid solution alone failed to substantially damage the mucosa (Fig 1). This dose of U-46619 caused an increase in gastric perfusion pressure of Δ 66 ± 5 mmHg ($n = 6$; $P < 0.001$), indicating marked vasoconstriction in the gastric circulation. When the mucosa was exposed to acid-taurocholate, extensive mucosal damage developed during the 30 min infusion of the thromboxane mimetic (Fig. 1). As found with TxA_2 itself, localized areas of blanching, engorgement, and stasis could clearly be observed during the infusion of the thromboxane mimetic. These areas often were the initial or predominant sites for necrosis and punctate bleeding, which became apparent within 10 to 15 min of the infusion. Sloughing of the mucosal epithelial tissue led to extensive bleeding from the exposed underlying tissue following termination of the infusion.

Protective Actions of a Thromboxane Synthase Inhibitor

To investigate the role of locally generated TxA_2 in the pathogenesis of gastric mucosal damage, the protective actions of the thromboxane synthase inhibitor, 1-benzyl imidazole, against ethanol-induced lesions was studied. Gastric mucosal lesions in male rats which had been starved 18 h previously (but allowed water) were induced by the oral administration of 1 ml of an acidified ethanol mixture (40% ethanol in 100 mM HCl) via a rubber intragastric tube [12]. The degree of gastric damage was assessed 2 h after treatment, with each mucosa being coded to avoid observer bias and assigned a lesion score based on the incidence and severity of the macroscopic lesions, visible as discrete haemorrhagic erosions.

Pre-treatment with 1-benzyl imidazole as the fumerate salt (BZI, Wellcome Research Laboratories) at doses of 1.25–20 mg kg^{-1} administered by an intragastric tube (0.1 ml/100g body weight) 30 minutes prior to challenge, reduced the incidence and severity of the gastric erosions seen 2 h after acid-ethanol treatment, as shown in Fig. 2. The ID_{50} (dose inhibiting gastric lesions by 50%) was calculated to be 3.2 mg kg^{-1}. BZI 1–10 mg kg^{-1} s.c. was also effective following parenteral administration,

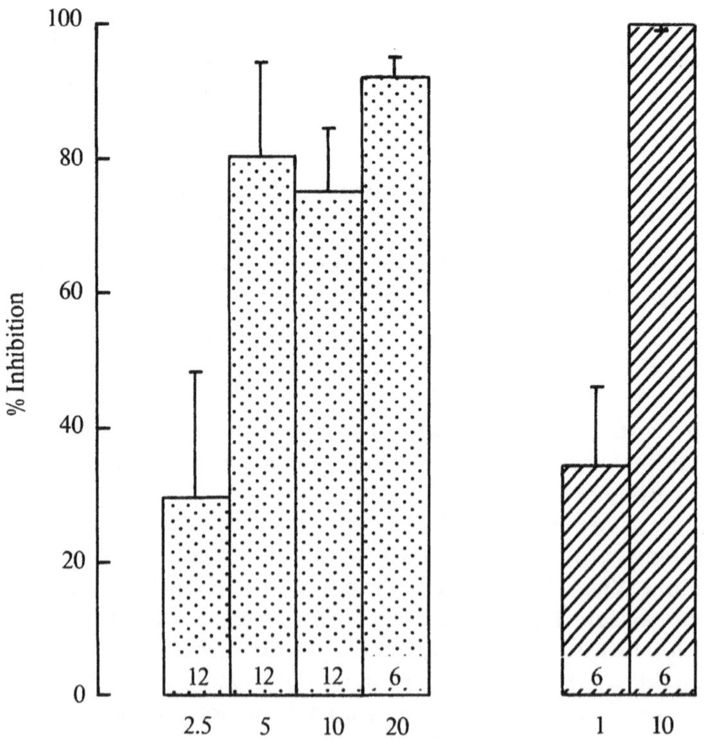

Fig. 2. Inhibition of gastric mucosal damage induced by intragastric administration of acidified ethanol (40% in 100 mM HCl) by 1 hour pre-treatment with the thromboxane synthase inhibitor, 1-benzyl-imidazole (BZI; 1–20 mg kg^{-1}), in the rat. Results are shown as mean ± s.e.m. from (n) rats. Data are adapted from [12]

administered 1 hour prior to challenge (ID_{50} 3.8 mg kg^{-1}). This indicates that the protective action was not the result of a local buffering action of BZI in the gastric lumen or from a local weak-irritant action, which has been shown to confer some protection to the gastric mucosa.

Microcirculatory Actions of the Thromboxane Mimetic and Leukotriene C_4

To understand further the pro-ulcerogenic actions of the thromboxane mimetic, its actions on the gastric microcirculation were investigated. In addition, the vasoactive effects of the peptido-lipid lipoxygenase product, leukotriene C_4 (LTC_4), were likewise determined.

The *in vivo* microscopy technique described by Guth and colleagues [2, 3] was used to study gastric submucosal arteriolar and venular responses in the pentobarbital-anaesthetized rat. A fibre-optic light carrier rod was inserted into the gastric lumen via an incision in the forestomach to transilluminate the stomach wall. After removal of the serosal and muscle layers, a shallow disk with a 5 mm orifice was sealed over the exposed submucosa for the local application of Krebs' solution and the compounds under investigation. This system allowed direct microscopic visualization and measurement of the submucosal vascular networks, which were video-recorded via a T.V. camera. Arterioles and venules of resting diameter 20 and 50 μm were selected for study. Changes in the diameter of the microvessels were subsequently determined by an image-splitting monitor.

Topical application of U-46619 (1–1000 nM) to the exposed submucosal vascular bed reduced vessel diameter in both arterioles and venules, reaching plateau responses

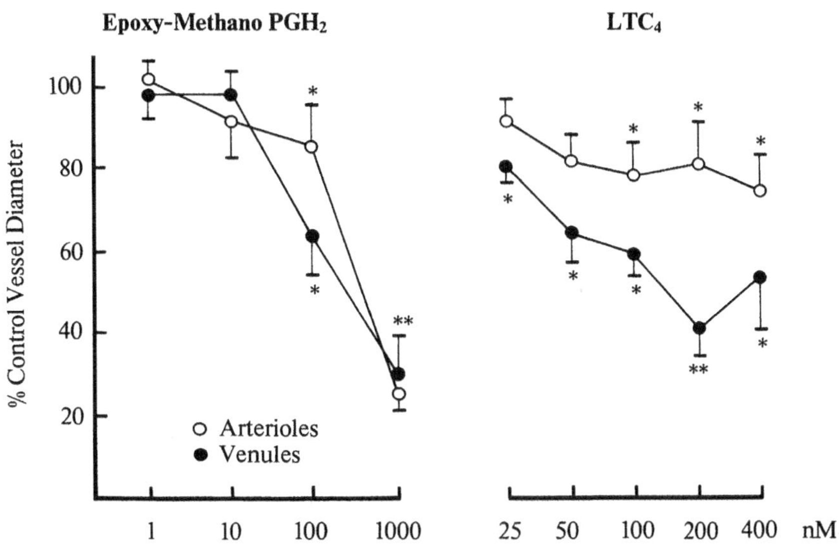

Fig. 3. Vasoconstrictor effects of the thromboxane mimetic U-46619 (1–1000 nM) and leukotriene C_4 (25–400 nM) on the gastric submucosal arterioles (○——○) and venules (●---●) of the rat. Results are shown as % change in vessel diameter from control value, mean ± s.e.m. of 6–11 experiments, where $^*P < 0.05$; $^{**}P < 0.01$. Data are adapted from [16]

within 2 min of application (Fig. 2). At the highest concentration studied, the reduction in vessel diameter was comparable for both arterioles and venules. Application of LTC_4 (25–400 nM) induced extensive vasoconstriction in the venules, which was more pronounced than in the arterioles, reaching peak responses within 1.5 min (Fig. 3). With both LTC_4 and the thromboxane mimetic, intense focal vasoconstriction in the venules was clearly demonstrated, leading to sluggish blood flow and stasis within the vessels.

Actions of the Lipoxygenase Inhibitor BW755C

The role of lipoxygenase metabolites in gastric damage was further explored using the lipoxygenase inhibitor BW755C. Although in many tissues including inflammatory cells and platelets, this experimental anti-inflammatory agent inhibits the formation of both cyclo-oxygenase and lipoxygenase metabolites [4, 10], BW755C fails to inhibit the cyclo-oxygenase enzyme in rat gastric mucosal tissue [7, 14]. BW755C may therefore be a useful selective probe for elucidating the involvement of the lipoxygenase products.

Rats were pretreated orally or subcutaneously with BW755C (3-amino-[m-(trifluoromethyl)-phenyl]-2-pyrazoline) as the dihydrochloride (Wellcome Research Laboratories) or with indomethacin, 1 hour prior to oral challenge with 1 ml acid-ethanol (40% ethanol in 100 mM HCl and 1 hour later the gastric mucosa was assessed for damage.

Pre-treatment with indomethacin (5 mg kg^{-1} s.c.) significantly ($P < 0.01$) augmented the degree of macroscopically apparent mucosal damage induced by the acid ethanol (Fig. 4). Thus removel of endogenous prostanoids makes the mucosa more susceptible to damage. In contrast, BW755C (10 mg kg^{-1} s.c.) significantly ($P < 0.05$) reduced the degree of mucosal damage. In other studies, oral administration of BW755C (10–100 mg kg^{-1}) significantly reduced both macroscopically and histologically-assessed gastric damage [11]. Likewise, BW755C (50 mg kg^{-1}) significantly reduced the incidence and severity of the gastric lesions induced by indomethacin (20 mg kg^{-1} s.c.) which developed over a three hour period; the erosion score being reduced from 34 ± 8 to 7 ± 3 ($P < 0.02$).

Discussion

As found with TxA_2, the chemically stable epoxy-methano analogue of PGH_2 (U-46619) which acts as a thromboxane mimetic, was a potent vasoconstrictor in the canine gastric circulation following local intra-arterial infusion. Studies on the rat gastric microcirculation demonstrated vasoconstriction in both the submucosal arterioles and venules, the vessels that regulate mucosal blood flow. In the presence of a weak topical irritant, sodium taurocholate, in a concentration which itself caused minimal damage to the canine gastric mucosa, U-46619 caused extensive necrotic damage supporting the studies with endogenously generated TxA_2. Thus these thromboxanes reduce the ability of the mucosa to withstand challenge from normally-mild

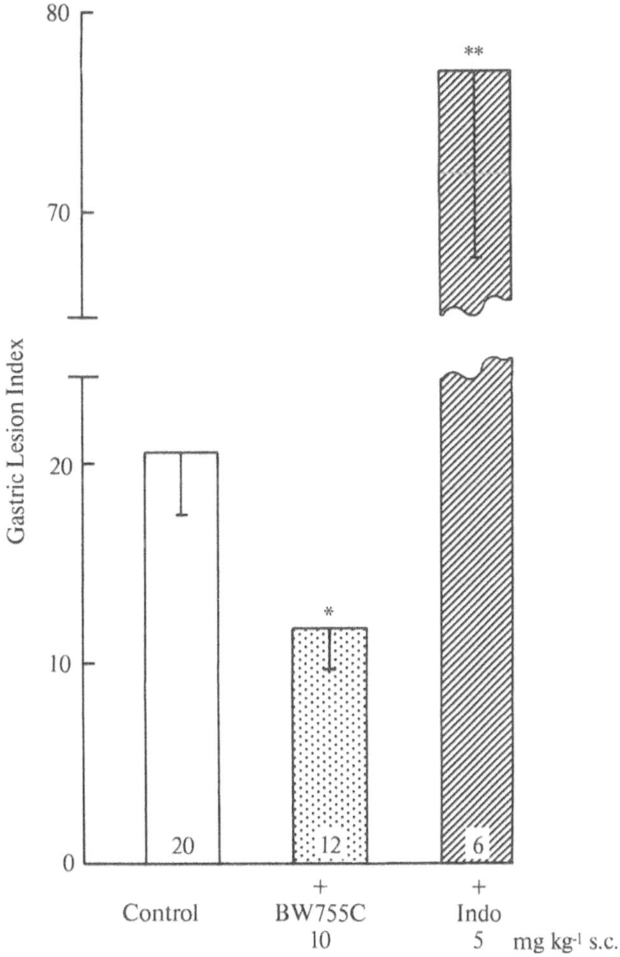

Fig. 4. Effects of 1 hour pretreatment with indomethacin (5 mg kg^{-1} s.c.) or the lipoxygenase inhibitor BW755C (10 mg kg^{-1} s.c.) on the gastric mucosal damage induced by acidified ethanol (40% in 100 mM HCl) in the rat. Results are shown as the erosion index, mean ± s.e.m. of (n) experiments, where *$P < 0.05$; **$P < 0.01$

irritants, an action which may be related to their vasoconstrictor properties, although direct cytolytic actions on the mucosal cells cannot be entirely excluded.

These potent actions of the thromboxanes raise the possibility that local generation of TxA_2, perhaps following platelet activation in the microcirculation or as a result of local trauma or general shock may be involved in the pathogenesis of gastric ulcerogenesis. Studies with selective thromboxane synthase inhibitors in experimental models give some support to this concept. Thus OKY-1581 reduced bile-salt induced gastric necrosis, although it failed to inhibit that induced by ethanol [5]. Further, while the thromboxane synthase inhibitor, benzyl-imidazole [14], substantially inhibited gastric damage induced by acid-ethanol, it also inhibited indomethacin-induced erosions [12]. Since the dose of indomethacin used would inhibit cyclo-oxygenase, and therefore would reduce TxA_2 formation, the mechanisms of its protective action are not fully clear. However, the involvement of TxA_2 in gastric damage resulting from local ischaemia and other microcirculatory disorders requires further consideration.

The finding that locally-applied LTC_4 was a potent vasoconstrictor in the gastric microcirculation, especially in the submucosal venules, identifies this arachidonate product as a further endogenous mediator with pro-ulcerogenic potential [16]. The predominant venular constriction led to vasocongestion and stasis in the microcirculation, histological characteristics of several forms of gastric damage including that induced by local application of ethanol [3, 6]. Indeed, recent studies have identified the release of LTC_4 from the rat gastric mucosa following ethanol challenge [8]. The ability of BW755C to prevent such gastric damage may therefore reflect the inhibition of the biosynthesis of these pro-ulcerogenic lipoxygenase products [11]. The less specific lipoxygenase inhibitor NDGA has also been demonstrated to reduce ethanol-induced gastric necrosis [8]. Other products of the lipoxygenase enzymes, such as the hydroperoxy intermediates, 5-, 12- or 15-HPETE and the free-radicals which they can produce, may also be involved in tissue destruction.

It is apparent that unlike the protective prostanoids, the cyclo-oxygenase product, TxA_2, and the 5-lipoxygenase product, LTC_4, may exert potent pro-ulcerogenic actions on the gastric mucosa. Elucidation of the involvement of these arachidonate metabolites, as well as the related phospholipid platelet-activating factor (PAF) which is the most potent ulcerogen yet described [9], in various forms of mucosal damage will provide a greater understanding of the pathogenesis of peptic ulceration and its therapy.

References

1. Coleman RA, Humphrey PPA, Kennedy I, Levy GP, Lumley L (1981) Comparison of the actions of U-46619, a prostaglandin H_2-analogue, with those of prostaglandin H_2 and thromboxane A_2 on some isolated smooth muscle preparations. Br J Pharmac 73: 773–778
2. Guth PH, Moler TL (1982) The role of endogenous prostanoids in the response of the rat gastric microcirculation to vasoactive agents. Microvasc Res 25: 336–342
3. Guth PH, Paulsen G, Nagata H (1984) Histologic and microcirculatory changes in alcohol-induced gastric lesions in the rat. Effect of prostaglandin cytoprotection. Gastroenterology 87: 1083–1090
4. Higgs GA, Flower RJ, Vane JR (1979) A new approach to anti-inflammatory drugs. Biochem Pharm 28: 1959–1961
5. Konturek SJ, Brzozowski T, Piastucki I, Radecki T, Dembinska-Kiec A (1983) Role of prostaglandin and thromboxane biosynthesis in gastric necrosis produced by taurocholate and ethanol. Dig Dis Sci 28: 154–160
6. Morris GP, Wallace JL (1981) The role of ethanol and of acid in the production of gastric mucosal erosions in rats. Virchows Arch (Cell Pathol) 38: 23–38
7. Peskar BM, Weiler H, Peskar BA (1982) Effect of BW755C on prostaglandin synthesis in the rat stomach. Biochem Pharmac 31: 1652–1653
8. Peskar BM, Large K, Hoppe U, Peskar BA (1986) Ethanol stimulates formation of leukotriene C_4 in the rat gastric mucosa. Prostaglandins 31: 283–293, 1986
9. Rosam AC, JL Wallace, BJR Whittle (1986) Potent ulcerogenic actions of platelet-activating factor of the stomach. Nature 319: 54–56
10. Salmon JA, Simmons PM, Moncada S (1983) The effects of BW755C and other anti-inflammatory drugs on eicosanoid concentrations and leucocyte accumulation in experimentally-induced acute inflammation. J Pharm Pharmacol 35: 808–813
11. Wallace JL, Whittle BJR (1985) Role of prostanoids in the protective actions of BW755C on the gastric mucosa. Eur J Pharmacol 115: 45–52
12. Whittle BJR (1984) Cellular mediators in gastric damage: Actions of thromboxane A_2 and its inhibitors, in: Mechanisms of Mucosal Protection in the Upper Gastrointestinal Tract, eds. A Allen, G Flemstrom, A Garner, W Silen, LA Turnberg (Raven Press, New York) p 295–301

13. Whittle BJR, Higgs GA, Eakins KA, Moncada S, Vane JR (1980) Selective inhibition of prostaglandin production in inflammatory exudates and gastric mucosa. Nature 284: 271–273
14. Whittle BJR, Kauffman GL, Moncada S (1981) Vasoconstriction with thromboxane A_2 induces ulceration of the gastric mucosa. Nature 292: 472–474
15. Whittle BJR, Moncada S (1983) Ulceration induced by an endoperoxide analogue and by indomethacin in the canine stomach. In: Advances in Prostaglandin, Thromboxane and Leukotriene Research vol 12, ed. B Samuelsson, R Paoletti, P Ramwell, Raven Press, New York, pp 373–378
16. Whittle BJR, Oren-Wolman N, Guth PH (1985) Gastric vasoconstrictor actions of leukotriene C_4, prostaglandin $F_{2\alpha}$ and a thromboxane mimetic (U-46619) on the rat submucosal microcirculation in vivo. Am J Physiol 248: G580–586

Discussion Following the Report of Dr. Whittle

FORD-HUTCHINSON

It appeared that during your infusion of LTC_4 into the rat stomach a rebound phenomenon was occurring. This reminds me of some cardiovascular studies in the pig carried out in our laboratory. In these studies a vasoconstriction was initially observed, followed by a subsequent phase of dilatation. The vasodilatation is due to the secondary release of other mediators, in the pig from the platelets. Do you think you are getting similar effects in your studies?

WHITTLE

This is an interesting point; in the concentration I demonstrated, you do see this fade of the vasoconstriction. At higher concentrations, this fade was less pronounced. We do not know whether it is the result of the release of other opposing mediators. It is certainly not due to the release of cyclo oxygenase products, because these experiments can be performed in the presence of indomethacin, and we still get this pronounced vasoconstriction.

FORD-HUTCHINSON

Yes, it is not due to cyclo oxygenase products in the pig either. Does the rebound phenomenon occur with LTD_4?

WHITTLE

In our hands and with the batch of LTD_4 that we had available, we obtained much less pronounced effects than with LTC_4 in this preparation.

FLEMSTRÖM

I have very much the same question, and this is the general physiological question: Do you think that there is autoregulation of blood flow in the gastric mucosa as thought for other parts of the intestine, and in such case, is this overruled by your thromboxane mimetic? How long-lasting are your effects?

WHITTLE

When we infused PAF-acether for a period of 20 min, there were predominant changes in the capillary circulation with a slowing of blood flow, until after about 20 min blood flow has almost completely ceased in this superficial circulation. Under these conditions, any autoregulation of the microcirculation is completely overruled. With the thromboxane mimetic we have measured perfusion pressure in the dog chamber preparation, and this remained elevated during the 30 min period of infusion, indicating prolonged vasoconstriction.

SOLL

My question concerns the mechanism of action of thromboxane and leukotrienes. Do these agents act directly on smooth muscle producing receptor-mediated vasoconstriction? Is there hydrolysis of phosphatidylinositol, with subsequent effects due to calcium-mediated or diacylglycerol-mediated mechanisms?

WHITTLE

So far we have investigated in detail only the effects of thromboxanes, and certainly one can antagonize many of the effects of the thromboxane mimetic using selective thromboxane antagonists, suggesting that it is a receptor-mediated effect. As yet, we have not investigated in any detail the effects of LTC_4 and the receptors involved. However, as a pharmacologist, I have great hope that it would be a receptor-mediated effect. I certainly have not yet looked further at the cascade of biochemical events which may be involved, such as the phospatidylinositol cycle.

HAMMARSTRÖM

In the endotoxin experiments reported, do you have any direct evidence that PAF is involved, that is, by antagonists or inhibitors? During endotoxin shock there is also a massive leukotriene release which could contribute to the effects observed.

WHITTLE

The problem with studies on endotoxin is the potential number of different mediators. Most of these mediators have not fully stood the test of pharmacological intervention. For instance, if you treat a rat with lipoxygenase inhibitors, you cannot completely alleviate all the effects of endotoxin shock. We have recently had opportunity to use several structurally unrelated PAF-antagonists, and these have prevented the prolonged cardiovascular effects in endotoxin shock and, indeed, have prevented the gastrointestinal damage which we can observe both macroscopically and histologically. We feel therefore that in our particular model of endotoxin shock, in which *E.coli* or *Salmonella typhosa* lipopolysaccharide is used, these effects may be primarily through PAF release. We do not know whether PAF is the initial triggering agent for the other products. It could well be that PAF induces the release of leukotrienes, and indeed we have some evidence for this. Thus, if you can antagonize the action of PAF, you may block the whole sequel of events.

HAMMARSTRÖM

Did you try some leukotriene antagonists as well?

WHITTLE

Because of the potential for many different leukotrienes being released, we felt it was a better approach to use specific lipoxygenase enzyme inhibitors, which would inhibit the formation of the whole cascade of products.

O'BRIEN

I wish to pursue the site of action of the thromboxane mimetic. On the slide showing the diameters of the vessels, it appeared that the venules changed in diameter earlier than did the arterioles. I wonder whether you could comment on where the likely primary site of the effect is. Could it be in the capillaries, in the venules, or in the arterioles?

WHITTLE

We were concerned whether vasoconstriction in the arterioles, by reducing blood flow and thus the venous return, would simply result in venular collapse. However, using norepinephrine applied locally we obtained pronounced vasoconstriction in the arterioles with no change in vessel diameter in the venules. We therefore do not think the venular constriction is a consequence of arterial constriction. As to which comes first, I do not think the time course which we have is sufficiently detailed to be able to say. One of the problems of looking at venular constriction is the focal segmental nature. Obviously some areas are constricted far more than others, and unless you look specifically at one particular area, it would be difficult to know which event is first.

SOLL

Did smooth-muscle cell contraction produce vasoconstriction, or did a local inflammatory response mimick constriction? A second question is whether pretreatment with agents that relax smooth muscle will prevent vasoconstriction?

WHITTLE

We have not had opportunity to try such direct muscle relaxants. Whether it is a local inflammatory response, may be a question of terminology. The effects occur quickly, within 1 min, whereas inflammatory responses usually take longer with an influx of cells. Of course, it may well be that there is resident population of inflammatory cells which release their mediators, as your own studies may point towards.

Microvascular Injury and the Role of Leukotrienes and Prostaglandins in Acute Mucosal Damage and Protection

G. PIHAN, and S. SZABO

Introduction

The realization that damage to the surface gastric mucosal cells and injury to deep layers of the mucosa, in which vascular lesions are prominent, are related, yet to different phenomena, can be traced back to Davenport [1]. It has been well documented that mucosal protective agents such as prostaglandins and sulfhydryls prevent vascular injury and deep epithelial damage but are unable to modify injury to surface mucosal cells [2, 3].

Recent data indicate that the vascular endothelium is not a passive bystander and alterations within the vessel wall may actively participate in the pathogenesis of gastric mucosal injury. We review here our data on morphologic and functional changes in mucosal vessels after intragastric administration of damaging chemicals and on the effect of prostaglandins and leukotrienes upon these changes.

Mucosal vascular changes caused by ethanol, HCl or NaOH

Structural changes

Among the techniques available for studying the morphologic changes in the microvasculature the use of dyes or particles as vascular tracers is particularly informative. After intravenous injection, blue (monastral blue) or black (colloidal carbon) particles become trapped between the endothelium and the basement membrane in damaged blood vesssels. The particles can be visualized by stereomicroscopy after clearing the formaldehyde-fixed stomach by overnight immersion in glycerol, and the area of vascular injury may be quantitated by planimetry [3].

Intragastric administration of ethanol, HCl or NaOH to fasted Sprague-Dawley rats caused a rapidly developing vascular injury, as revealed by monastral blue-labelling of superficial mucosal capillaries of the gastric mucosa. The area of monastral blue-labelled vessels 1 min after 0, 25, 50, 75 or 100% ethanol (1 ml intragastrically – i.g.) was 0.01 ± 0.07; 2.1 ± 0.6; 13 ± 2.2, or 17.1 ± 2.3% of the mucosal surface area of the glandular stomach. Similarly 3 min after 0.6N HCl or 0.2N NaOH (1 ml i.g.) the labelled area was 25.7 or 47.9% of the surface area of the glandular mucosa. At this time only a few congested areas and hemorrhagic erosions were observed. These results indicate that vascular injury occurs early and precedes the development of hemorrhagic mucosal lesions.

Functional changes

The effect of luminal ethanol on the gastric mucosal microcirculation was studied using in vivo microscopy and laser-Doppler velocimetry (LDV) [4]. To observe the microcirculation in superficial mucosal capillaries the posterior wall of the stomach of fasted Sprague-Dawley rats was enclosed in a thermo-regulated chamber musocal side up and continuously bathed in saline (0.9% NaCl) at 37 °C. The transilluminated mucosa was observed with a compound microscope. Images were projected onto a television monitor via a television camera and stored on tapes through a video tape recorder for later play-back analysis. Five min after beginning the recordings, either saline (control) or ethanol was applied topically for 5 min. During analysis the time for red blood cells (RBC) to stop circulating in the superficial mucosal capillaries under observation was recorded. At the end of the experiment, the area of mucosa enclosed in the chamber was retrieved, fixed in 10% formalin and the areal density of hemorrhagic mucosal lesions measured [3].

Topical application of saline did not stop circulation of RBC in all 5 control trials (Table 1). On the other hand, ethanol had a concentration-dependent effect, stopping RBC circulation in 100, 88, and 0% of trials after 100, 50 and 25% ethanol, respectively (Table 1). RBC circulation stopped soon after ethanol application as indicated by a mean time to reach stasis of 54 and 85 sec after 100 of 50% ethanol, respectively (Table 1). There was a good correlation between the development of stasis and the occurence of hemorrhagic mucosal lesions as all 12 rats given 100% ethanol and all but one given 50% ethanol exhibited hemorrhagic mucosal lesions at autopsy. None of the 5 animals given 25% ethanol developed hermorrhagic erosions. 0.6 N HCl and 0.2 N NaOH induced similar changes to those described for 100% ethanol.

These results indicate that stasis in superficial mucosal capillaries is an early event in acute mucosal damage, and that it correlates with the development of extensive disruption of the mucosal lining as indicated by the presence of hemorrhagic mucosal lesions.

Since changes in superficial mucosal capillaries may not accurately reflect those in the whole mucosal vascular bed, experiments were carried out to assess whole mucosal perfusion after ethanol. To this end, we used LDV, a technique which unites spatial and temporal resolution of microcirculatory blood flow [5]. Animals were prepared and exposed to ethanol in a similar fashion as for in vivo microscopy, except that the

Table 1. Incidence and time of development of microcirculatory stasis in superficial gastric mucosal capillaries after graded concentrations of ethanol. Effect of 16,16-dimethyl PGE_2

				Microcirculatory stasis	
Treatment		Pretreatment	(n)	Incidence %	Time to stasis (sec)
Saline		–	(5)	0	N.S.
Ethanol 100%		–	(12)	100*	54
Ethanol 50%		–	(9)	88*	85
Ethanol 25%		–	(5)	0	N.S.
Ethanol 50%	+	16,16-Dimethyl PGE_2	(7)	0	N.S.

N.S. No stasis; * $P < 0.05$ (Fisher's exact test);

Table 2. Changes in mucosal blood flow after topical application of 50% ethanol and effect of pretreatment with 16,16,-dimethyl PGE_2

			Time after ethanol (min)				
Treatment	Pretreatment	(n)	1	3	5	10	15
Ethanol 50%	–	(8)	87 ± 10	82 ± 11	49 ± 9*	40 ± 10	36 ± 10*
Ethanol 50%	+ 16,16-Dimethyl PGE_2	(7)	101 ± 18	116 ± 14	95 ± 12	97 ± 13	85 ± 8

All values of blood flow are per cents of those obtained at the times shown in rats exposed to saline alone. * $P < 0.01$ versus saline control (Student's *t* test)

microscope was replaced by a LDV probe (LD 5000 MedPacific). Application of saline did not induce major changes in mucosal perfusion. Topical application of 50 or 100% ethanol, however, led to a progressive decrease of mucosal perfusion after 3 min. In those animals that develop hemorrhagic lesions after 50% ethanol, blood flow decreased markedly reaching values of 50–40% of control in 5–10 min (Table 2).

These results indicate that mucosal perfusion decreases early during acute mucosal damage, and that the magnitude of decrease correlates well with the extent of hemorrhagic damage.

Effect of prostaglandins or leukotrienes on gastric microvasculature

Effect of prostaglandins

To determine whether prostaglandins influence the microcirculatory changes induced by ethanol, rats were preteated with prostaglandins, and the extent of vascular injury was investigated by stereomicroscopy and the mucosal microvasculature was studied by in vivo microscopy and LDV.

In fasted rats pretreated by prostaglandin (PG) $F_{2\beta}$ (0.2 mg/100 g i. g.) 30 min before ethanol, HCl or NaOH (see above) the extent of vascular injury as revealed by monastral blue was markedly diminished. In vivo microscopy of superficial mucosal capillaries showed that none of 7 animals pretreated with 16,16-dimethyl PGE_2 (1 μg/100 g i. g.) and subsequently exposed to 50% ethanol had microcirculatory stasis (Table 1). Five of these 7 animals showed no hemorrhagic erosions. The remaining two had small lesions covering 1–2% of the challenged mucosa. LDV measurement of mucosal perfusion indicated that pretreatment with 16,16-dimethyl PGE_2 was able to totally prevent the mucosal hypoperfusion induced by 50% ethanol (Table 2) and the development of hemorrhagic mucosal lesions. Since prostaglandins fail to prevent damage of the surface epithelium [2], these results lead us to postulate that the mucosal microcirculation is an important mechanism in prostaglandin-induced protection.

Table 3. Effect of local intra-arterial infusion of leukotrienes on gastric hemorrhagic mucosal lesions and vascular injury as revealed by monastral blue staining

Treatment	(n)	Area of hemorrhagic mucosal lesions (% glandular stomach)	Area of dye staining (% glandular stomach)
Saline	(6)	0	0.9 ± 0.6
LTC_4	(6)	0.8 ± 0.3	70.1 ± 10.1*
LTD_4	(6)	0.1 ± 0.1	66.5 ± 3.0*

LTC_4 and LTD_4 were infused at 1 nmol/100g/min for 15 min. Monastral blue (3 mg/100g) was injected i.v. 3 min before commencing the infusions. * $P < 0.001$ (Student's *t* test)

Effect of leukotrienes

Leukotrienes (LT) are potent inflammatory mediators. To determine whether LT can induce gastric mucosal damage and/or vascular injury, LTC_4 or LTD_4 was infused into the gastric circulation of anesthetized rats at a rate of 1 nmol/100 g/min for 15 min [6]. To label damaged blood vessels monastral blue (3 mg/100 g) was given i.v. 3 min before starting the LT infusions. At the end of the infusions the stomachs were fixed in 10% formalin and the extent of hemorrhage erosions and blue labelling evaluated as previously described [3].

As shown in Table 3, saline infusion induced no hemorrhagic lesions and only negligible dye staining. On the other hand both LTC_4 and LTD_4 produced widespread vascular labelling, yet little if any hemorrhagic lesions. Collecting venules in the mucosa were preferentially labelled by monastral blue after LT infusion (Fig. 1). Interestingly, there was also widespread labelling of submucosal and muscular venules

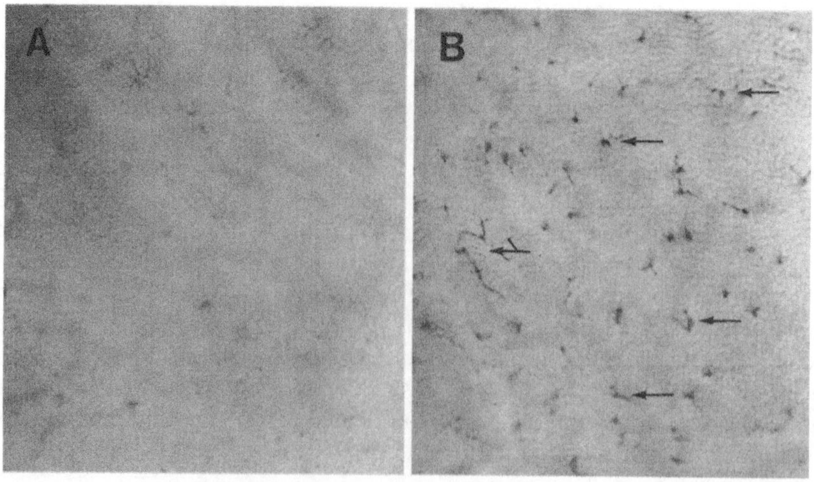

Fig. 1. En face view of gastric mucosa after the fixed stomach was cleared in glycerol. The rats were injected with monastral blue (3 mg/100 g i.v.) 3 min before starting the intra-arterial infusion. (A) Control rat infused with saline. (B) Rat infused with LTC_4 (1 nmol/100 g/min). Notice the labelling of collecting venules in B (arrows) (× 40)

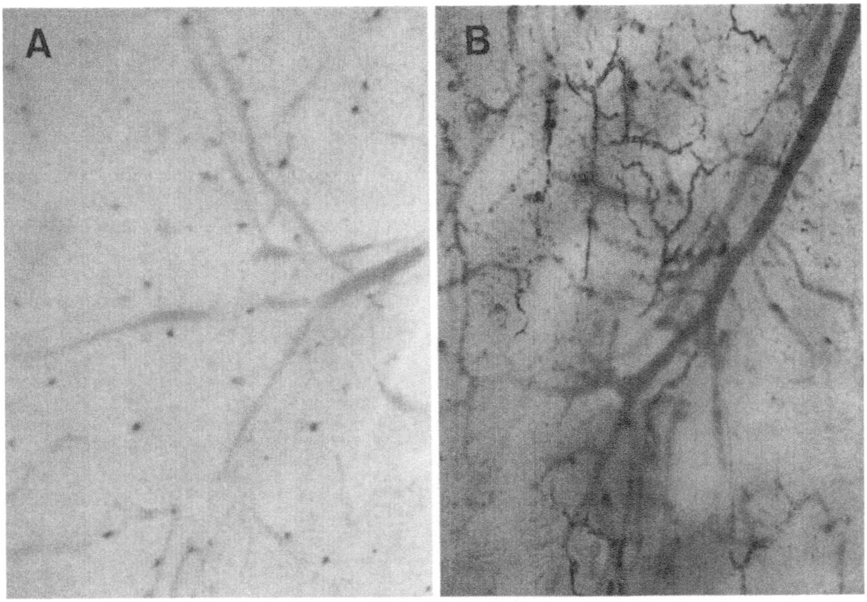

Fig. 2. En face view of the serosal side of the gastric wall after the stomach was cleared with glycerol. The rats were injected with monastral blue (3 mg/100 g i.v.) 3 min before starting the intra-arterial infusions. (A) Rat infused saline (B) Rat infused LTC_4 (1 nmol/100 g/min). Notice the widespread labelling of submucosal and muscularis propria venules in (B). (× 40)

after either LT (Fig. 2). Histologic examination of 1 um of thick section stained with hematoxylin and eosin indicated that short-term infusion of LT seldom if ever induced damage to epithelial cells yet produced extensive disruption of the mucosal microcirculation (Fig. 3).

To investigate whether LT can potentiate mucosal damage induced by ethanol or by near-physiologic concentrations of HCl, LTC_4 or LTD_4 was infused as described above and 5 min or 15 min before ending the infusions, 1 ml of ethanol or HCl, respectively, was given i.g. As shown in Table 4, LTC_4 or LTD_4 potentiated hemorrhagic mucosal lesions after all concentrations of ethanol tested. Similarly LTD_4 but not LTC_4 aggravated lesions induced by 0.2N HCl.

Table 4. Effect of local intra-arterial infusion of leukotrienes on gastric hemorrhagic mucosal lesions induced by graded concentrations of ethanol

		Ethanol %		
Treatment	(n)	25	50	100
Saline	(6)	6 ± 2	12 ± 4	17 ± 3
LTC_4	(6)	21 ± 4	24 ± 2*	38 ± 4**
LTD_4	(6)	15 ± 4	29 ± 4	40 ± 4**

LTC_4 or LTD_4 were infused at 1 nmol/100g/min for 15 min.
* $P < 0.05$, ** $P < 0.001$ experimental versus control (Student's *t* test)

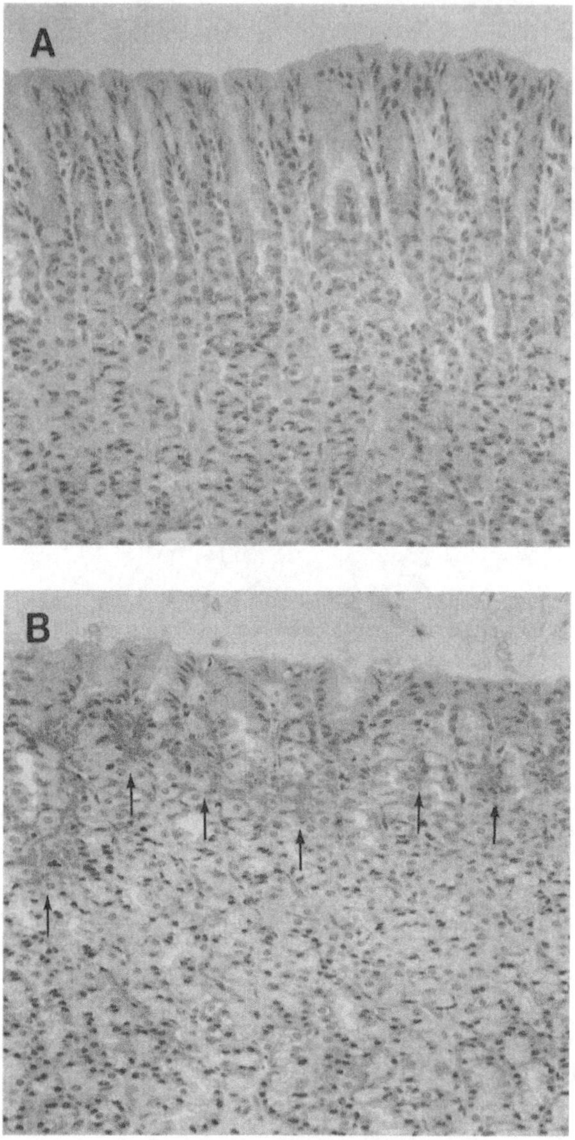

Fig. 3. Semithin sections of gastric mucosa stained with hematoxylin and eosin. (A) Control rat infused intra-arterially with saline. (B) Rat infused with LTC_4 (1 nmol/100 g/min). Subepithelial hemorrhage (shown by the vertical arrows) are evident in (B) ($\times$ 40)

Our results thus indicate that leukotrienes are potentially damaging mediators in the gastric mucosa acting almost exclusively, at least at first, on the gastric mucosal microcirculation, where they induce widespread congestion and hemorrhagic lesions. Since they cause no histologically evident epithelial damage, their potentiating effect on the damaging actions of ethanol or acid seems to depend on vascular factors. Furthermore, our preliminary results indicate that chronic administration of unsaturated fatty acids which act as false substrate for 5-lipoxygenase dose- and time-dependently decreased the hemorrhagic erosions caused by 100% ethanol or 0.6 N HCl in the rat [7].

These studies along with similar findings by others concerning the role of leukotrienes [8] and microvascular changes [9, 10] in the pathogenesis of ethanol-induced gastric mucosal changes strongly suggest a rate-limiting step for the microvasculature in the mechanism of gastric mucosal damage and protection. Structural and functional changes in blood vessels in the stomach may then actively contribute to development and prevention of mucosal lesions.

Summary

Morphologic studies have suggested that intragastric administration of damaging agents such as concentrated ethanol, HCl or NaOH produce two major types of damage; injury to the surface mucus cell and deep mucosal damage which consists of vascular lesions such as congestion, hemorrhage and necrosis of gastric glands often extending throughout the mucosa. From a clinical standpoint, only the latter type of musocal damage is important. Our results indicate that the gastric mucosal microcirculation is altered early both structurally and functionally during acute mucosal damage induced by ethanol. Prostaglandins prevent these early vascular changes and the subsequent development of hemorrhagic erosions suggesting that the effect of prostaglandins on the microcirculation is responsible for mucosal protection. Leukotrienes on the other hand, may act as mediators of damage partly reproducing the microvascular but not the epithelial alteration induced by ethanol. It is therefore likely that during mucosal challenge a balance between cyclooxygenase and lipoxygenase products modulates the microvasculature and crucially determines the presence or absence of mucosal damage.

References

1. Davenport HW (1975) Mayo Clin Proc *50* 507–514
2. Lacy ER (1985) Dig Dis Sci *30* Suppl: 835–945
3. Szabo S, Trier JS, Brown A, Schnoor J (1985) Gastroenterology *88:* 128–236
4. Pihan G, Majzoubi D, Haudenschield C, Trier JS, Szabo S (1986) Gastroenterology *91:* 1415–1426
5. Granger DN, Kvietys PR (1985) Gastroenterology *88:* 1073–1076
6. Pihan G, Rogers C, Szabo S Dig Dis Sci (in press)
7. Rogers C, Pihan G, Szabo S (1986) Gastroenterology *90:* 1797
8. Peskar BM, Lange K, Hoppe U, Peskar BA (1986) Prostaglandins *31:* 283–292
9. Leung FW, Robert A, Guth PA (1985) Gastroenterology, 1985, *88:* 1948–1953
10. Tarnawski A, Hollander D, Stachura J, Krause WJ, Gergely H (1985) Gastroenterology *88:* 334–352

Discussion Following the Report of Dr. Szabo

PESKAR

You have pointed out that endothelial damage is observed within 1 min of ethanol administration and within 3 min of acidified aspirin administration. Hemorrhagic lesions after ethanol develop within 1 min, but erosions after acidified aspirin are observed only after several hours. Do you have an explanation for this difference?

SZABO

It depends on the techniques and on the dose of aspirin. In our laboratory we see hemorrhagic erosion within 3–6 min after aspirin if we use acidified aspirin with the proper homogenizing agent which retains the aspirin in the stomach. We thus see a very rapid development of vascular injury and hemorrhagic erosions. So in our laboratory the aspirin is slightly slower acting than ethanol, but nevertheless it is acting within the first few minutes.

WHITTLE

I would like to ask you to expand on the events that occur following this initial endothelial damage. You say that there is endothelial cell damage, and subsequently you eventually get stasis. Do you think the stasis is simply due to transudation of plasma, ore are there some other phenomena occuring inside the vessels actually to cause this stasis?

SZABO

This is a crucial question and one which needs expansion. There is much more than just increased vascular permeability. We think that the plasma rushing out clearly contributes to hemoconcentration, but that this is not the only factor. The other possibilities we are considering are changes within the basement membrane, which becomes sticky and for one reason or another attracts red blood cells. We also think probably the red blood cells and not the white cells or the platelets are crucial for the initial development. I can tell this only in discussion and not in a regular presentation, because it was only a quick and dirty experiment which we did a few years ago. We wanted to see if a possible release of free radicals from white cells contributes to the development of lesions. So we depleted the white cells and platelets by giving cyclophosphamide to the rat, and we had histological evidence that the bone marrow was wiped out. However, the changes caused by ethanol were not reduced; if anything, they were almost aggravated. It remains to be seen what happens to the red blood cells. We have a few possible theories, but they are really very vague. Thus, we do not claim that it is only the hemoconcentration and endothelial changes, but additional factors such as alterations in the basement membrane and probably the red blood cells also contribute to the stickiness of the red blood cells to the damaged capillaries. Eventually the circulation is slowed down and results in standstill without any vasoconstriction. Late venular constriction may also develop.

GRAHAM

We cannot afford rats in our laboratory and are forced to work with people. With Dr. SZABO's continued urging we finally did an experiment that we had talked about. If I get this wrong, Karen, please give the correct data, because Dr. Woods is the one who did the experiment. We gave people Evan's blue and acidified aspirin and then looked into the stomach by a gastric washing technique. As in the animal experiments, we found that the Evans blue appeared in the gastric washings significantly before there was any bleeding. So the observations in animals seem to be also relevant to the human situation, at least with aspirin.

SZABO

Thank you for mentioning this. I was considering giving a brief reference, but I would feel it inappropriate to release your results. But, if you say so, it is very assuring that vascular injury occurs in humans as well.

SOLL

It is good to see traditions preserved; it is good to see that your Hungarian accent and flavor are still very viable. Another tradition deserves to be preserved and that is Davenport's gastric barrier. Although it is very clear that the target of the agents you are using is the endothelial cell, these agents first will have to break the barrier to get to the endothelial cell. Under many physiological conditions, the barrier may be an important rate-limiting step in protecting the mucosa.

SZABO

This is true, but I purposely left out the epithelial damage because we take for granted that so far nothing protects against epithelial injury. And although nothing protects against surface injury, this surface damage is not as crucial as we initially thought because mucosal epithelium regenerates easily. Of course, you are right; this also implies that for severe damage to occur, the epithelial layer must be destroyed most of the time. There are two additional reasons why we think the mucosal barrier is not crucial in *acute* lesions. Dr. Guth's studies with aspirin and Dr. Robert's studies with labeled ethanol showed that the concentrations of damaging agents in the gastric mucosa were the same in protected and nonprotected stomachs. There are methodological difficulties and criticisms of both studies, but all this would suggest that the preservation of epithelial barrier is not crucial for *acute* protection. Or, maybe moving the barrier around the blood vessels in what really counts, and we should speak about vascular barrier and not epithelial barrier. Furthermore, we have very recent studies conducted mostly by Dr. Pihan, suggesting the development of vascular injury without marked epithelial damage. Namely leukotrienes infused intra-arterially and indomethacin given subcutaneously cause vascular injury within minutes, and hemorrhagic erosions develop much later. So we think that there are situations in which the initial event is endothelial damage. This does not deny that the epithelial barrier is also important, especially in *chronic* safeguarding of the mucosa.

SOLL

You are using somewhat extreme models that are overriding normal defense mechanisms. Possibly the epithelial barrier is important under many physiological conditions but not under the conditions that you use.

SZABO

This is what people used to say, and this is the reason that we shifted to use of 0.1–0.2 HCl, close to physiological concentrations. We leave the extreme 100% ethanol or perform dose-response studies with low concentrations of ethanol.

Inhibition of Prostaglandin Synthesis and Proliferation of the Gastric Mucosa

F. HALTER, A. BAUMGARTNER, and H. R. KOELZ

Introduction

High doses of natural prostaglandin E_2 (PGE_2) or various methylated PGE_1 or PGE_2 analogues, exert trophic effects on all parts of the gastrointestinal tract including the pancreas. It has been proven both in experimental animals and in man that these trophic effects are reversible after discontinuation of the treatment [1–7]. There are indications that both cell proliferation [3, 9] and especially prolongation of the life cycle of individual epithelial cells [4, 7, 8] contribute to the substantial increase of mucosal volume following such treatment.

Most of the changes in the gastric mucosa have only been observed after administration of high, antisecretory PG doses. However, hyperplasia of the superficial mucus-producing cells is also observed following the administration of small "cytoprotective" doses [1]. The latter observation does not exclude that PGS might play a physiological role in the regulation of the growth of the gastric mucosa. It is therefore of interest to evaluate to what degree inhibition of PG synthesis counteracts these PG effects.

Information available so far on this subject is scanty and conflicting. Early observations made by Croft and Wood in 1967 [10] have demonstrated that aspirin treatment induces an increase of cell desquamation into the gastric lumen. More recent studies have clearly demonstrated that in the rat both aspirin and indomethacin induce an increase in cell proliferation predominantly in the gastric corpus [11, 12].

Since in previous studies cell shedding and cell proliferation were not assessed concomitantly, we performed a combined histomorphometric and cell kinetic study in which rats were treated for up to 2 weeks with a nonulcerative dose of indomethacin. In some of these experiments the effect of indomethacin was directly compared to the changes observed following prostaglandin treatment.

Studies on Cell Proliferation

Two groups of eight rats were treated with indomethacin 2 mg/kg (8 a.m. and 5 p.m.) or solvent for 3 days. During the last 24 h the rats were fasted. Six h after the last dose the animals were killed and tissue samples of ~5 mm in diameter were then immediately incubated in a medium containing [^{3}H]thymidine (10 μCi/ml) according to a method described in detail elsewhere [13]. The results were expressed as disintegrations per minute per microgramme DNA (μg DNA). [^{3}H]thymidine incorporation after 3-days treatment was increased by 86% in the corpus and 32% in the antrum ($P < 0.05$) (Table 1).

Table 1. Cell proliferation and cell shedding after treatment with indomethacin 2 mg/kg s.c., b.d. (INDO) or solvent (Solv)

	Corpus		Antrum	
	Solv	INDO	Solv	INDO
Cell proliferation (n = 8)				
DPM/μg DNA after 3-day treatment	43 ± 8	80 ± 13*	111 ± 10	146 ± 8*
Cell shedding (n = 5)				
DNA-DPM/organ × 10^{-2} after 14 day treatment	1073 ± 90	532 ± 24*	132 ± 14	71 ± 25*

* $P < 0.05$

Studies on Cell Shedding

These studies were measurements of DNA-bound, residual radioactivity. The fasted animals were injected at midnight with [^{3}H]thymidine (1 μCi/g) intra peritoneally. In this study five animals each were treated in the same way as for autoradiography. On days 7 and 14 all rats of each group were killed. The whole glandular stomach was removed and separated along the microscopically visible border between antrum and corpus. These two parts of the stomach were separately homogenized and specific radioactivity of mucosal DNA was then determined and expressed as DNA bound disintegration per min per total corpus or antrum – DNA/organ x10^{-2} [13]. At the end of the observation period the residual, DNA-bound radioactivity of both the corpus and antrum was reduced in the indomethacin treated groups by a mean of 68% ($P < 0.5$) and 46% ($P < 0.06$) respectively (Table 1).

Studies on Cell Migration

In these studies rats were fasted for 20 h with free access to water and were injected at midnight with [^{3}H]thymidine (1 μCi/g intraperitoneally). 8 h later the rats were refed and treatment with indomethacin (2 mg/kg, b.i.d.) or solvent was started. After 1 and 3 days, five animals of each group were killed and histological sections were obtained from the corpus and antrum. These sections were processed for autoradiographic studies according to techniques previously described [13]. The number of labelled nuclei was counted in each compartment and mean values are shown in histogrammes (Fig. 1).

Fig. 1. Histograms of labelled cells after 1 and 3 days of treatment with indomethacin (*closed circles*) or solvent (*open circles*). Animals were injected with [^{3}H]thymidine intraperitoneally before treatment. *MP*, Median position of labelled cells as distance from surface: Means ± SE of 5 rats; *$P < 0.05$; **$P < 0.01$

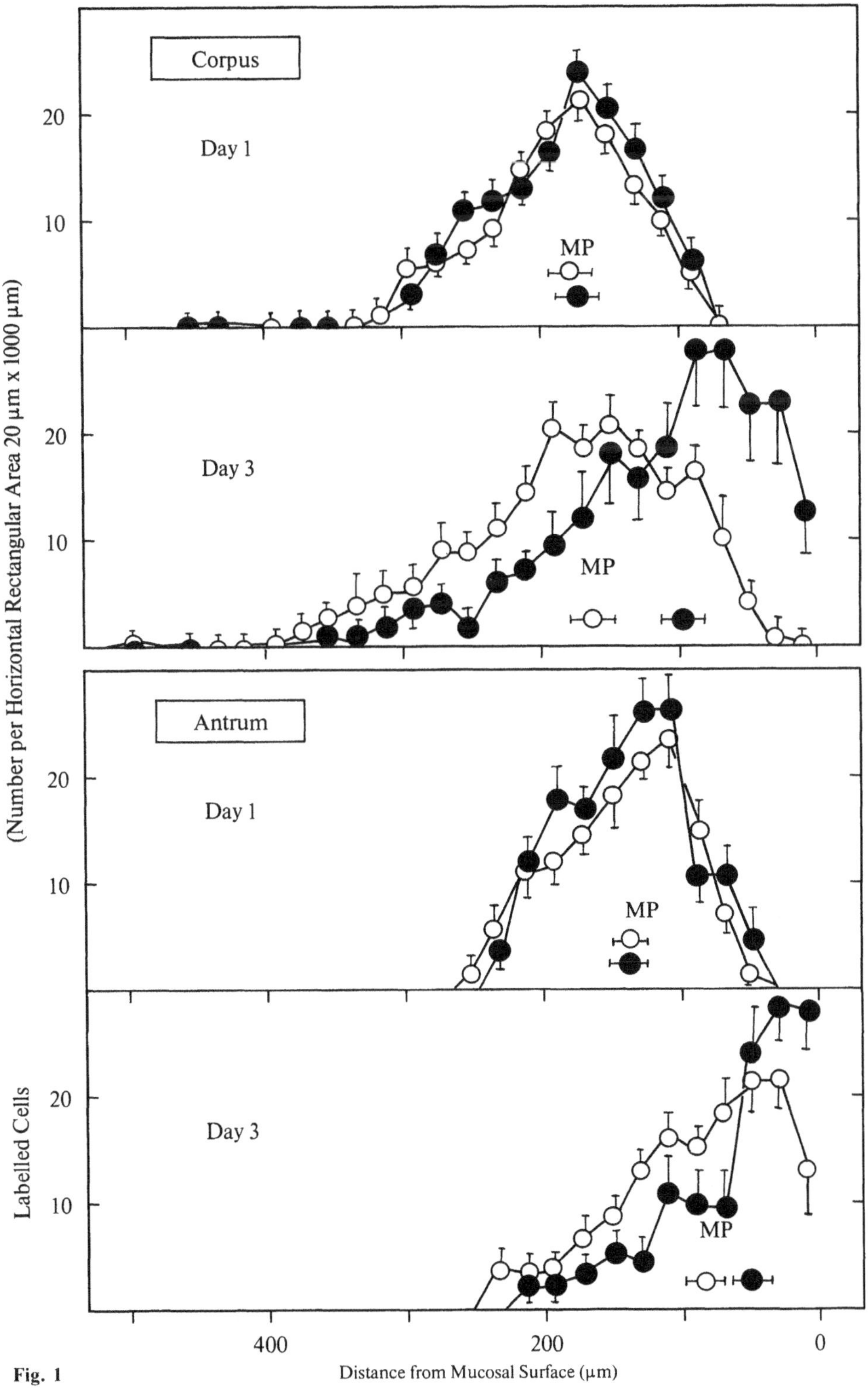
Corpus
Day 1
MP
Day 3
MP
Antrum
Day 1
MP
Day 3
MP
20
10
20
10
20
10
20
10
Labelled Cells
(Number per Horizontal Rectangular Area 20 μm x 1000 μm)
400
200
0
Distance from Mucosal Surface (μm)

Fig. 1

On day 1 the distribution of labelled cells in the corpus and antral mucosa was similar in the two groups. From day 1 to day 3 the medium position of labelled cells in control animals had migrated towards the surface in the corpus by 10 μm (1.8% of the mean mucosal height) and by 61 μm (29% of the mean mucosal height) in the antrum. On day 3 the front of labelled cells had nearly reached the surface in the antrum but not in the corpus.

Comparing indomethacin-treated animals with the control group, an increased shift of labelled cells towards the surface after 3 days treatment was observed, an effect which was more pronounced in the corpus than in the antrum. The median position of labelled cells was displaced in the corpus of indomethacin-treated animals by 65 μm ($P < 0.01$) and the antrum by 32 μm ($P < 0.05$).

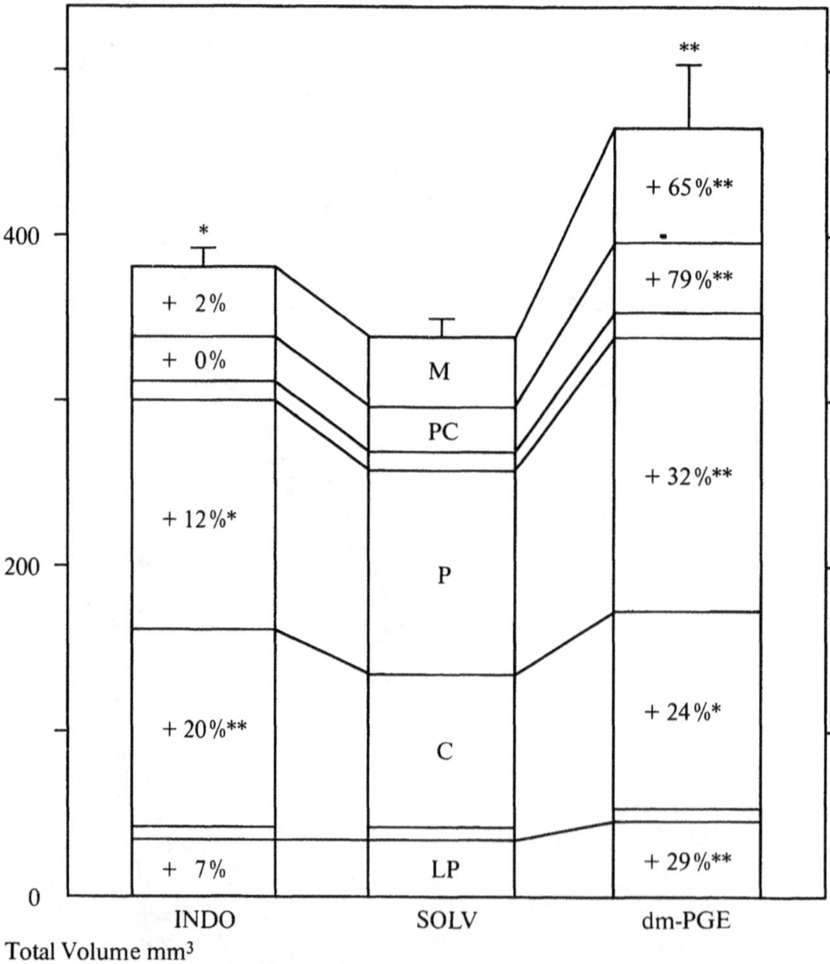

Fig. 2. Gastric corpus: total mucosal volume and total volume of different mucosal cell types after 14 days of treatment with indomethacin (*INDO*), solvent (*SOLV*), or 16,16-dimethyl prostaglandin E_2 (*dm-PGE*). *M*, Mucous cells; *PG*, progenitor cells; *MN*, mucous neck cells; *P*, parietal cells; *C*, chief cells; *E*, endocrine cells; *LP*, lamina propria. Means ± SE of 8 animals; $^*P < 0.05$; $^{**}P < 0.01$

Morphometric Studies

Three groups of eight rats were treated as above for 14 days with indomethacin, 2 mg s.c., b.i.d, 16,16-dimethyl PGE_2 (dm PGE), 100 μg, i.g., b.i.d., or solvent. Two h after the last dose the rats were killed and the stomach was submitted to detailed morphometric analysis with the methodology previously described in detail [1].

In the corpus, indomethacin treatment increased the basal volume by 11% ($P < 0.05$) resulting from an increased parietal cell and chief cell mass by 12% ($P < 0.05$) and 21% ($P < 0.01$) respectively (Fig. 2). The total volume of other cell types especially mucus cells was unchanged. Parietal and chief cells showed an increase in total cell number of 15% ($P < 0.05$) and 44% ($P < 0.01$) respectively. With PGS all the changes were considerably more pronounced (Fig. 2). In addition surface mucus cells were increased by 65%. In the antrum of indomethacin treated animals a tendency

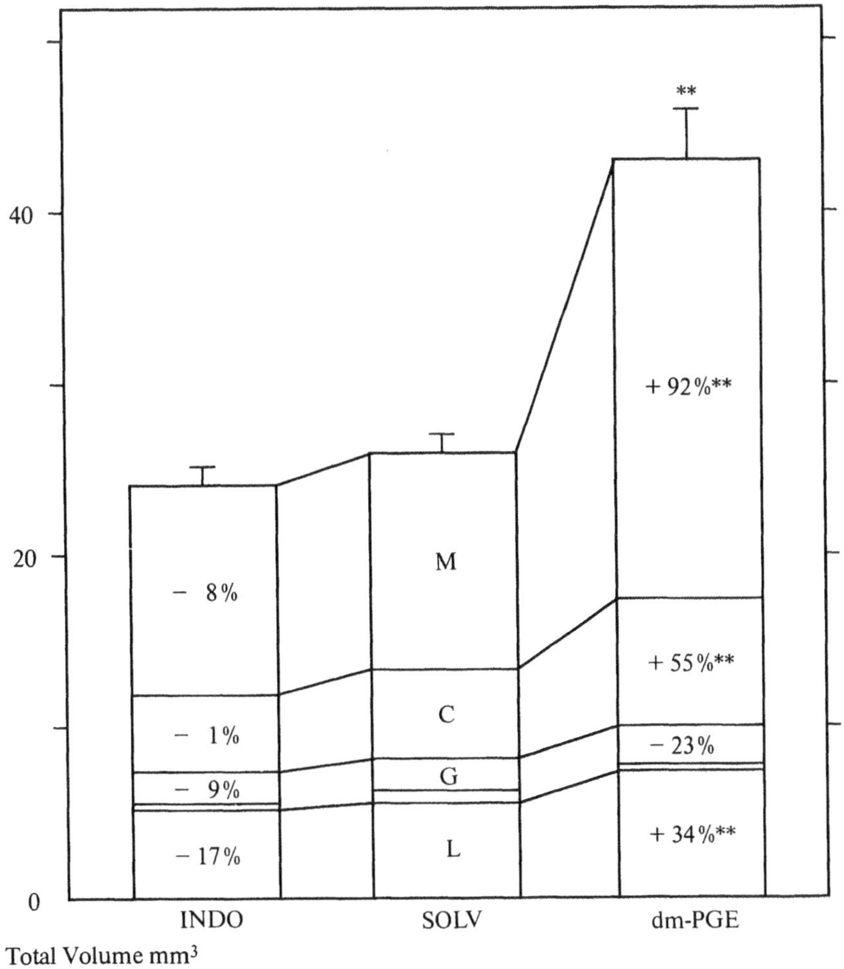

Fig. 3. Gastric antrum: same treatment as given in Fig. 2. *M*, Mucous cells; *PG*, progenitor cells; *E*, endocrine cells; *G*, antral gland cells; *L*, lamina propria. Means ± SE of 8 animals; $^{**}P < 0.01$

towards decreased volume of all different cell types did not reach statistical significance. In contrast, a more than 30% increase in mucosal cell mass was observed following dm PGE treatment (Fig. 3), mainly resulting from an increase in surface mucus cells (92%).

Estimation of Mucosal PGE_2

In these studies eight rats per group were treated for 14 days with indomethacin or solvent with the same treatment as mentioned under morphometric studies. Corpus and antral mucosa scrapings were obtained immediately after dissecting the stomach and frozen at $-80\,°C$. The mucosa was processed later according to methods described for estimation of PG formation [14, 15]. Mucosal PGE generation 2 h after the last dose was reduced by 63% in the corpus and by 81% in the antrum following indomethacin treatment (Fig. 4). PG treatment resulted in a 41% inhibition of PG formation in the gastric corpus mucosa. This was not influenced by the latter treatment in the gastric antrum.

Serum Gastrin Levels

Serum gastrin measured in rats given the treatment for 2 weeks was unchanged (as for estination of mucosal PGE_2).

Discussion

Our studies have confirmed earlier observations [11, 12] that inhibition of cyclooxygenase by the highest indomethacin doses tolerated by rats during prolonged treatment exerts a trophic effect on the gastric mucosa, especially in the gastric corpus. The cell kinetic studies suggest that in the gastric corpus the increase in cell shedding is overcompensated by a massive increase in cell proliferation. So paradoxically, both PG [2, 9] and indomethacin [11, 12] treatment can stimulate cell proliferation in the gastric mucosa [1–8]. The morphological changes are different however. The massive hyperplasia of the surface and foveolar-mucosa cells, which is highly specific for PG treatment [1, 7] is absent following indomethacin treatment. It can not be excluded that the changes in cell proliferation, especially those observed after prostaglandin treatment represent a secondary phenomenon following modification of the life cycle of the individual cell. Since PGS and indomethacin influence cell shedding in an opposite manner the possibility remains open that regulation of the growth of superficial epithelial cells is a physiological property of PGS. As PGS enhance bicarbonate and mucus production in the same cell types such a regulation would be a meaningful phenomenon actively contributing to the defense function of the gastric mucosa. Of interest is the observation in these studies that exogenous PG application diminishes PG synthesis in the gastric corpus mucosa. It is likely that this represents a feed back mechanism aimed at limiting trophic effects following PG treatment.

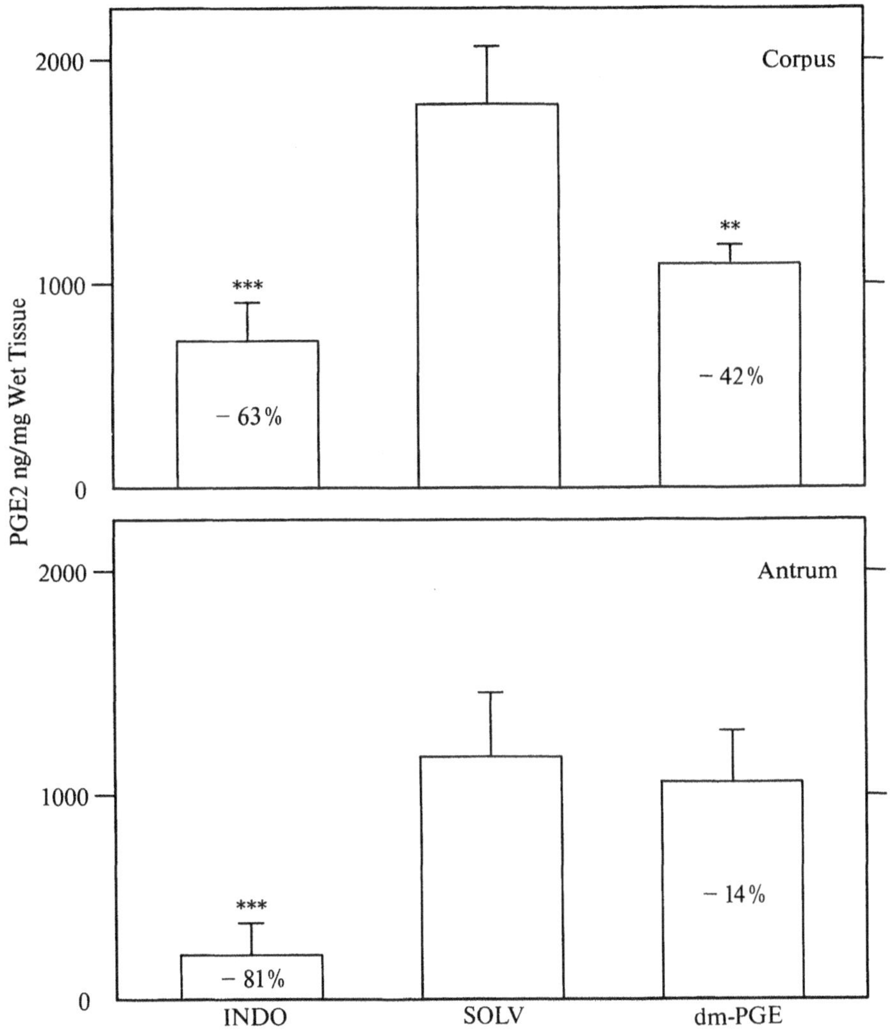

Fig. 4. Ex vivo PGE_2 generation after 2-week treatment with indomethacin *(INDO)* solvent *(SOLV)*, or 16,16-dimethyl PGE_2 *(dm-PGE)* in corpus and antrum mucosa as measured 2 h after the last dose. Means ± SE of 8 animals; $^{**}P < 0.01$; $^{***}P < 0.005$

References

1. Reinhart WH, Müller O, Halter F (1983) Influence of long-term 16,16-dimethyl prostaglandin E_2 treatment on the rat gastrointestinal mucosa. Gastroenterology 85: 1003–1010
2. Halter F, Meyrat P, Fritsche R, Müller O, Lentze MJ, Koelz HR (1984) Both topical and systemic treatments with 16,16-dimethyl prostaglandin E_2 are trophic to rat gastric mucosa. Scand J Gastroenterol 19 (Suppl. 101) 47–54
3. Meyrat P, Kappeler M, Halter F (1984) A simple gastroscopy technique in the rat. Dig Dis Sci 29: 327–329

4. Fich A, Arber N, Sestieri M, Zajicek G, Rachmilewitz D (1985) Effect of misoprostol and cimetidine on gastric cell labelling index. Gastroenterology 89: 57–61
5. Helander HF, Johansson C, Blom H, Ulribe A (1985) Trophic action of E_2 prostaglandins in the rat gastrointestinal mucosa. A quantitative morphological study. Gastroenterology 89: 1303–1399
6. Koelz HR, Fritsche R, Müller OM, Lentze MJ, Varga L, Halter F (1986) Structure and function of gastric corpus mucosa in suckling rats after treatment with 16,16-dimethyl prostaglandin E_2. Prostaglandins 31: 133–141
7. Tytgat GNJ, Offerhaus GJA, van Minnen AJ, Everts V, Hensen-Logmans SC, Samson G (1986) Influence of oral 15(R)-15-methyl prostaglandin E_2 on human gastric mucosa. Gastroenterology 90: 1111–1120
8. Uribe A, Johansson C, Rubio C (1985) Effects of prostaglandin E_2 on cell kinetics of the rat gastrointestinal mucosa. Gastroenterology 88: 1621 (abstract)
9. Dembinski A, Konturek SJ (1985) Effects of E, F and I series prostaglandins and analogs on growth of gastroduodenal mucosa and pancreas. Am J Physiol 248: G170–G175
10. Croft DW, Wood DHN (1967) Gastric mucosa and susceptibility to occult gastrointestinal bleeding caused by aspirin. Br Med J 1: 137
11. Eastwood GL, Quimby GF (1982) Effect of chronic aspirin ingestion on epithelial proliferation in rat fundus, antrum, and duodenum. Gastroenterology 82: 852–856
12. Kuwayama H, Eastwood GL (1973) Effects of water immersion, restraint, stress and chronic indomethacin ingestion on gastric antral and fundic epithelial proliferation. Gastroenterology 64: 421–428
13. Baumgartner A, Koelz HR, Halter F (1986) Indomethacin and turnover of gastric mucosal cells in the rat. Am J Physiol 250: G830–G835
14. Whittle BJR, Higgs GA, Eakins KE, Moncada S, Vane JR (1980) Selective inhibition of prostaglandin production in inflammatory exudates and gastric mucosa. Nature Lond 284: 271–273
15. Bauminger S, Zor U, Kinder HR (1973) Radioimmunological assay of prostaglandin synthetase activity. Prostaglandins 4: 313–324

Discussion Following the Report of Prof. Halter

PESKAR

Nonsteroidal anti-inflammatory compounds such as indomethacin have two distinct actions: they inhibit prostaglandin formation, and in addition they break the mucosal barrier when given orally. Is the effect of indomethacin on cell migration due to inhibition of prostaglandin formation, or could it possibly be the consequence of breaking the barrier resulting in damage to the mucosa even in the absence of macroscopically visible lesions?

HALTER

It is difficult to say, because in our studies we injected indomethacin. But in the study of Eastwood it was given orally. So obviously both of these mechanisms are of importance.

BERNIER

You conclude that indomethacin increases cell renewal. I agree with your conclusion; however, on your first slide you show that there is a difference between the 7-day treatment and the 14-day treatment. How do you explain the change?

HALTER

I have some difficulties with your question, because there was an increase in cell proliferation shown on day 7. No, it is not true. We only looked at cell proliferation on day 3, but this may be a misunderstanding. We looked at *cell shedding* on day 7 and day 14. As a matter of fact, the differences shown on day 7 were not statistically significant. They were only significant on day 14. Although one has the impression that the differences were larger on day 7, due to the larger variation, significant levels were not achieved.

SZABO

You have probably said this but I missed it. There was a dramatic cell proliferation caused by indomethacin early in your treatment. As indomethacin can cause lesions even after parenteral administration, my question is whether this proliferation was due to some local erosions, or whether it was a phenomenon without any lesions being apparent? And the corollary of this, are these cell proliferations a general phenomenon detected in all areas of the gastric mucosa or only on certain areas of the stomach? I learned namely during the Brazil meeting from Dr. Uribbe, Dr. Johansson's coworker, that these proliferations are often localized in certain areas of the gastric mucosa only.

HALTER

The answer to the second questions first: We had the impression that the proliferations were generalized. Maybe the investigation of Dr. Uribbe was more detailed because we did not assess the effect quantitatively. And to the first question: In preliminary experiments we gave various dosages of indomethacin to the rat and found that the

2 mg/kg dose twice daily was the highest dosage not producing lesions. In none of the animals did we see any macroscopic or microscopic lesions.

RACHMILEWITZ

You have mentioned that indomethacin stimulates cell turnover. I agree with what Professor Peskar said, that this may not be related to its effect on gastric prostaglandins. Furthermore, you suggested that prostaglandins stimulate cell turnover to compensate for the increased cell shedding. This does not combine well. I would like to mention that, as you know, we have shown that in humans treated for 4 weeks with synthetic prostanoids cell turnover in the stomach was decreased. How can you reconcile these divergent data?

HALTER

I showed only the data on cell shedding obtained in animals treated with solvent or indomethacin. We also had a third group included that was treated with a high prostaglandin dose. However, in contrast to your studies we could not find a significant decrease in cell shedding following prostaglandin treatment. In our study the content of labelled DNA was similar in PGE- and placebo-treated animals. As prostaglandin-induced changes occur predominantly in the gastric antrum, you may be particularly interested in that region. Maybe in the gastric antrum mucosa there was a tendency towards less cell shedding after prostaglandin treatment as compared to placebo. Thus, there is a difference between the prostaglandin and the indomethacin data. I agree that, if one cannot demonstrate a phenomenon in an experiment, this is no proof that it may not occur. If we had lesser variations in the data, we would have found a highly significant difference. You may also be aware of data from our group and from Professor Konturek's group showing that at least in the initial phase prostaglandin treatment significantly enhances proliferation.

LANGMANN

Did you measure outside the stomach? Did you get the same sort of thing in the intestine?

HALTER

We did not look at the intestine.

RUPPIN

Did you perform the prostaglandin measurements at the same time as the measurements of proliferation and cell shedding? I could imagine that there is a rebound phenomenon of prostaglandin production by the tissue after challenge with indomethacin.

HALTER

It was indeed not measured at the same time. Prostaglandin synthesis was measured after 2 weeks treatment, cell proliferation after 3 days, and cell shedding after 7 and 14 days.

WHITTLE

I understand the technical complexities of doing these experiments, but one way of knowing whether this effect relates to inhibition of prostaglandin biosynthesis or to a specific action of indomethacin would obviously be to use nonsteroid anti-inflammatory drugs, other than indomethacin. Since it is quite likely that most of these drugs will inhibit prostaglandin biosynthesis, did you attempt to do any studies with such agents?

HALTER

Unfortunately not. As you know, these studies are very time-consuming, especially if you do morphometric studies, but this is, of course, a very good suggestion.

GRAHAM

One of the problems we have with this whole field is that we cannot make people act like rats. If you do the studies again, you should try to use a drug that does not have an enterohepatic circulation. You then eliminate the problem of potential reflux of the active drug into the stomach, which may occur even if it is given parenterally. There are now monoclonal antibodies available that will identify cells in the proliferative cycle. You can use them for immunohistochemical staining, which is much easier than radiography.

HALTER

I just wanted to suggest that you should come to Bern and do it for us.

MÜLLER

Somatostatin has some antitrophic effects on gastrointestinal organs. Have you measured the correlation between somatostatin content in the gastric mucosa and the effects on cell proliferation?

HALTER

We have not studied it.

Role of Prostaglandins in Intestinal Fluid Secretion

E. BEUBLER

Introduction

In the late 1960s endogenous prostaglandins (PGs) were assumed to be related to certain types of human diarrhea, diarrhea being one of the most prominent side effects associated with the clinical use of PGE and PGF. Meanwhile, secretory as well as motor functions have been shown to be involved in PG-induced diarrhea. Despite the well documented effects of PGs on intestinal smooth muscle, which may partly contribute to diarrhea and particularly to the abdominal colics that accompany it, the probably more important properties are those responsible for intestinal secretion.

Biosynthesis of PGs

PGs are present in the gastrointestinal wall of man and animals [1] and the biosynthesis of PGs is easily stimulated by physical disturbances such as mechanical stimulation [2], ischemia or irradiation [3]. Also hormones like thyroxine and pentagastrin [4], neurotransmitters like serotonin and chemical laxatives like ricinoleic acid, bisacodyl and anthraquinones [4, 6] are able to stimulate PG synthesis in the gut. Furthermore, diarrhea caused by infections with *Salmonella typhimurium, Escherichia coli* and *Vibrio cholera* [4] have been discussed as being associated with enhanced biosynthesis of PGs. In humans and laboratory animals, in vivo administration of PGE or PGF elicits the net secretion of fluid and sodium, potassium, chloride and bicarbonate ions and inhibits absorption of sodium and glucose [4]. Addition of PGs to small intestine and colonic mucosa preparations in vitro results in increased potential difference and short-circuit current, in inhibition of sodium and chloride absorption and in stimulation of chloride secretion similar to the effect of cyclic AMP, proving that the diarrheagenic effects of PGs are due to the stimulation of an active electrolyte secretion [1].

Inhibition of PG Biosynthesis

Inhibition of PG biosynthesis in vivo by pretreatment with indomethacin affects blood flow and net fluid transport, results which are opposite to those observed after exogenous administration of PGs. This suggests that endogenous PGs may be considered as physiological local regulators of blood flow and fluid and ion transport in the intestine [7]. The observation that pretreatment of stripped human jejunum with indomethacin increased the sensitivity of the tissue to exogenous PGE_2 and at the same time abolished the artificial in vitro formation of endogenous PGs supports the concept of a physiological role for eicosanoids in the regulation of intestinal ion transport [8].

Stimulation of Adenylate Cyclase by PGs

The cellular mechanisms by which PGs induce intestinal secretion are still a matter of discussion. It is generally accepted that stimulation of adenylate cyclase and accumulation of cyclic AMP result in active intestinal secretion [9]. Since PGs, in concentrations from 10^{-7} *M* upwards, stimulate adenylate cyclase [10] and in high concentrations increase mucosal cyclic AMP content [11], and, as the secretory effects of PGs are indistinguishable from those caused by cyclic AMP, the likely explanation was that PGs exert their effect via stimulation of the adenylate cyclase-cyclic AMP system.

This widely held belief has recently been questioned because of several reasons. Stimulation of adenylate cyclase by PGs and intestinal secretion accompanied by enhanced mucosal cyclic AMP levels has been observed only in response to supraphysiologic concentrations of exogenous PGs.

However, in vitro evcidence of secretion can be obtained with PG concentrations 100–1000 times below those required for activation of the adenylate cyclase [8]. Furthermore, in vivo studies have shown that endogenous 5-hydroxytryptamine (5-HT) mediates colonic secretion, in morphine withdrawal diarrhea, through stimulation of endogenous PGE_2 formation without any change in mucosal cyclic AMP levels. This secretion is prevented not only by indomethacin, but also by the selctive 5-HT receptor antagonist ketanserin. Hence 5-HT may be an external signalling system that acts through stimulation of local PG formation without involving cyclic AMP [12].

The secretory effect of physiologically low doses of PGE_2 is also prevented by verapamil (Fig. 1), whereas the effect of high doses of PGE_2 which increase mucosal cyclic AMP levels is not affected by verapamil [5], thus providing further support for the notion that low doses of PGE_2 increase intracellular Ca^{2+} by facilitating Ca^{2+} entry rather than by activating the adenylate cyclase. This hypothesis is strengthened by the observation that a cyclic AMP dependent secretagogue like vasoactive intestinal polypeptide does not increase PGE_2 output into the lumen and that neither indomethacin nor verapamil change its secretory effect [5].

The dissociation between the effect of PGs and cyclic AMP levels is further supported by the observation that cholera toxin induced fluid secretion is reduced by indomethacin without lowering the elevated cyclic AMP levels [13]. Recent experiments have shown that cholera toxin stimulates 5-HT and PGE_2 release into the gut lumen and that the dose response curve of cholera toxin induced secretion is shifted to the right by indomethacin and by the $5\text{-}HT_2$ receptor antagonist ketanserin. The finding that verapamil also inhibits cholera toxin induced secretion supports the concept outlined above [14].

Summary

To date two major pathways can be defined for the stimulus-secretion coupling in the intestine, namely, that using cyclic nucleotides as second messengers (e.g. vasoactive

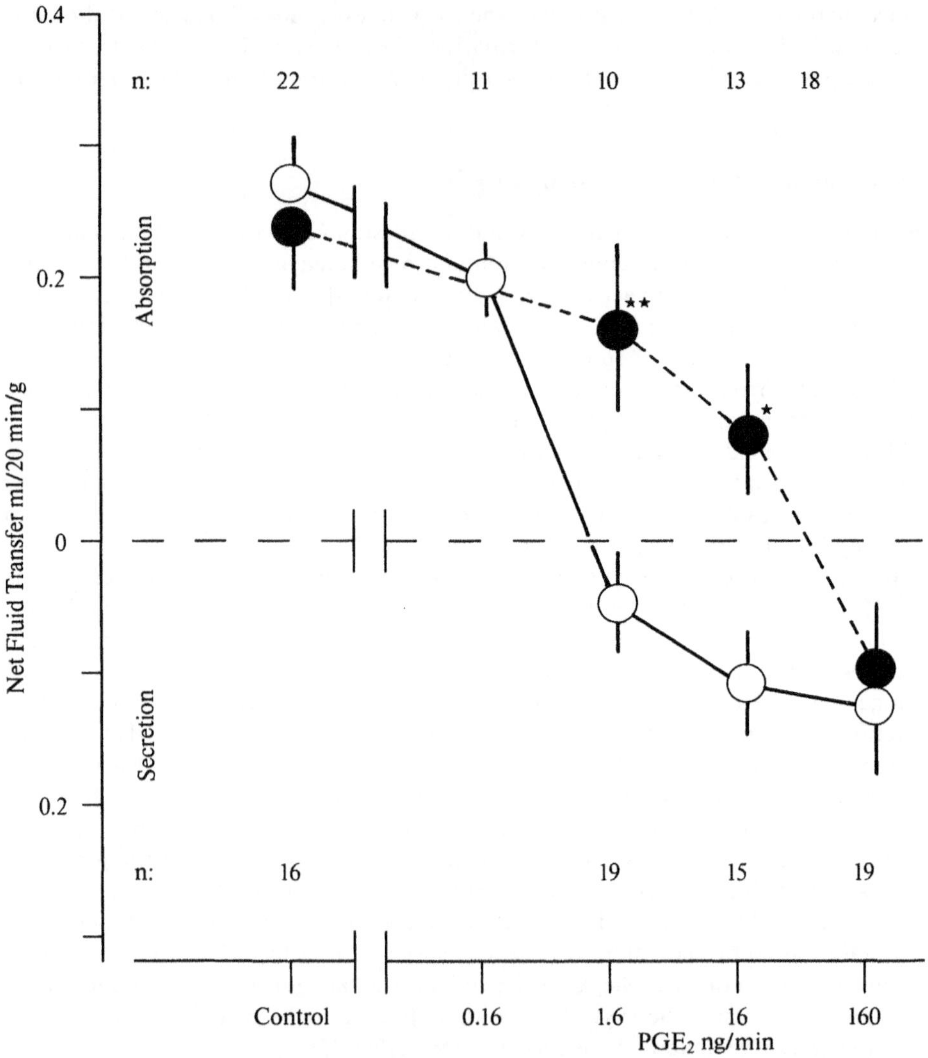

Fig. 1. Effect of verapamil (9.5 μg/min i.a.) on intestinal fluid secretion induced by close intraarterial infusion of PGE_2 in the rat jejunum in vivo; +verapamil, (●); −verapamil, (○)

intestinal polypeptide, heat stable *Escherichia coli* enterotoxin) and that using inositol lipids as part of a transduction mechanism which raises intracellular Ca^{2+} without involving cyclic nucleotides (e.g. 5-HT, acetylcholine). Because the production of eicosanoid mediators is limited by the release of arachidonic acid (probably from diacylglycerol as a result of phosphoinositide turnover), eicosanoids may be important physiological and pathophysiological intermediates involved in the mediation of secretory response.

References

1. Field M (1981) Role of prostaglandins in the regulation of intestinal electrolyte transport. Prostaglandins (Suppl) 21: 73–79
2. Beubler E, Juan H (1978) PGE-release, blood flow, and transmucosal water movement after mechanical stimulation of the rat jejunal mucosa. Naunyn-Schmiedeberg's Arch Pharmacol 305: 91–5
3. Rask-Madsen J, Bukhave K (1981) The role of prostaglandins in diarrhea. Clin Res Rev 1 (Suppl 1): 33–4
4. Hawkey CJ, Rampton DS (1985) Prostaglandins and the gastrointestinal mucosa: Are they important in its function, disease, or treatment? Gastroenterology 89: 1162–88.
5. Beubler E, Bukhave K, Rask-Madsen J (1986) Significance of calcium for the prostaglandin E_2-mediated secretory response to 5-hydroxytryptamine in the small intestine of the rat in vivo. Gastroenterology 90: 1972–7
6. Beubler E, Kollar G (1985) Stimulation of PGE_2 synthesis and water and electrolyte secretion by senna anthraquinones is inhibited by indomethacin. J Pharm Pharmacol 37: 248–51
7. Beubler E, Juan H (1977) The function of prostaglandins in transmucosal water movement and blood flow in the rat jejunum. Naunyn-Schmiedeberg's Arch Pharmacol 299: 89–94
8. Bukhave K, Rask-Madsen J (1980) Saturation kinetics applied to in vitro effects of low prostaglandin E_2 and $F_{2\alpha}$ concentrations on ion transport across human jejunal mucosa. Gastroenterology 78: 32–42
9. Field M (1981) Secretion of electrolytes and water by mammalian small intestine. In: Johnson LR, ed Physiology of the gastrointestinal tract. New York: Raven Press 963–82.
10. Kimberg DV, Field M, Johnson J, Henderson A, Gershon E (1971) Stimulation of intestinal mucosal adenylcyclase by cholera enterotoxin and prostaglandins. J Clin Invest 50: 1218–30
11. Kimberg DV, Field M, Gershon E, Henderson A (1974) Effects of prostaglandins and cholera toxin on intestinal mucosal cyclic AMP accumulation. J Clin Invest 53: 941–9.
12. Beubler E, Bukhave K, Rask-Madsen J (1984) Colonic secretion mediated by prostaglandin E_2 and 5-hydroxytryptamine may contribute to diarrhea due to morphine withdrawal in the rat. Gastroenterology 87: 1042–8
13. Wals A, Gotterer GS, Rajendra GR et al (1977) Effect of indomethacin on cholera-induced fluid movement, unidirectional sodium fluxes, and intestinal cAMP. Gastroenterology 72: 106–10
14. Beubler E, Kollar G, Saria A, Bukhave K, Rask-Madsen J (1987) Role of 5-hydroxytryptamine and PGE_2 in cholera-induced fluid secretion by the rat jejunum in vivo. J Physiol 382:46P

Discussion Following the Report of Dr. Beubler

SIMON

Do you postulate a second receptor for the effect of prostaglandin on calcium influx?

BEUBLER

It is hard to talk about receptors without having any results in this direction. You need binding studies at least. So I cannot answer the question.

SOLL

We had a lot of trouble working with verapamil on fundic musocal cells. We see nonspecific effects even in concentrations as low as 1 μ *M*. Is there other evidence for a role of calcium influx in mediating prostaglandin effects on intestinal secretion?

BEUBLER

I see the problems using verapamil. A major point is that you can stimulate fluid secretion with prostaglandins using a concentration of 10^{-9} *M*, and this concentration is unable to increase adenylate cyclase activity. Concerning the verapamil studies, we work with a calculated local concentration of verapamil of 10^{-5} *M*; this is the border concentration in talking about calcium transport. We cannot look into the cell to see whether it is really the calcium entrance, but the results rather support this hypothesis. We cannot find any nonspecific effect concerning fluid transport with this concentration of verapamil.

SOLL

The role of cyclic AMP is very difficult to determine. Because of methodological problems we may not be able to characterize cyclic AMP turnover, so I would be somewhat cautious in the interpretation from that standpoint.

BEUBLER

I know the problems as you do.

RACHMILEWITZ

You did not discuss at all the possible effects of prostaglandins on absorptive mechanisms. The net accumulation of fluid in the intestine is the result of secretion and absorption. We have demonstrated together with Dr. Sharon that prostanoids inhibit intestinal sodium-potassium ATP-ase activity, which may be involved in possible effects on intestinal fluid transport.

BEUBLER

Actually, we tried to reproduce your results on sodium-potassium ATP-ase but failed; I do not know why. What is known is that prostaglandins increase absorption, and I think my introductory slides have shown that sodium-chloride absorption is enhanced by prostaglandins. This may be due to an effect on the sodium-potassium ATP-ase.

RACHMILEWITZ

By the way, Dr. Moszik from Hungary showed that prostanoids inhibit gastric sodium-potassium ATP-ase as well.

FLEMSTRÖM

When you are measuring cyclic AMP, do you have a chance to distinguish between villous cells and crypt cells?

BEUBLER

Not with our method, no.

Novel Leukotriene D_4 Receptor Antagonists and 5-Lipoxygenase Inhibitors: Implications in Human Disease

A. W. FORD-HUTCHINSON

Introduction

The leukotrienes are a group of mediators derived from arachidonic acid through the action of the 5-lipoxygenase enzyme [1, 2]. The initial enzymic step involves insertion of molecular oxygen into arachidonic acid to produce the unstable intermediate 5-hydroperoxyeicosatetraenoic acid. This intermediate is converted in a dehydrase step by the same enzyme (5-lipoxygenase) to the 5,6-epoxide, leukotriene A_4. The term leukotriene derives from

1. the fact that these compounds were first isolated out of leukocytes and
2. the presence of the triene conjugated system within the molecule which gives these compounds their characteristic ultraviolet spectra.

Leukotriene A_4 may be metabolized by two specific enzymes to produce biologically active compounds or may undergo nonenzymatic hydrolysis to dihydroxy fatty acids with little biological activity. The first of these enzymes is leukotriene A_4 hydrolase which inserts water to produce a dihydroxy fatty acid, leukotriene B_4, with a precise stereochemistry (5[S],12[R]-dihydroxy-6,14-cis-8,10-trans eicosatetraenoic acid) [3, 4]. Further metabolism of leukotriene B_4 involves ω-oxidation to produce 20 OH-leukotriene B_4 and 20 COOH-leukotriene B_4 [5]. This metabolism results in loss of biological activity [6]. The second route of conversion of leukotriene A_4 involves insertion of glutathione by another specific enzyme leukotriene C_4 synthetase. This results in the production of a peptidolipid conjugate, leukotriene C_4. Leukotriene C_4 may be rapidly metabolized with loss of glutamic acid to produce leukotriene D_4 which in turn can lose glycine to produce leukotriene E_4. These leukotrienes collectively account for the biological activity known as slow-reacting substance of anaphylaxis [1, 2].

Biological Activities

Leukotriene B_4 has high affinity, structurally specific receptors on leukocytes, activation of which is associated with induction of a number of leukocyte functions [7–9]. Thus, leukotriene B_4 has been shown to be a potent chemokinetic, chemotactic and aggregating substance for polymorphonuclear leukocytes [7], effects mediated through the presence of high affinity, structurally-specific receptors. This is reflected in vivo where injection of leukotriene B_4 induces neutrophil migration in a number of systems [8]. Leukotriene B_4 may also modulate vascular permeability [10, 11] and pain responses in vivo [12] and both these responses have been shown to be secondary to the initial induction of leukocyte migration. In addition to effects of leukotriene B_4 on neutrophil function, there is evidence that this leukotriene may also have effects on lymphocyte function mediated through high affinity receptor sites on these cells [13]. For example, leukotriene B_4 has been shown to induce suppressor cell activity [14], to stimulate natural cytotoxic cells [15] and to replace interleukin 2 or helper cell requirement for γ-interferon production [16]. Thus, it has been suggested that leukotriene B_4 might be an important modular of lymphocyte function [17].

Leukotriene D_4 has high affinity, structurally specific receptor sites on smooth muscle membranes which are associated with smooth muscle contraction (e.g. bronchoconstriction and vasoconstriction) [18]. In most systems, leukotriene C_4 is rapidly converted to leukotriene D_4 and thus the effects of this leukotriene are mediated through the leukotriene D_4 receptor. However, under certain circumstances leukotriene C_4 may also interact with its own recognition unit, the function of which is not entirely clear. Leukotriene E_4 interacts with the leukotriene D_4 receptor with a somewhat lower affinity. Because of their potent constrictor activity on respiratory smooth muscle both in vitro and in vivo following administration by aerosol to man, peptido-lipid leukotrienes have been postulated as important mediators of diseases such as human bronchial asthma [8, 18].

Therapeutical approache

Two therapeutic approaches to the production or action of leukotrienes have been intensively investigated by the pharmaceutical industry. These are, first, 5-lipoxygenase inhibitors which by inhibiting the initial oxygenation step will prevent the further production of both leukotriene B_4 and thus its effects on leukocytes, and the smooth muscle contracting agents, leukotrienes C_4, D_4, and E_4. The socond approach is to produce highly selective, potent leukotriene D_4 receptor antagonists which will block the action of this autocoid on smooth muscle preparations and hence prevent, for example, bronchoconstriction. An example of a potent orally active and selective 5-lipoxygenase inhibitor is L-651,392(4-bromo-2,7-dimethoxy-3H-phenothiazine-3-one) [19]. For this compound, the IC_{50} values for rat peritoneal polymorphonuclear leukocytes incubated with ionophore A23187, mouse CXBG mastocytoma cells incubated with ionophore A23187, mouse peritoneal macrophages incubated with zymosan, and human polymorphonuclear leukocytes incubated with cytochalasin B and f-met-leu-phe were 0.6, 2.5, 2.5 and 2.6 $\times 10^{-7}$ M. In the presence of NADH the compound produced significant inhibition of a crude 5-lipoxygenase from rat basophil leukemia cells (mean IC_{50} 0.8 $\times 10^{-7}$ M). The compound failed to inhibit preparations of the 12-lipoxygenase from human platelets or porcine leukocytes, the 15-lipoxygenase from soybean, cytochrome P450 from rat liver microsomes, or the cyclooxygenase enzyme from ram seminal vesicle microsomes. The potent inhibitory effects of L-651,392 on the 5-lipoxygenase enzyme in vitro were manifested in vivo through inhibition of antigen-induced bronchoconstriction in inbred rats and squirrel monkeys [20] and antigen-induced changes in vascular permeability in the guinea-pig conjunctiva [21]. Thus, compounds such as L-651,392 may be important for assessing the role of 5-lipoxygenase products in physiological and pathological processes both in vitro and in vivo.

Two examples of specific leukotriene D_4 receptor antagonists are L-648,051 (sodium 4-(3-(4-acetyl-3-hydroxy-2-propyphenoxy)propylsulfonyl)-γ-oxo-benzene butanoate) [22] and L-649,923 (sodium βS*, γR*)-4-(3-(4-acetyl-3-hydroxy-propylphenoxy)-propylthio)-γ-hydroxy-β-methyl-benzene butanoate) [23]. L-648,051 is a competitive inhibitor of [^{3}H]leukotriene D_4 (K_i 6 μM) binding in guinea-pig lung homogenates but it is less effective as an inhibitor of [^{3}H]leukotriene C_4 binding (K_i 37 μM). The compound competitively antagonized the contractions of guinea-pig ileum induced by leukotriene D_4 (pA_2 7.7) and contractions of guinea-pig trachea induced by leukotriene D_4 (pA_2 7.3) and leukotriene E_4 (pA_2 7.4). The compound does not significantly antagonize contractions induced by other contractile agonists on respiratory tissues. L-648,051 is rapidly metabolized in vivo, shows significant activity when tested by the aerosol route and is being tested in man using this route of administration. L-649,923 is an orally active leukotriene D_4 receptor antagonist which is an inhibitor of [^{3}H]leukotriene D_4 (K_i 0.4 μM) and to a lesser extent [^{3}H]leukotriene C_4 (K_1 9.0 μM) binding to guinea-pig lung homogenates. The compound selectively antagonizes contractions of the guinea-pig trachea induced by leukotrienes but not other agonists. Competitive inhibition of contractions of the guinea-pig ileum induced by leukotriene D_4 (pA_2 8.1) and the guinea-pig trachea induced by leukotriene E_4 (pA_2 7.1) were obtained. Following oral administration, L-649,923 inhibits antigen-induced dyspnea in inbred rats and leukotriene D_4- and ascaris-induced bronchoconstriction in squirrel monkeys [20]. In man, L 649,923 produces a 3.8 fold shift in the dose response curve to leukotriene D_4 without affecting histamine-induced bronchoconstriction [24].

Leukotriene B_4 may have pathological implications in deseases where neutrophil infiltration is a predominant event. Thus, therapy with 5-lipoxygenase inhibitors has been proposed for the treatment of psoriasis and ulcerative colitis [8]. Leukotriene D_4 receptor antagonists have been primarily proposed for treating allergic diseases such as bronchial asthma. In addition, there have been suggestions that leukotrienes may have a role in the gut. Thus peptido-lipid leukotrienes can evoke smooth muscle contractions or certain preparations obtained from the gastrointestinal tract. For example, leukotrienes C_4 and D_4 induce contractions of isolated rat stomach and colon strips but do not cause contractions on the rat duodenun or ileum [25]. On the other hand, the guinea-pig ileum is highly responsive to leukotrienes C_4 and D_4 [26]. These contractions of gastrointestinal tissue are blocked by specific leukotriene receptor antagonists suggesting the presence of specific receptors for leukotrienes on tissues such as the rat stomach. Thus, in theory leukotrienes could be involved in gastric mucosal damage through induction of gastric stasis, decreased gastric mucosal blood flow and ischemia. Following infusion of leukotrienes D_4, C_4 and E_4 into the cat stomach a lowering of transgastric potential difference, an increase in pepsin secretion but no effect on gastric acid secretion was observed [27]. Of the leukotrienes tested, leukotriene C_4 was the most potent, suggesting possibly an involvement of a leukotriene C_4 rather than a leukotriene D_4 receptor in the response. When such cats were treated with the leukotriene D_4 receptor antagonist, L-649,923, inhibition of pepsin secretion was observed but no effect on the transgastric potential difference [28]. This has been interpreted to indicate different leukotriene receptor subtypes mediating each response. L-649,923 has also been studied in the rat where in one study it was shown to inhibit lesions induced by indomethacin and other non-steroidal anti-inflammatory drugs (M. M. Goldenberg, D. Rosen, S. Luell, D. Keller: The gastric protective activity of a novel leukotriene antagonist, L-649,923 in the rat, unpublished work) and in another to inhibit lesions induced by ethanol in the rat (see the chapter by Peskar in this volume). In addition, Peskar has demonstrated that the rat stomach produces increased levels of leukotriene C_4 following ethanol stimulation and a correlation between inhibition of leukotriene C_4 production and inhibition of ethanol-induced ulcers has been observed [29]. These effects of L-649,923 are only observed at relatively high doses and could be due either to leukotriene D_4 receptor antagonism, to leukotriene C_4 receptor antagonism or to some other unidentified property of the compound. Further studies with other inhibitors and antagonists of defined mechanism of action will be required to ascertain the exact mechanisms of inhibition observed with compounds such as L-649,923.

Conclusion

In conclusion, leukotrienes have been shown to have potent biological activities and have been suggested as possible mediators of diseases such as bronchial asthma, psoriasis and ulcerative colitis. A putative role for leukotrienes in induction of gastrointestinal lesions in the rat has been suggested from preliminary data with one leukotriene D_4 receptor antagonist. The use of selective antagonists and inhibitors in man will define the true role of such biologically active compounds in human disease.

References

1. Samuelsson B (1982) The leukotrienes: an introduction. In: Samuelsson B, Paoletti R (eds) Adv in Prostaglandin, Thromboxane Leukotriene Res. Raven Press, New York, vol 9, pp 1-17
2. Samuelsson B (1983) Leukotrienes: A new class of mediators of immediate hypersensitivity reactions and inflammation. Adv in Prostaglandin Thromboxane Leukotriene Res. Raven Press, New York, vol 11, pp 1-13
3. Borgeat P. Samuelsson B (1979) Arachidonic acid metabolism in polymorphonuclear leukocytes: Effects of ionophore A23187. Proc Natl Acad Sci USA (76): 2148-2152
4. Borgeat P, Samuelsson B (1979) Transformations of arachidonic acid by rabbit polymorphonuclear leukocytes. Formation of novel dihydroxyeicosatetraenoic acids. J Biol Chem 154: 2643-2646
5. Powell WS (1984) Properties of leukotriene B_4 20-hydroxylase from polymorphonuclear leukocytes. J Biol Chem 258: 3082-3089
6. Camp RDR, Wollard PM, Mallet AJ, Fincham NJ, Ford-Hutchinson AW, Bray MA (1982) Neutrophil aggregating and chemokinetic properties of 5,12,20-trihydroxy-6,8,10,14-eicosatetraenoic acid isolated from human leukocytes. Prostaglandins 23: 631-641
7. Ford-Hutchinson AW, Bray MA, Doig MV, Shipley MF, Smith MJH (1980) Leukotriene B, a potent chemokinetic and aggregating substance released from polymorphonuclear leukocytes. Nature 286: 264-265
8. Ford-Hutchinson AW (1985) Leukotrienes: Biological properties, evidence for specific receptor sites and evidence for the involvement of leukotrienes in pathological situations *In:* Lands WEM (ed) Biochemistry of Arachidonic Acid Metabolism. Boston, Nijhoff, pp. 269-285

9. Goldman DW, Goetzl EJ (1982) Specific binding of leukotriene B_4 to receptors on human polymorphonuclear leukocytes. J Exp Med 129: 1600–1604
10. Bray MA, Cunningham FM, Ford-Hutchinson AW, Smith MJH (1981) Leukotriene B_4: A mediator of vascular permeability. Br J Pharmacol 72: 483–486
11. Wedmore CV, Williams TJ (1980) The control of vascular permeability by polymorphonuclear leukocytes in inflammation. Nature 284: 646–650
12. Rackham A, Ford-Hutchinson AW (1983) Inflammation and pain sensitivity: effects of leukotrienes D_4, B_4, and prostaglandin E_1 in the rat paw. Prostaglandins 25: 193–203
13. Payan DG, Missirian-Basteian A, Goetzl EJ (1984) Human T-lymphocyte subset specificity of the regulatory effects of leukotriene B_4. Proc Natl Acad Sci USA 81: 3501–3505
14. Rola Pleszczynski M, Borgeat P, Sirois P (1982) Leukotriene B_4 induces human suppressor lymphocytes. Biochem Biophys Res Commun 108: 1531–1537
15. Rola-Pleszczynski M, Gagnon L, Sirois P (1983) Leukotriene B_4 augments human natural cytotoxic cell activity. Biochem Biophys Res Commun 113: 531–537
16. Johnson HM, Torres BA (1984) Leukotrienes: positive signals for regulation of γ-interferon production. J Immunol 132: 413–416
17. Goodwin JS, Atluru D, Sierakowski S, Lianos EN (1986) Mechanism of action of glucocorticosteroids. Inhibition of T cell proliferation and Interleukin 2 production by hydrocortisone is reversed by leukotriene B_4. J Clin Invest 77: 1244–1250
18. Piper PJ (1984) Formation and action of leukotrienes: Physiol Rev 64: 744–761
19. Guindon Y, Girard Y, Maycock A, Ford-Hutchinson AW, Atkinson JG, Bélanger PC, Dallob A, DeSousa D, Dougherty H, Egan R, Goldenberg MM, Ham E, Fortin R, Hamel P, Hamel R, Lau CK, Leblanc Y, McFarlane CS, Piechuta H, Thérien M, Yoakim C, Rokach J (1984) L-651,392, A Novel, Potent, and Selective 5-Lipoxygenase Inhibitor. Adv in Prostaglandin, Thromboxane and Leukotriene Res (Eds B Samuelsson, R Paoletti, and PW Rumwell) Raven Press, New York, pp 554–557
20. Letts LG, McFarlane CS, Piechuta H, Ford-Hutchinson AW (1987) The effects of a 5-lipoxygenase inhibitor (L-651,392) and leukotriene D_4 antagonist (L-649,923) in two animal models of immediate hypersensitivity. Adv in Prostaglandin, Thromboxane and Leukotriene Res (Eds. B Samuelsson, R Paoletti, and PW Rumwell) Raven Press, New York, pp 1007–1011
21. Garceau D, Ford-Hutchinson AW The role of leukotrienes in allergen-induced vascular permeability changes in the guinea-pig conjunctiva. Adv in Prostaglandin, Thromboxane and Leukotriene Res (Eds B Samuelsson, R Paoletti, and PW Rumwell) Raven Press, New York, pp 167–170
22. Jones TR, Guindon Y, Young R, Champion E, Charette L, DeHaven RN, Denis D, Ethier D, Ford-Hutchinson AW, Fortin R, Letts G, Masson P, Maycock A, McFarlane C, Piechuta H, Pong SS, Rokach J, Yoakim C (1986) L-648,051, Sodium 4-[3-(4-acetyl-3-hydroxy-2-propylphenoxy) propylsulfonyl]-γ-oxo-benzenebutanoate: A leukotriene D_4 receptor antagonist. Can J Physiol Pharmacol, 64: 1535–1542
23. Jones TR, Young R, Champion E, Charette L, Denis D, Ford-Hutchinson AW, Frenette R, Gauthier J-Y, Guindon Y, Kakushima M, Masson P, McFarlane C, Piechuta H, Rokach J, Zamboni R (1986) L-649,923, sodium (βS*, γR*)-4-(3-(4-acetyl-3-hydroxy-2-propylphenoxy)-propylthio)-γ-hydroxy-β-methyl-benzenebutanoate, a selective orally active leukotriene receptor antagonist. Can J Physiol Pharmacol 64: 1068–1075
24. Barnes N, Piper PJ, Costello J (1987) The effect of an oral leukotriene antagonist L-649,923 on histamine and leukotriene D_4-induced bronchoconstriction in normal man. J Allergy Clin Immunol 79: 816–821
25. Goldenberg MM, Subers EM (1983) The effect of leukotriene D_4 on the isolated stomach and colon of the rat. Life Sciences 33: 2121–2127
26. Holme G, Brunet G, Masson P, Girard Y, Rokach J (1980) The activity of synthetic leukotriene C-1 on guinea-pig trachea and ileum. Prostaglandins 20: 717–721
27. Pendleton RG, Shepherd-Rose AJ, Stavorski JM (1986) Leukotriene effects upon the transgastric potential difference and pepsin secretion. Europ J Pharmacol 123: 29–30
28. Pendleton RG, Stavorski JR (1986) Evidence for differing leukotriene receptors in gastric mucosa. Europ J Pharmacol 125: 297–299
29. Peskar BM, Lange K, Hoppe U, Peskar BA (1986) Ethanol stimulates formation of leukotriene C_4 in rat gastric mucosa. Prostaglandins 31: 283–293

Discussion Following the Report of Dr. Ford-Hutchinson

FLEMSTRÖM

May I make a comment? The basal potential difference is usually some 50–60 mv in the cat. Therefore, I guess that the small changes you were seeing were related to some changes in ion transport rather than in protection.

SZABO

A comment and a question. I am not surprised at the relatively vague cytoprotective effect of the leukotriene antagonist because at least in our hand it was really not very active, although we have not finished all the dose and time responses. My question is whether there are any leukotriene receptors in the gastric tissue? The elegant studies you show were all done in the lung. Do you have any similar receptor studies in gastric tissue?

FORD-HUTCHINSON

No, we have not looked at gastric tissues for leukotriene receptors.

WHITTLE

I wonder whether you are concerned about giving such a dose of leukotriene as 1 μ/kg per minute? Surely not even under pathophysiological conditions could such concentrations be achieved?

FORD-HUTCHINSON

The doses of leukotrienes were high, but it is difficult to relate these to the local concentrations due to the rapid metabolism and elimination of these products. the high dose may also explain the difficulty in blocking the response with the LTD_4-receptor antagonist.

WHITTLE

When you give the leukotrienes intravenously, presumably there is a myriad of effects in different tissues, such as perhaps the heart. Are the effects on the stomach indirect, resulting from changes in circulatory parameters?

FORD-HUTCHINSON

Fortunately, the cat is relatively insensitive to LTD_4 in terms of cardiovascular and respiratory actions. Pendleton observed changes in local blood flow associated with the infusion of leukotrienes. Another problem with these types of studies is the species variations observed. It is difficult to say which is the appropriate species for man. The cat certainly is not a good one in terms of airway and cardiovascular changes.

PESKAR

Would you prefer a 5-lipoxygenase enzyme inhibitor or a leukotriene-receptor antagonist for the treatment of human diseases?

FORD-HUTCHINSON

That depends on the clinical disease. If your interest is in terms of asthma, a key mediator would be leukotriene D_4, and the approach would be effective. If you are interested in such deseases as inflammatory bowel diseases or psoriases where a potential role for leukotriene B_4 has been postulated, you clearly need a 5-lipoxygenase inhibitor.

Protective Effects on the Gastrointestinal Mucosa. New Aspects of the Last Two Years

"Aggressive" and "Protective" Factors in the Pathogenesis of Peptic Ulcer Disease

W. D. W. REES, and C. J. SHORROCK

Introduction

A popular model of peptic ulcer pathogenesis depicts the disease as arising from an imbalance in the equilibrium that normally exists between the stomach's "protective" barriers and "aggressive" luminal factors such as acid, pepsin, refluxed bile salts and ingested drugs. Clearly such aggressive factors are important but whether or not they instigate gastroduodenal damage remains controversial. We know acid and pepsin outputs are within the normal range in the majority of ulcer patients and non-steroidal anti-inflammatory drugs, while being important, are only relevant to a proportion of the total ulcer population. The obvious implication is that patients with peptic ulcer disease have abnormal mucosal resistance or defence to damaging luminal factors.

Components of Mucosal Defence (Fig. 1)

Mucus Bicarbonate Barrier

The "first line" defence against intraluminal contents is provided by the "mucus-bicarbonate" barrier, which consists of a thick layer of adherent mucus gel into which is

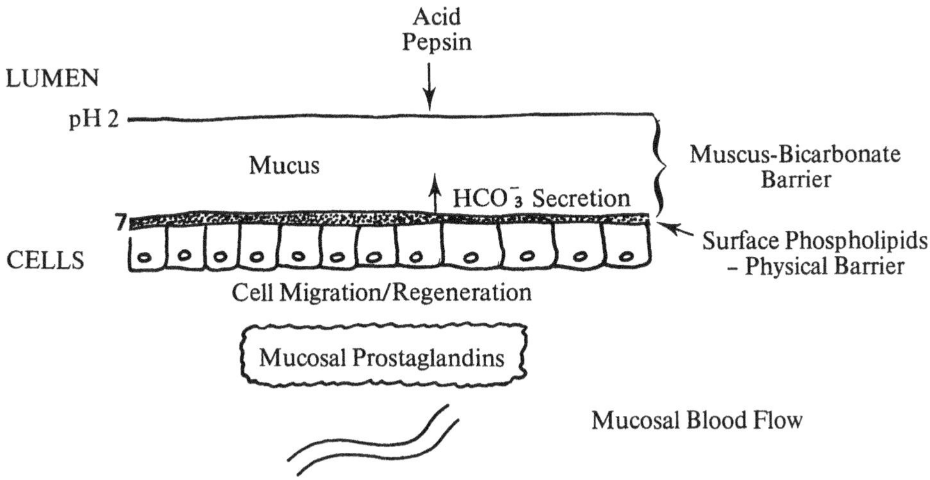

Fig. 1. Gastric mucosal barriers and protective mechanisms

secreted bicarbonate by underlying epithelial cells. The basal rate of bicarbonate secretion is around 5 to 10% of maximal acid output, while proximal duodenal mucosa secretes alkali at twice the rate of basal gastric output. Therefore, in the absence of a mucus gel layer which confines neutralisation to the cell surface, the small amounts of alkali produced would be completely overwhelmed by acid secretion if delivered directly into the lumen.

The presence of a thick layer of mucus gel adherent to the gastroduodenal epithelium by its visco-elastic properties produces an unstirred layer which confines acid-bicarbonate interaction close to the mucosal surface. The glycoprotein matrix of the mucus substantially reduces the rate of diffusion of small ions across it. The end result is an unstirred layer of mucus gel where acid diffusing across from the lumen is neutralized by bicarbonate secreted by surface cells diffusing in the opposite direction. The gel therefore sustains a pH gradient with the cell surface at pH 7–8 despite luminal pH's of 2–3 and this dynamic barrier is the first line of defence in the healthy stomach. Recent evidence suggests that another type of mucus-bicarbonate barrier may be just as important in the damaged stomach. Damaged mucosa is covered by a thick layer of mucus gel, fibrin and sloughed cells into which diffuses large quantities of bicarbonate from plasma and interstitial fluid. The resultant zone buffers surviving cell nests from further damage from luminal acid and pepsin, thus allowing regeneration and re-epithelialization of the damaged mucosa.

Surface Epithelial Cells

Epithelial cells play an important role in the first line defence of the stomach by the delivery of mucus gel and transport of bicarbonate. However, there is evidence that the epithelial cells have intrinsic barrier properties. Early studies by Davenport and Code in the 1960's suggested that the apical membrane and "tight junctions" between epithelial cells were relatively impermeable to H^+ ions and therefore formed a barrier to diffusion. Some evidence suggests that fixed charges are present in channels within surface epithelium which impede the movement of positively charged ions such as H^+. More recent studies have documented the existence of surface active phospholipids providing the surface epithelium with a hydrophobic lining. This lining allows molecules of high lipid solubility to pass freely into the mucosa but retards the passage of water soluble ions such as H^+. Agents such as NSAIDs and bile salts increase mucosal permeability to H^+ ions and virtually eliminate surface hydrophobicity and these effects may be important in mediating their damaging action.

The ability of surface epithelial cells to rapidly migrate across denuded lamina from cells in the gastric pits appears to be an important part of the mucosal defence system. After extensive destruction of superficial epithelial cells, experiments have shown complete re-epithelialization within an hour. The repair process is protected from the damaging luminal environment by the above mentioned layer of mucus gel and passive diffusion of bicarbonate. The mechanisms for regulating this re-epithelialization process as yet remain unknown.

Blood Flow

Mucosal blood flow, by delivering oxygen, nutrients and bicarbonate to the surface epithelium and removing H^+ ions which have penetrated the mucus-bicarbonate and epithelial "barriers", plays a vital role in protecting the gastric mucosa. There is considerable evidence that reduction in blood flow is important in mediating mucosal damage and duodenal mucosa appears more susceptible to reduction in blood flow than gastric mucosa. Prostaglandins can reduce or prevent the changes in gastric microcirculation produced by damaging agents and may thus be important in regulating mucosal blood flow.

The Role of Prostaglandins

The importance of prostaglandins in modulating mucosal defence mechanisms is implied from observations that NSAIDs, which cause gastric mucosal damage, are potent inhibitors of prostaglandin synthesis, and that exogenous prostaglandins protect mucosa from a variety of damaging agents including NSAIDs. Although prostaglandins do inhibit gastric acid secretion some of their protective actions occur at concentrations which do not influence acid output.

Several types of prostaglandins have been identified from gastric mucosa and gastric juice, namely those of the F, E, and I series, and enzymes for their biosynthesis and degradation can be found in gastric mucosa. Exogenous application of prostaglandins has favourable effects on virtually every component of mucosal defence.

Aggressive Factors (Fig. 2)

A number of luminal factors have been implicated in the production of gastroduodenal mucosal damage, in particular acid, bile acids and ingested drugs such as NSAIDs or ethanol. Dietary ingredients and smoking may also affect mucosal integrity either by a direct action on the epithelium or by influencing the concentrations of damaging

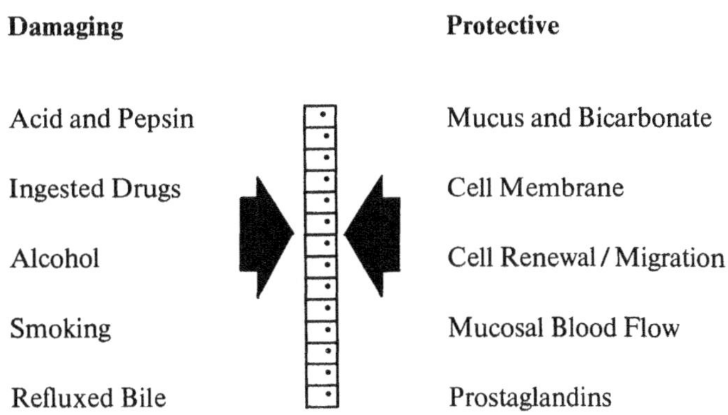

Fig. 2. Factors involved in damaging and protecting gastric mucosa

luminal factors. In recent years, interest has been aroused by the demonstration of a bacterium, Campylobacter Pylori, at the mucus-cell interface of damaged mucosa, although the role it plays in producing gastroduodenal damage remains uncertain.

Gastric Acid

Schwartz's dictum of "no acid, no ulcer" still holds true today and there is no doubt that luminal acid is necessary for the production of gastric and duodenal ulcers.

Basal and nocturnal acid secretion are normal in the majority of peptic ulcer patients, although suppression of nocturnal output is important in ulcer healing. The most consistent abnormality of acid secretion observed in duodenal ulcers is meal stimulated output, being increased in about two thirds of patients. In gastric ulcer stimulated acid output ranges from being increased in pre-pyloric ulcers, to decreased in main body ulcers. However, in all these groups there is a large overlap between normal controls and ulcer patients. The duodenum has pH sensitive receptors which regulate gastric acid emptying by an undefined mechanism and there is evidence that a defect in acid inhibition of gastric emptying occurs in some duodenal ulcer patients.

Pepsin

The role of pepsin in the pathogenesis of peptic ulceration is far from being clear. Pepsin is a powerful proteolytic enzyme at low pH and in theory would contribute to mucosal disruption by other factors. Abnormal serum pepsinogen levels have been detected in DU and GU patients and are indicative of increased chief cell mass and gastritis, respectively. Increased pepsin output has been demonstrated in a proportion of DU patients. At present, these findings contribute little to our understanding of ulcer pathogenesis.

Duodenogastric Reflux and Bile Salts

Certain constituents of duodenal contents such as bile salts and lysolecithin have been shown to damage gastric mucosa and hence chronic reflux of duodenal juice into the stomach has been implicated in the pathogenesis of gastric ulcer. High concentrations of bile salts cause gastric mucosal damage, inhibition of gastric bicarbonate secretion, disruption of mucus gel, reduction of the pH gradient across mucus gel and increase in the permeability of the epithelial layer to H^+ ions. However, there is some doubt as to the relevance of these findings to the low concentrations of bile salts found in the stomach of ulcer patients. Furthermore, the demonstration of abnormal bile reflux in GU patients is unconvincing.

Non-steroidal Anti-inflammatory Drugs

As in the case of bile salts there is ample evidence that acute exposure of gastric or duodenal mucosa to aspirin or other NSAIDs disturbs mucosal function causing damage to the surface epithelium. Aspirin and indomethacin are potent inhibitors of gastroduodenal alkali secretion and reduce the pH gradient across the mucus gel layer. They also disrupt surface active phospholipids and increase cell exfoliation. Many of these actions are prevented by pretreatment with prostaglandins and since the drugs inhibit cyclo-oxygenase activity, it has been postulated that their damaging action is due to depletion of local tissue prostaglandins.

Recent work suggests that in 30% of patients over the age of 60 admitted to hospital with upper gastrointestinal bleeding the haemorrhage is attributable to NSAIDs and that these agents account for the maintained or rising incidence of peptic ulcer in this age group.

Dietary factors

There is little evidence that avoidance of certain foods plays a role in maintaining mucosal integrity. A high fibre diet may reduce duodenal ulcer relapse but there are no convincing data that ulcer healing is improved. Increased intake of polyunsaturated essential fatty acids has recently been linked to the decline in peptic ulcer incidence over the last decade or so. These may act as precursors for mucosal prostaglandin synthesis and this hypothesis may have major implications for ulcer therapy and prevention of relapse. Ingestion of ethanol in high concentrations damages gastric mucosa and disturbs mucosal defence mechanisms, although there is little epidemiological evidence that alcohol plays any role in the pathogenesis of peptic ulcer disease.

Smoking

There is evidence that cigarette smoking harms the balance that normally exists between aggressive luminal factors and defence mechanisms. Smokers are more likely to develop peptic ulcers and respond less well to treatment. It has been shown that smoking adversely affects mucosal prostaglandin production and increases gastroduodenal reflux of bile, although the evidence is far from convincing. Smoking does stimulate nocturnal acid secretion which may be particularly important in producing mucosal damage.

Gastric microflora

The finding of *Campylobacter pylori* in the mucus gel overlying damaged mucosa has stimulated much interest in the role of bacteria in causing mucosal damage. The mechanism by which these organisms damage gastroduodenal mucosa remains uncertain. Disturbance of mucus production by surface epithelial cells has been demonstrated with *C. pylori* and the organism also possesses powerful urease activity. These properties may therefore disturb the "mucus-bicarbonate" barrier and expose the epithelium to a damaging acidic environment.

References

1. Crampton JR, Rees WDW (1986) Gastroduodenal bicarbonate secretion: Its role in protecting the stomach and duodenum. In: Recent Advances in Gastroenterology; Ed Pounder RE. Churchill Livingstone. 35–50
2. Flemstrom G, Turnberg LA (1984) Gastroduodenal defense mechanisms. Clinics in Gastroenterology: Vol 13, no 2, 327–354
3. Guth PH (1984) Local metabolism and circulation in mucosal defense. In: Allen A, Flemstrom G, Garner A, Silen W, Turnberg LA (eds). Mechanisms of mucosal protection in the upper gastrointestinal tract. Raven Press, New York 253–258
4. Hills BA, Butler BD, Lichtenberger LM (1983) Gastric mucosal barrier: Hydrophobic lining to the lumen of the stomach. American Journal of Physiology 244 (Gastrointest Liver Physiol 7): G561–G568
5. Lacy ER, Ito S (1984) Ethanol-induced insult to the superficial rat gastric epithelium: A study of damage and rapid repair. In: Allen A, Flemstrom G, Garner A, Silen W, Turnberg LA (eds). Mechanisms of mucosal protection in the upper gastrointestinal tract. Raven Press, New York 49–55
6. Rathbone BJ, Wyatt JI, Heatley RV (1986) Campylobacter pyloridis – A new factor in peptic ulcer disease? Gut 27, 635–641
7. Venables CW (1986) Mucus, pepsin, and peptic ulcer. Gut 27, 233–238

Discussion Following the Report of Dr. Rees

GRAHAM

One of the problems that we all have is the philosophy that if we can measure something in the laboratory, it must have something to do with the disease. Recently we have been able to measure the presence of the *Campylobacter pylori* organism in patients' stomachs. We note that they swim in the mucus, and they probably alter its structure and function. They are clearly associated with altered surface of the gastrointestinal mucosa and with polymorphonuclear cell infiltration. To renew themselves they should induce some other alterations in the cells' abilities. Would you discuss this? How does this fit with the other information that you have given us?

REES

Yes, certainly, I think that perhaps it would have been wise to have included *Campylobacter* in the first slide, although I must admit that as yet I am a little unclear myself as to what role it precisely plays. As you say quite clearly, evidence is accumulating to suggest that this organism actually does produce mucosal damage. Even talking to people who actually work in this area it is still unclear as to what comes first, "the horse or the cart," because it is quite possible that the environment created by damaged mucosa allows these organisms to infiltrate the mucus gel layer and to exist at that site.

GRAHAM

It has been clearly shown that normal mucosa is transformed to abnormal by the organisms, and that it returns to normal when you eliminate them. Thus it can be concluded that mucosal alterations are caused by *Campylobacter pylori.*

REES

Yes, I think there is some evidence for this. I think evidence is coming along to suggest that this organism does produce gastric mucosal damage, but the evidence is still thin on the ground. This organism's very potent urease activity may be important. There are publications suggesting that perhaps local production of urea at the cell-mucus interface may well be an important damaging mechanism. I do not doubt, that in the case of gastritis *Campylobacter* is important. What I find very difficult to understand, is how it produces local peptic ulcer disease.

FLEMSTRÖM

Did the indomethacin or metabolic inhibition reduce aluminum-increased alkali secretion?

REES

I did not show a slide on it. We have completed work on sucralfate. Indomethacin abolishes in our laboratory the effects of sucralfate on alkali secretion. With aluminum we have not completed the experiments but the evidence suggests that it does the same. Our preliminary experiments using 10^{-5} *M* indomethacin show inhibition.

Heartburn and Mucosal Barrier Weakness

J. J. BERNIER, and CH. FLORENT

Introduction

Most of the patients who suffer from illness of the digestive tract do not show any signs of lesion after a careful examination. They are classified as "dyspentic" or of "psychosomatic" patients; many cases seem to have a functional disorder somewhere in the digestive tract. Our aim is to show that some patients have a mucosal defect which we shall call "mucosal barrier weakness." The rationale of this hypothetic mechanism is:

1. Experimental cytoaggression by different drugs is clearly established.
2. The major symptom of many dyspeptic patients is epigastric heartburn (quite different from pyrosis, which is a retrosternal and ascending pain), which appears shortly after ingestion of some beverages (white wine, coffee) or meals (jam or spices). These nutrients may possibly act as cytoaggressors.
3. We have found [2] in normal subjects that montmorrillonnite, an inert and neutral clay, reduces the aggressive effect of aspirin not only when they are both ingested at the same time, but also when aspirin is ingested 24 h after the clay (Tarnasky et al. have observed the same with glucagon [8]).
4. According to the general law linking pathological and physiological mechanisms (the first being either an enhancement or a diminution of the second), one may hypothesize that if some substances are able to increase the resistance of the mucosa, some others could produce the opposite: a weakening of the mucosal barrier.

We shall show that patients suffering from epigastric heartburn have 1. an abnormal gastric potential difference; 2. some surface mucosal lesions detected by scan electron microscopy [4].

Methods

Subjects and Patients

We have studied two groups:

a) One hundred asymptomatic young volunteers were tested, 54 of whom were checked by endoscopy.
b) 45 patients (28 males, 17 females, mean age 35 years, range 19–76) complained of early postprandial heartburn, usually related to some nutrients (coffee, wine, alcohol, jam).

Patients with pyrosis were disregarded. Some suffered from other digestive complaints (bloating, belching) and a few had colonic symptoms. An esogastroduodenoscopy had been performed in each case disregarding any mucosal lesion (ulcer, cancer, oesophagitis or gastritis); some biopsies were performed in fundus and antrum.

Potential Difference Measurements

Gastric potential difference (PD) was measured by the technique described by Florent et al. [3]. One electrode (a flow of saline through a catheter connected with an agar-K Cl bridge) was located in the antrum. The other one was connected with a subcutaneous needle. PD was measured during three periods: 30 min, basal; after intragastric instillation of 500 mg of aspirin in 100 ml saline; after intragastric instillation of 100 ml alcohol (10% v/v). The order of periods 2 and 3 were randomized.

Histological Studies

In all patients a light microscopic examination was done using conventional techniques. In 10 controls and nine patients, gastric mucosa biopsies were immediately fixed by immersion in fixative [9]. After 48 h delay, specimens were dehydrated in ethanol gradients, then dessicated by critical point drying, and coated with goldpalladium. After mounting on aluminium stubs, the biopsies were examined with a Jeol Scan 100 CX:

Results

Basal PD was significantly lower in patients than in controls (controls, -39.3 mV $\pm$ 3.3; patients, 26.6 $\pm$ 6.3). Basal PD was not different from controls in duodenal ulcers and in irritable colon. The effect of aspirin in patient differs from that in controls (Fig. 1); the magnitude of the PD drop is the same in both cases, but the return to basal value is longer in dyspeptic patients. Alcohol (10%), which was a weak aggressor in controls, was in contrast as aggressive as aspirin in patients. Figures 2 and 3 show the diagnostic efficacy of PD measurements (basal PD and 30 min after alcohol).

On scanning electron microscopy, antral and fundic biopsies of patients show more or less deep alterations of the mucosa: mucus hypersecretion, small ulcer craters in which erythrocytes, platelet aggregates, lymphocytes and necrotic cells can be viewed. These lesions were observed in all nine patients and in four out of 10 controls ($P < 0.005$. χ^2 test).

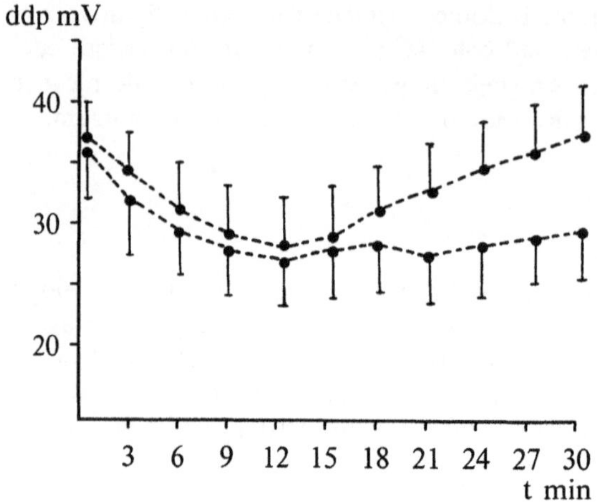

Fig. 1. Variations in PD after 500 mg of aspirin in controls (●) (n=100), and in dyspeptic patients (▼) (n=45).

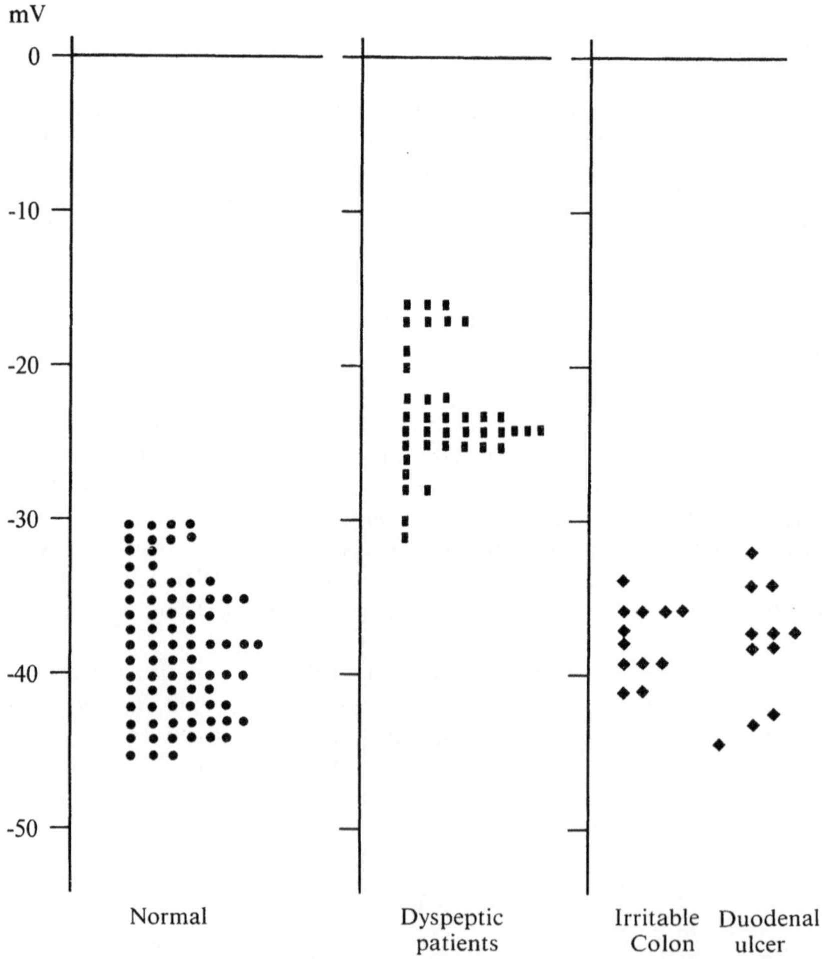

Fig. 2. Individual values of basal PD in controls (● in dyspeptic patients (■) and in patients with irritable colon and duodenal ulcer (◆)

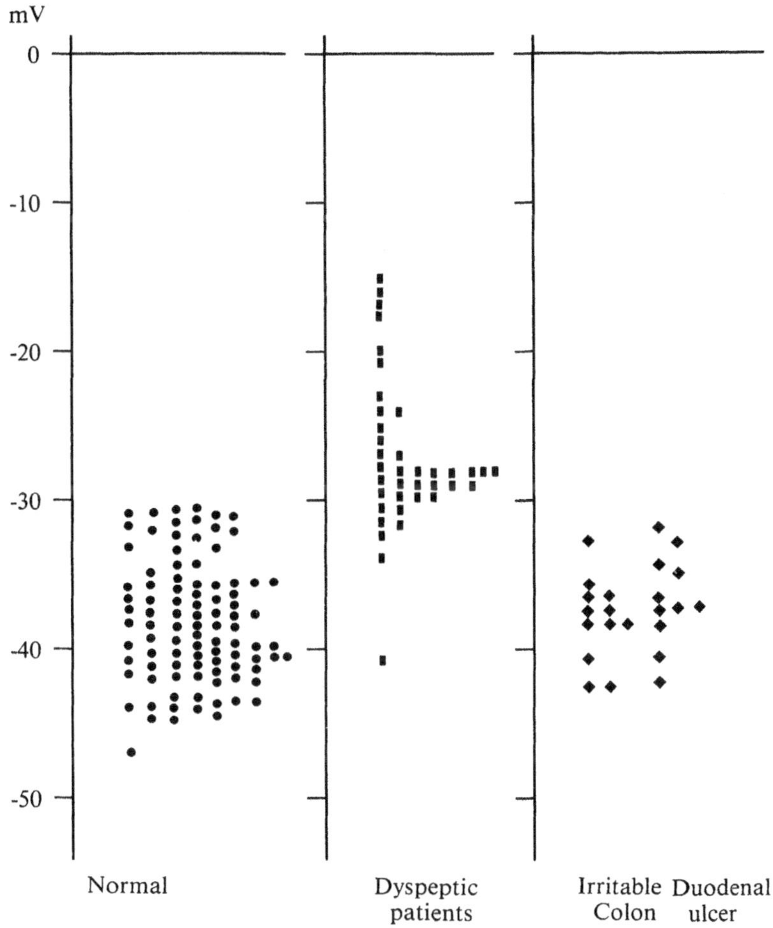

Fig. 3. Individual values of PD 30 min after alcohol 10% v/v in controls and in patients. Symbols see Fig. 2

Discussion

Definition of the Patient Group

The dyspeptic patients were selected on the following criteria: epigastric early post-prandial heartburn, without pyrosis, related to some food or beverages. These criteria are less numerous than those included in the "nonulcerous dyspepsia" of the English literature [5] and are quite different from those described in Malagelada's "dyspepsia" [7]. It is well known that it is difficult to link the site of an abdominal pain to an organ of the digestive tract [6].

One may criticize the homogeneity or our group of patients. We can say that

a) patients have been included in the study by agreement of two trained gastroenterologists and

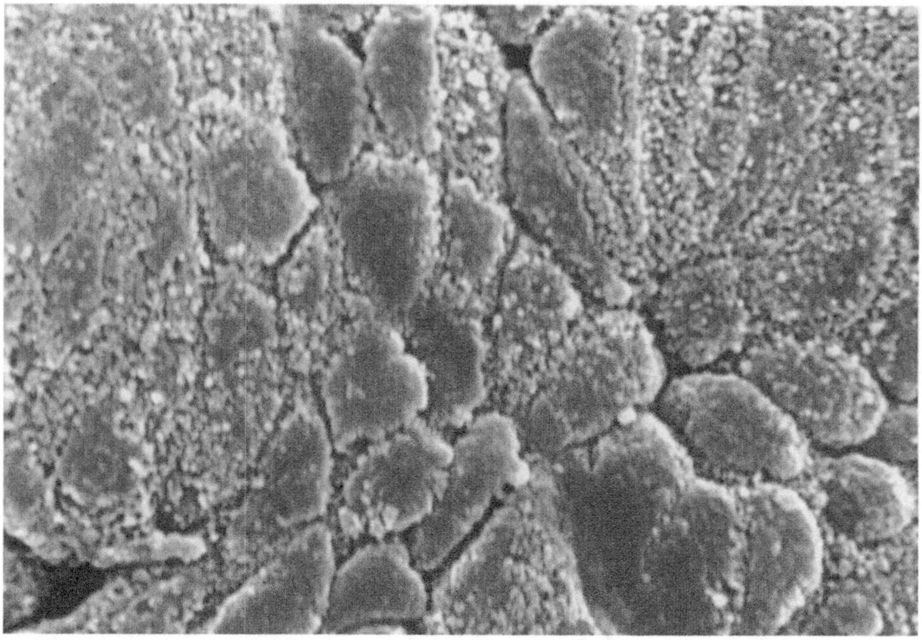

Fig. 4. Scanning electron microscopy (×2000). Normal

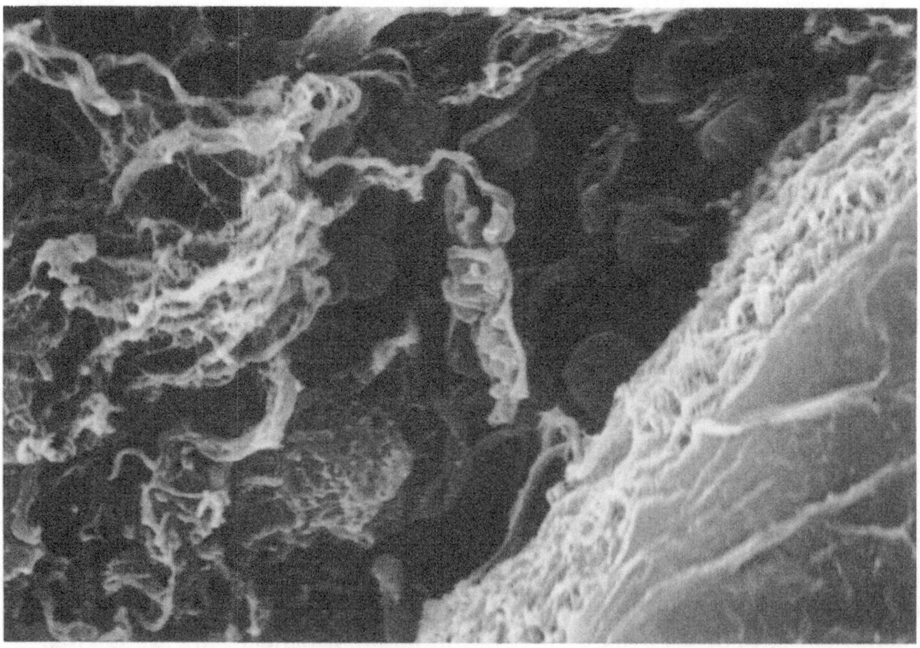

Fig. 5. Scanning electron microscopy (×1500). Heartburn dyspeptic patient; ulceration with erythrocytes, modification of the mucus

b) a systematic gastroscopy (with biopsies) had shown that the upper digestive tract appeared normal (no visible esophagitis or gastritis, no ulcer, no cancer).

No special study had been performed in order to test gastro-oesophageal reflux; this may be questioned as Blum at al. [1] said that heartburn and gastroesophageal reflux are frequently associated.

Value of PD Variations

PD measurement is not easy, but technical artifacts produce a sudden drop of the line. A slow and continuous drop of the base line may cause some difficulties in the lecture of the curves.

What Distinguishes the Patients with Regard to the PD Variations?

In patients, compared to controls,
a) basal PD is lower;
b) variations after aspirin are longer;
c) variations after alcohol are greater and longer. This combination is constant.

Looking at the individual data, we have observed that:
1. Basal PD value (normal limit −32 mV) classifies 100 controls and 45 patients except eight (9%) (three controls and five patients).
2. All except four patients with a low basal PD show an abnormal response to aspirin and alcohol; the four patients who differ from the others are not in opposition to the general concept; their PD was so low that it could not drop further.
3. Using the PD 30 min after aspirin or alcohol (normal limit −30 mV) there were only three errors (2%), one control and two patients. One may conclude that PD is a good screening test.

Which Mucosal Lesions are Associated with the Electrical Abnormalities? Do patients have Gastritis?

To the second question the answer is no. Endoscopists have never seen either mucosal aspects of gastritis or small erosions as seen in patients using NSAIDs. Biopsies performed in 45 cases have shown interstitial gastritis in nine cases only. It is clear that these conclusions are questionable, as there is great discussion among endoscopists and pathologists about gastritis criteria.

Nevertheless, it seems that constant superficial lesions of the mucosa exist as shown by scan microscope, i.e., changes in mucus aspect, small erosions, appearance of numerous blood cells. The pathologist, Mme Droy-Lefay, who is well trained in experimental work on the rat, thinks that these lesions look like the findings seen in experience with weak aggressors. During a blind test she correctly classified 15 among 19 patients or controls.

We suggest to call this syndrome "mucosal barrier weakness" because
a) basal PD is lower than normal and it is correlated to surface alterations,
b) aspirin has more aggressive effects than in controls.
c) 10% alcohol which has weak aggressive effects in controls has an effect as aggressive as aspirin in patients.

What Causes the Mucosal Barrier Weakness?

The first hypothesis is bile reflux, but with respect to gastric juice and noting the yellow color of bilirubin, there was no difference between controls and patients. Our hypothesis, yet unproved, is that the deleterious agents are nutrients. Heartburn after white wine ingestion correlates well with PD abnormalities observed with 10% alcohol. The same effect after jam ingestion may be an osmotic cytoaggression. The main fact is that the mucosa reacts abnormally to beverages or food which are weak aggressors in controls. The most interesting hypothesis is that the mucosal defect is chronic and that the patients suffer for a long period of time. Is this defect related to an insufficiency of local prostaglandins? This is an unsolved problem, as is the question of a possible benefit from treatment with synthetic prostaglandins.

Conclusion

Gastric PD measurements (basal and after alcohol 10%, v/v) allow us to describe a mucosal barrier weakness in dyspeptic patients. It could be an accurate tool in therapeutic trials.

References

1. Blum A, Heartburn and gastrooesophageal reflux. Personal communication
2. Florent C, Flourie B, Bernier JJ (1985) Effets d'un pansement anti-acide sur les modifications de la différence de potential gastrique induite par l'aspirine chez l'homme. Gastroenterol Clin Biol 8: 359-363
3. Florent C, Flourie B, Pfeiffer A, Bernier JJ (1985) Mesure de la différence de potential transépitheliale gastrique. Gastroenterol Clin Biol 9: 58-64
4. Florent C, Pfeiffer A, Bernier JJ (1985) La faiblesse de la barrière muqueuse gastrique: un nouveau concept. Gastroenterol Clin Biol 9: 65-71
5. Jorgensen LS, Bonlokke L, Wamberg P (1985) Non-ulcer upper dyspepsia. Aspect of pain. Scand J Gastroenterol 20: 46-50
6. Kingham GC, Dawson AM (1985) Origin of chronic right upper quadrant pain. Gut 26: 783-788
7. Malagelada J (1986) Dyspepsia, Workshop World Congress São Paulo
8. Tarnawski A, Krause WJ, Kevin JI (1978) Effect of glucagon on aspirin-induced gastric mucosal damage in man. Gastroenterology 74: 240-245
9. Trump BF, Mac Dowell EM (1976) Histologic fixatives suitable for diagnostic light and electron microscopy. Arch Path Lab Med 100: 405-414

Discussion Following the Report of Prof. Bernier

HOLTERMÜLLER

Your patients were symptomatic when you studied them. Was there a difference in the findings when the same patients being asymptomatic were examined again?

BERNIER

Yes, we have performed some trials with various drugs. Montmorrillonite (a kind of clay), which is an old drug, leads to symptomatic relief after 3 weeks of treatment. It normalizes variations of the potential difference, i. e. basal value, and is the answer to aspirin and/or alcohol.

RASK-MADSEN

Using the electrical potential difference as a single marker of mucosal barrier weakness alone, there may be a problem of interpretation, which might explain the differences you observed by using this technique. You have to measure the pH as well and correct for the diffusion potential occuring as a consequence of hydrogen ion flux.

BERNIER

Yes, I agree. In fact we have checked the pH in each sample. In the mean there were no differences between controls and patients.

COHEN

Not only is PD affected by both active and passive ionic movement, but the PD can also change merkedly, in fact up to 30 mV, depending on precisely where in the gastroduodenum your position the electrode. So my first question is: How do you place the tube accurately, so that it is in the same position for all subjects? My second question is: Does the investigator know whether the patient has non-ulcer dyspepsia or is a control?

BERNIER

Yes, the investigator knows the clinical situation. The electrode was introduced into the antrum. Its accurate position was checked by radioscopy.

GRAHAM

I hate to come back to the *Campylobacter pyloridis* again. Dr. ALA TOUKON in Jordan showed last year that patients with non-ulcer dyspepsia almost always had polymorphonuclear infiltrates in antral mucosa biopsies. Previous studies by Greenlow and others indicate that this is a universal finding. Your studies suggest the same phenomenon. The reasons for this are pyloric *Campylobacter* and altered mucosa. I assume that you are doing your PDs with fluid in the stomach before you obtain an average PD and not the focal PD that Dr. COTTEN was talking about. *Campylobacter pyloridis* would also probably explain the response to clay. Heavy metals such as bismuth will eradicate these organisms at least temporarily, and restore histology to normal. This would explain the change of potential difference. I would recommend to repeat PD measurements shortly after your experiments with DeNol as the drum sticks will come back again if you wait too many days. PD will then be normal, and you have found another way to measure the presence of pyloric *Campylobacter* in the stomach. This is my hypothesis.

BERNIER

Of course, we were interested in finding *Campylobacter* in our patients, but looking carefully the biopsy material we have found only one case.

GRAHAM

I will send you some of our test materials so that you can find it in everyone.

The Functional Role of Prostanoids in the Gastroduodenal Mucosa

G. BERTACCINI, and G. CORUZZI

Introduction

The term prostanoids embraces compounds derived from the action of cycloxygenase on arachidonic acid, that is prostaglandins (PGs) and thromboxanes (TXs). Human gastric mucosa can synthesize PGD_2, PGE_2, $PGF_{2\alpha}$, 6-keto $PGF_{1\alpha}$ and TXA_2; however, the sources of these products and their role in gastric functions have not been fully elucidated. We do not know exactly which cells produce these substances; for instance, it is uncertain to what extent the thromboxanes and PGI_2 are released from blood platelets or blood vessels into the gastric mucosa. Some discrepancies may arise from different methods of evaluation, from "in vivo" vs "in vitro" studies, different species etc.

The Physiological Role of Prostanoids

The role of prostanoids can be mainly deduced from the observed action of exogenously administered PGs (especially synthetic derivatives) or from inhibitors of their synthesis. The two main effects of PGs are the inhibition of acid secretion and protection of the mucosa from noxious stimuli, whereas thromboxanes predominantly affect blood vessels, causing a potent vasoconstriction in the gastric vasculature and a remarkable proaggregatory action.

There are many doubts about the possible physiological role of PGs in the control of gastric secretion. Tepperman et al. [40] suggested that endogenous PGs are not physiological regulators of acid secretion, after observing the inability of indomethacin to alter acid output, though reducing PGs synthesis and release in the dog stomach. More recently Mogard and Walsh [28] showed that basal acid secretion and the secretory response to a pepton meal in humans were not affected by indomethacin pretreatment and had no effect on plasma gastrin levels.

These results, of course, cast some doubts on a physiological role of PGs in the control of acid secretion. However, the recent demonstration of a receptor for E-type PGs on the parietal cell membrane is suggestive of a specific function for endogenous PGs in the secretory process [41].

A physiological role for PGs in mucosal protection appears more likely; the effects on mucus and bicarbonate production both in the stomach and in the duodenum have been demonstrated in a variety of mammalian species, including humans (for review

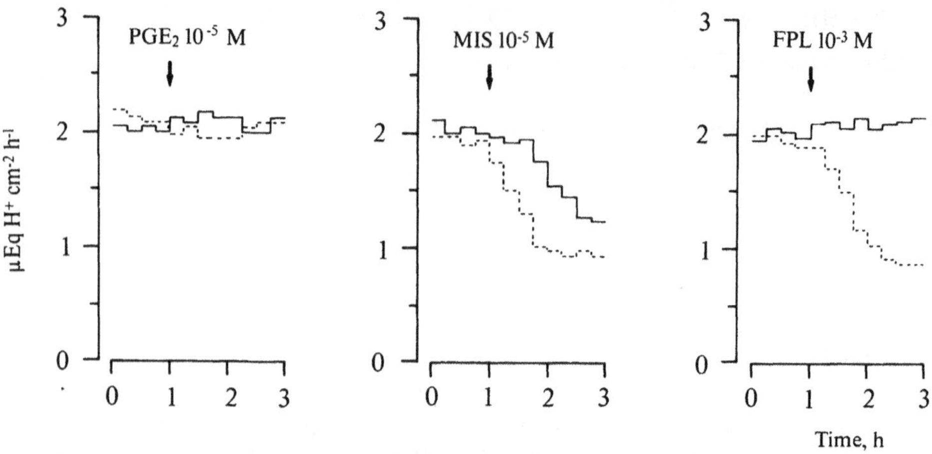

Fig. 1. Isolated gastric fundus from immature rat. Effect of different compounds on basal acid secretion, administered at *arrows. MIS,* misoprostol; *FPL,* FPL 52694; *continuous line,* administration of the drugs on the serosal side; *dashed line,* administration on the mucosal side

see [13]). Also the PG effects of gastric microcirculation, gastric mucosal sulfhydryl compounds, surface-active phospholipids and macromolecular synthesis (with a definite increase in DNA and RNA synthesis) are well known [27]. According to recent findings some synthetic PGs are also able to stabilize the mast cell membrane [35], however, it is still unknown whether or not this interesting property is also shared by natural PGs. However, it is interesting that other mast cell stabilizers may have gastric cytoprotective properties [11] or may actually inhibit gastric acid secretion [7, 10]. Preliminary experiments performed in our laboratory seem to demonstrate that the synthetic PGE analog misoprostol, like the mast cell stabilizing agent FPL 52694 [10], can inhibit basal acid secretion in the rat isolated stomach, whereas PGs do not ([12], Coruzzi and Bertaccini, unpublished; Fig. 1).

Prostanoids and Gastric Pathology

Interesting findings have been made concerning pathological conditions, like gastric (GU) and duodenal (DU) ulcer. In GU patients the PGE content of the stomach was found to be significantly lower than in healthy subjects [44]. Konturek [19] reported also that 6-keto-$PGF_{1\alpha}$ and TXB_2 were significantly reduced in GU patients, whereas the reduction was not statistically significant in DU patients. However, data concerning DU patients are not uniform, since both a reduction and an increase in PG content have been reported [1, 25, 33]. Moreover, in DU patients, in contrast to healthy subjects, the secretory response after ingestion of a meal resulted in a definite decrease in PG synthesis. A significant reduction in the synthesis of PGE_2 from antral biopsy specimens (from 616 $\pm$ 166 to 253 $\pm$ 94 pg/mg of mucosa) was also found in subjects suffering from reflux gastritis [9].

Thromboxanes and PGI_2 are important modulators of gastric acid secretion and blood flow. As a consequence, an imbalance in their relative synthesis could result in an increase in gastric secretion and a decrease in gastric blood flow and finally in gastric ulceration. In fact Hillier et al. [16] showed that in DU patients the ratio of PGI_2 to thromboxane formation was significantly reduced. Since PGI_2 is cytoprotective [29] whereas thromboxanes are ulcerogenic [43], it seems reasonable to expect that an imbalance in the PGI_2 : TX ratio should favour tissue damage and then ulcerogenesis. On the contrary, a favourable PGI_2 : TX ratio should be cytoprotective. Accordingly, it was reported that imidazole or other thromboxane biosynthesis inhibitors are indeed highly cytoprotective [20, 42].

Gastric Mucosal Synthesis of Prostanoids and the Effects of Drugs

The effects of drugs on prostanoid synthesis in the gastric mucosa are controversial, probably because of different methods of evaluation and variable conditions of the samples and species examined. The observation that some drugs (probanthine, omeprazole, pirenzepine etc.) may be cytoprotective at non-antisecretory doses or irrespective of whether they can affect prostanoid synthesis indicates that other mechanisms must be involved in the beneficial effects of these drugs. Results obtained with some compounds involved in the control of gastric secretion and/or in mucosal protection are shown in Table 1.

Table 1. Effect of different drugs on prostanoid synthesis in the gastric mucosa

Drug	PGs	TXs	Species
H^2 antagonists	↑ [34, 8], ↓ [14], 0 [23]	0 [33]	Rat, Man
Histamine	↑ [2]		Rat
Pirenzepine	0 [18, 21]	↓ [38]	Rat, Man
De-Nol	↑ [22]		Rat
Carbachol	↑ [30]		Dog
Omeprazole	0 [26], ↑ [36]		Dog, Rat
Antacids	↑ [37]		Rat
Carbenoxolone	0 [5], (↓) [31]	0 [5], ↓[32]	Rat, Man
Sucralfate	0 [34], ↑ [22]	↓ [22]	Man
Somatostatin	↑ [17]		Man, Rat
NSAID	↓ [34]	↓ [34]	Man

↑ increase; ↓ decrease; 0 no effect; superscripts, references

A revolutionary concept was recently proposed by Japanese investigators [2, 14] who claimed that histamine exerts PG-induced cytoprotection through histamine type 2 (H_2) receptor stimulation (Table 2). Consequently, H_2-receptor blockers could reduce the mucosal content of PGs and the gastric mucosal integrity and could possibly favour the occurrence of a peptic ulcer relapse at the end of treatment. Another possible explanation for the relatively high incidence of peptic ulcer recurrences after

Table 2. Effects of histamine on the mucosal PG levels in normal rat stomach and HCl-induced lesions (modified after [2])

	Dose (mg/kg)	PGE_2 (ng/g)	Gastric lesions
Saline		559 ± 82	10.8 ± 1.6
Histamine	4	774 ± 57*	6.1 ± 1.5*
	20	1957 ± 160**	0.8 ± 0.5**

* $P < 0.05$; ** $P < 0.001$

H_2-antagonist treatment is the upregulation of gastrin and H_2-receptors, as reported by Bertaccini and Coruzzi [6].

However, controversies exist on the effect of cimetidine on prostanoid synthesis in the gastric mucosa. Both a decrease and an increase in PG content were described by different authors. In acute experiments performed in the rat [3, 14] a decrease in $PGE_{1\alpha}$ and PGE_2 content was reported, whereas after chronic treatment with cimetidine in humans (1 month) a definite increase in PGE_2, $PGF_{1\alpha}$ and PGI_2, with no change in TXB_2, was found [8, 33]. Tarnawski et al. [39] reported an increase in haemorrhagic changes due to ethanol administration with both cimetidine and ranitidine and concluded that inhibition of H_2-receptors may negatively interfere with cytoprotection by PGs.

Part of the mucosal protection induced in man by a synthetic PG was shown to be mediated by somatostatin, which significantly increased in the gastric juice (from 34.34 to 75.79 pg/ml) after treatment with PGs. However, cimetidine also caused a remarkable increase in somatostatin in the gastric juice, whereas the degree of mucosal protection was definitely lower than that for PGs. Therefore it was concluded that somatostatin was only one of the factors responsible for mucosal protection [15].

Conclusions

From the above data it seems that evidence for, rather than against a physiological role of prostanoids in the gastric mucosa is more likely, PGs acting in an antisecretory and cytoprotective role and thromboxanes acting as pro-ulcerogenic agents. Therefore one can consider synthetic analogs of the natural PGs and thromboxane synthesis inhibitors as agents capable of maintaining gastric mucosal integrity.

Acknowledgement, Original work of the authors was supported by a grant from the C. N. R., Rome.

References

1. Ahlquist DA, Dozois RR, Zinsmeister AR, Malagelada JR (1983) Duodenal prostaglandin synthesis and acid load in health and duodenal ulcer disease. Gastroenterology 85: 522–528

2. Arakawa T, Fukuda T, Nakamura H, Kobayashi K (1986) Endogenous prostaglandin-mediated cytoprotection by histamine and its abolition by cimetidine in rat gastric mucosa. 6th Int Conf on Prostaglandins and Related Compounds. Florence, June 3–6, p 18
3. Basso N, Materia A, Forlini A, Di Marco M, Rossi P, Jaffe B (1981) Gastric mucosal prostaglandin (PG) content in rats following cimetidine administration. Gastroenterology 80: 1105
4. Bauer RF (1986) Misoprostol, pre-clinical pharmacology: gastric antisecretory effects. 6th Int Conf on Prostaglandins and Related Compounds. Satellite Symposium. Florence, June 4
5. Bennett A (1984) Gastric mucosal formation of prostanoids and the effects of drugs. Acta Physiol Hungarica 64: 215–217
6. Bertaccini G, Coruzzi G (1987) Prostaglandins and acid peptic disease: State of the art. Prostaglandins 33 (Suppl): 1–16
7. Boyd EJS, Wilson JA, Wormsley KG, Richards MH, Langman MJS (1985) Effects of a mast cell stabilizer (FPL 52694) on human gastric secretion. Agents Actions 16: 462–467
8. Branski D, Sharon P, Karmeli F, Rachmilewitz D (1983) Effect of cimetidine on human gastric and duodenal prostanoid synthesis. Isr J Med Sci 19: 690
9. Calcamuggi G, Mingozzi R, Dughera L, Emanuelli G (1986) Mucosal PGE release in reflux gastritis. 6 Int Conf on Prostaglandins and Related Compounds, Florence 3–6 June, abs 22
10. Canfield SP, Coruzzi G, Curwain B, Rundell T (1985) The action of two mast cell stabilizing agents and verapamil on rat gastric acid secretion in vitro. Eur J Pharmacol 116: 89–95
11. Colton DG, Reiffenstein JC, Buyniski JP (1985) BMY – 26517 – 31, a mast cell stabilizer with cytoprotective properties. Gastroenterology 88: 1354
12. Coruzzi G, Adami M, Bertaccini G, Canfield SP (1986) Pharmacological study of basal acid secretion by the rat isolated fundus preparation. Arch int Pharmacodyn 282: 140–150
13. Flemstrom G (1986) Gastroduodenal mucosal secretion of bicarbonate and mucus. Am J Med 81 (Suppl 2A): 18–22
14. Fukuda T, Arakawa T, Nakamura H, Kobayashi K (1986) Effect of long – term administration of cimetidine on mucosal prostaglandins, acid secretion, and mucosal integrity in rat stomach. 6th Int Conf on Prostaglandins and related compounds. Florence, June 3–6, p 20
15. Godiwala T, Agrawal N, Groot K, Arimura A, Dajani E (1986) Is cytoprotection by misoprostol against ethanol induced gastric mucosal injury in man mediated by somatostatin? 6th Int Conf. on Prostaglandins and Related Compounds. Satellite Symposium. Florence June 4
16. Hillier K, Smith CL, Jewell R (1984) Abnormal duodenal mucosa (DM) prostanoid and thromboxane synthesis in duodenal ulcer (DU) patients. IUPHAR 9th Int Congr Pharmacol, London, p 160
17. Jaffe BM, Mariani P, Silecchia G, Genco A, Bagarani M, Basso N (1986) Effect of somatostatin on prostaglandin E_2 gastric intraluminal release in man. 6th Int Conf on Prostaglandins and Related Compounds Florence June 3–6, p 21
18. Jeremy JY, Dandona P (1984) The effect of pirenzepine on in vitro prostaglandin synthesis by human and rat gastric tissue. Proc Symp Pirenzepine: New aspects in research and therapy. Excerpta Medica: 41–47
19. Konturek SJ (1985) Prostaglandins in pathophysiology of peptic ulcer disease. Dig Dis Sci 30 (Suppl): 105S–108S
20. Konturek SJ, Brzozowski T, Piastucki I, Radecki T, Dembinska-Kiec A (1983) Role of Prostaglandin and thromboxane biosynthesis in gastric necrosis produced by taurocholate and ethanol. Dig Dis Sci 28: 154–160
21. Konturek SJ, Brzozowski T, Radecki T, Piastucki I (1982) Gastric cytoprotection by pirenzepine. Role of endogenous prostaglandins. Sc J Gastroenterol 17 (Suppl 72): 255–259
22. Konturek SJ, Kwiecien N, Obtulowicz W, Kopp B, Olewsky J (1986) Double-blind placebo-controlled study on the effect of sucralfate on gastric biosynthesis of prostaglandins (PG) and microbleeding in normal and aspirin-treated humans. 6th Int Conf on Prostaglandins and Related Compounds, Florence June 3–6, p 20
23. Konturek SJ, Radecki T, Brzozowski T, Piastucki I, Dembinska-Kiec A, Zmuda A (1981) Gastric cytoprotection by prostaglandins, ranitidine and probanthine in rats. Sc J Gastroenterol 16:7–12
24. Konturek SJ, Radecki T, Piastucki I, Drozdowicz D (1986) Advances in the understanding of the mechanism of cytoprotective action by colloidal bysmuth subcitrate. Sc J Gastroenterol 21 (Suppl): 6–10
25. Malagelada JR, Ahlquist DA, Moore SC (1986) Defects in prostaglandin synthesis and metabolism in ulcer disease. Dig Dis Sci 31: Suppl 205–275

26. Mattsson H, Andersson K, Larsson H (1983) Omeprazole provides protection against experimentally induced gastric mucosal lesions. Eur J Pharmacol 91: 111-114
27. Miller TA (1983) Protective effects of prostaglandins against gastric mucosal damage: Current knowledge and proposed mechanism. Am J Physiol 245: G601-G623
28. Mogard MH, Walsh JH (1986) Evidence against a physiological role of prostaglandins in the regulation of basal or meal-stimulated gastric acid secretion. VIII World Congress of Gastroneterology, São Paulo, September 7-12, abs 904
29. Mózsik G, Morón F, Jávor T (1982) Cellular mechanism of the development of gastric mucosal damage and of gastrocytoprotection by prostacyclin in rats. A pharmacological study. Prostaglandins, Leukotrienes and Medicine 9: 71
30. Payne NA, Gerber JG (1986) Stimulation of prostaglandin E release in canine gastric parietal cells. 6th Int Conf on Prostaglandins and Related Compounds. Florence, June 3-6
31. Peskar BM (1977) On the synthesis of prostaglandins by human gastric mucosa and its modification by drugs. Bioch Bioph Acta 487: 307-314
32. Peskar BM, Weiler H (1983) Carbenoxolone inhibits thromboxane B_2 synthesis by human gastric mucosa. Gut 24: A480
33. Rachmilewitz D (1984) Endogenous gastric and duodenal prostanoid synthesis: Effect of cimetidine and possible role in the pathogenesis and therapy of duodenal ulcer. Drug Therapy. Special Suppl 27-32
34. Rachmilewitz D, Ligumski M, Fich A, Goldin E, Eliakim A, Karmeli F (1986) Role of endogenous gastric prostanoids in the pathogenesis and therapy of duodenal ulcer. Gastroenterology 90: 963-969
35. Reimann HJ, Wendt P, Blueml G, Schmidt U, Ohe MVD, Dajani EZ, Wehrschuetz E (1986) Misoprostol prevents damage to the gastroduodenal mucosa by stabilizing the mast cells. 6th Int Conf on Prostaglandins and Related Compounds, Satellite Symposium, Florence, June 4
36. Schulman N, Bank S, Kranz V (1984) Effects of omeprazole on ethanol and cold-restaint stress induced gastric ulcers. Gastroenterology 86: 1239
37. Szelenyi I (1984) Functional cytoprotection by certain antacids. Acta Physiol Hungaria 64: 259-268
38. Takeda F, Kitagawa H, Kohei H (1985) Gastric cytoprotection by pirenzepine in rats: evaluating method for cytoprotective activity by antisecretory agents. Japan J Pharmacol 38: 337-346
39. Tarnawski A, Stachura J, Ivey KJ, Mach T (1981) Cimetidine and ranitidine increase ethanol-induced gastric mucosal damage in rat and partially abolish prostaglandin "cytoprotection". Gastroenterology 80: 1300
40. Tepperman BL, Ali M, McDonald JWD (1981) Gastric mucosal synthesis and release of prostaglandin E_2 6-keto prostaglandin $F_{1\alpha}$ and thromboxane B_2. Effect of pentagastrin stimulation. Gastroenterology 80: 1301
41. Tsai BS, Kessler LK, Conway RG, Butchko GM, Bauer RF (1986) Correlation of [^{3}H] misoprostol free acid binding and antisecretory activity in enriched canine parietal cells. Dig Dis Week, San Francisco May 18-21, abs 169
42. Vinegar R, Mehta NB, Truax JF, Selph JL, Lea A (1977) Imidazole as an inhibitor of the gastric damage produced by some anti-inflammatory drugs. Fed Proc 36: 1037
43. Whittle BJR, Kauffman GL, Moncada S (1981) Vasoconstriction with thromboxane A_2 induces ulceration of the gastric mucosa. Nature 292: 472-474
44. Wright NA, Young GO, Klaff LJ, Weers LA, Price SK, Marks IN (1982) Gastric mucosal prostaglandin E levels in patients with gastric ulcer disease and carcinoma. Gastroenterology 82: 263-267

Role of Leukotrienes in Gastric Mucosal Damage and Protection

B. M. PESKAR

Introduction

Contrary to the vasodilating properties of prostaglandin (PG)E_2 and PGI_2, which are major cyclooxygenase-derived arachidonic acid metabolites in the gastric mucosa, the 5-lipoxygenase product leukotriene (LT)C_4 has been found to constrict gastric submucosal vessels, particularly the venules, leading to sluggish blood flow and vasocongestion [1]. Furthermore, LTC_4 provokes plasma leakage in a number of vascular beds [2, 3]. Microcirculatory changes, such as capillary stasis, reduced mucosal blood flow, and plasma exudation have been described as prominent features of acute gastric mucosal damage caused by noxious agents such as ethanol [4–6]. 16,16-dimethyl-PGE_2 and sodium thiosulfate, which protect against gastric injury caused by ethanol, also prevent its effect on mucosal capillaries [6] suggesting that the microcirculation plays a crucial role in the pathogenesis of acute gastric mucosal damage.

Rat gastric mucosa has a high capacity to synthesize LTC_4 from endogenous substrate [7]. Intragastric instillation of ethanol leads to a pronounced stimulation of formation of this arachidonate metabolite by gastric mucosa incubated ex vivo [7]. The stimulatory action on mucosal LTC_4 synthesis is dose-dependent for ethanol and closely parallels the development of hemorrhagic mucosal lesions. Furthermore, stimulation of LTC_4 formation occurs rapidly and can be demonstrated within 1 min after contact of the noxious agent with the gastric surface (Fig. 1). Contrary to the pronounced effect on formation of the 5-lipoxygenase-derived arachidonate metabolite, mucosal synthesis of the cyclooxygenase product thromboxane (TX)B_2 is not affected by ethanol. Although TXA_2, the biologically active precursor of TXB_2, has been found to be a potent vasoconstrictor in the canine gastric circulation [8], increased formation of this cyclooxygenase product does not seem to contribute to the microcirculatory events in acute gastric mucosal damage [7, 9].

Gastroprotection by Agents that Inhibit Leukotriene Formation

Pretreatment of rats with the lipoxygenase inhibitor nordihydroguaiaretic acid inhibits gastric mucosal LTC_4 formation and simultaneously protects against mucosal damage caused by ethanol [7]. The degree of gastroprotection induced by nordihydroguaiaretic acid is comparable to that of well-known protective agents such as prostaglandins.

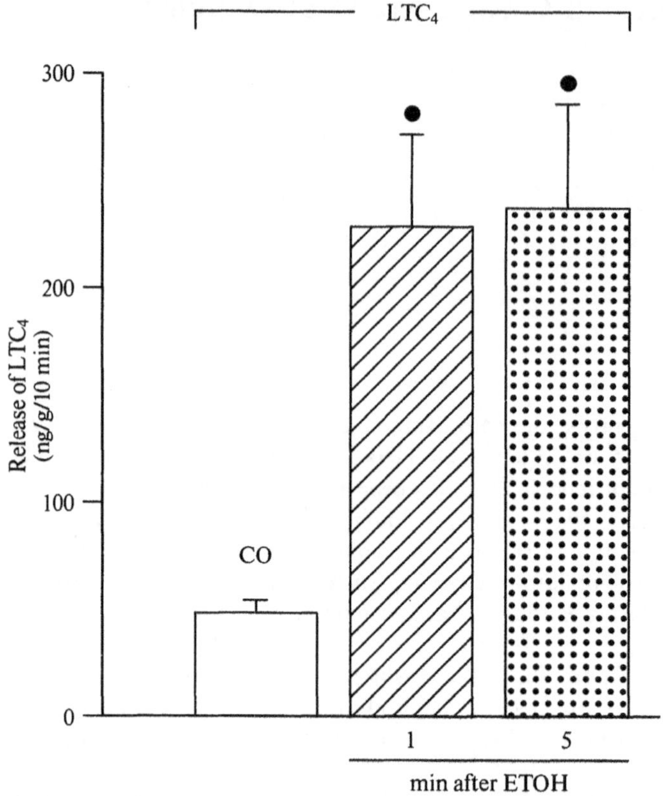

Fig. 1. Effect of ethanol on mucosal formation of LTC_4 and development of hemorrhagic mucosal lesions in rats. One or five minutes after intragastric instillation of 1.5 ml ethanol, the stomachs were removed in ether anesthesia. Controls *(CO)* received 1.5 ml water and were killed five minutes later. An ulcer index was evaluated as previously described [7]. Then mucosal tissue was excised and incubated in Tyrode solution at 37 °C. Release of LTC_4 into the medium was determined by radioimmunoassay as described elsewhere [7]. Results represent the mean ± SEM of six experiments. ● $P < 0.01$ as compared to controls (Student's *t* test)

Carbenoxolone, which was the first drug reported to accelerate the healing of gastric and duodenal ulcers by a mechanism not involving inhibition of acid secretion, was shown to inhibit prostaglandin-degrading enzymes [10] and to increase release of PGE_2 by human gastric mucosa in vitro [11]. In addition, the drug inhibits formation of TBX_2 in this tissue [11]. In duodenal ulcer patients carbenoxolone treatment enhances release of PGE_2 into the gastric juice [12]. In contrast to man, in the rat carbenoxolone does not affect formation of gastric mucosal cyclooxygenase products ex vivo [7, 13]. Carbenoxolone treatment prevents, however, the ethanol-induced stimulation of rat gastric mucosal LTC_4 formation [7]. Furthermore, carbenoxolone inhibits release of sulfidopeptide leukotrienes and LTB_4 from human gastric mucosa in vitro [14] suggesting that modulation of the 5-lipoxygenase pathway may be an additional mechanism underlying the protective and ulcer-healing action of the drug.

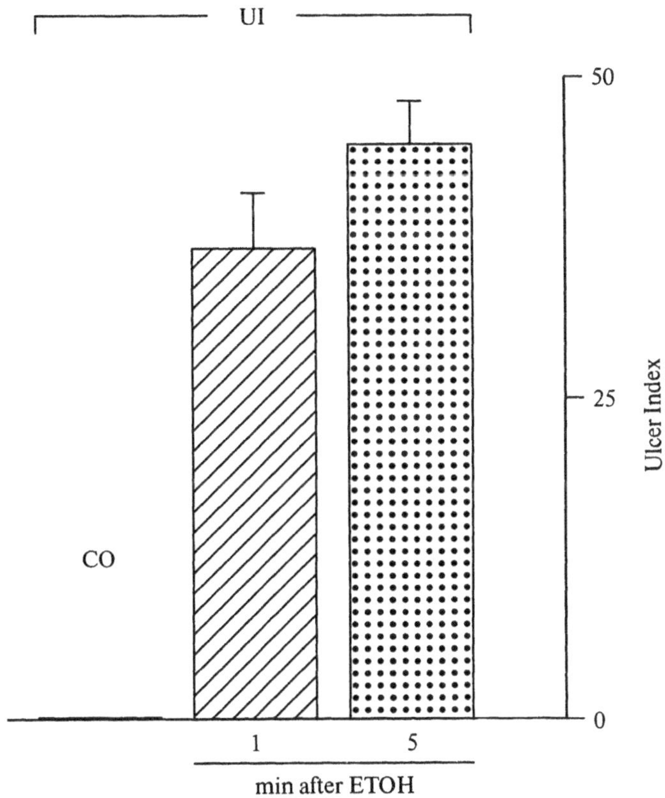

Fig. 1

Both sulfhydryl-containing agents such as cysteamine and sulfhydryl blockers such as diethyl maleate have been found to protect the gastric mucosa against injury caused by ethanol [15, 16]. Pretreatment of rats with cysteamine or diethyl maleate prior to intragastric instillation of ethanol dose-dependently inhibits gastric mucosal LTC_4 formation ex vivo [17]. The inhibitory action of cysteamine and diethyl maleate on mucosal LTC_4 synthesis (IC_{50} 26 and 9 mg/kg, respectively) closely parallels their gastroprotective activity (IC_{50} 20 and 5 mg/kg. respectively). In contrast, both compounds have divergent effects on formation of gastric mucosal cyclooxygenase-derived arachidonate metabolites. While diethyl maleate increases formation of 6-keto-$PGF_{1\alpha}$ and TXB_2, but inhibits release of PGE_2, cysteamine reduces mucosal release of all three cyclooxygenase products [17]. Thus, inhibition of gastric mucosal LTC_4 formation may be more important as a common mechanism of the protective activity of agents modulating gastric mucosal sulfhydryl levels than effects on the gastric prostaglandin system [15].

Table 1. Quotient of PGE_2/LTC_4 released by gastric mucosa of control and indomethacin-treated rats

Treatment	Mucosal PGE_2/LTC_4
Vehicle	22.2 ± 7.4
Indomethacin (5 mg/kg)	14.1 ± 6.6
Indomethacin (10 mg/kg)	5.3 ± 1.5*
Indomethacin (20 mg/kg)	3.9 ± 1.8*

Rats were treated with graded doses of indomethacin or vehicle and were killed 30 min later. Mucosal fragments were incubated in Tyrode solution at 37 °C for 10 min, and release of PGE_2 and LTC_4 was determined as described elsewhere [7]. Results represent the mean ± SEM of six experiments. (Student's t test). $P < 0.05$ compared to vehicle treated rats

Effect of Nonsteroidal Anti-inflammatory Drugs on Rat Gastric Mucosal Leukotriene Formation

It has been suggested that side effects of nonsteroidal anti-inflammatory drugs might be related not only to reduced formation of protective prostaglandins, but also to increased biosynthesis of leukotrienes. We have investigated the effect of nonsteroidal anti-inflammatory compounds on release of cyclooxygenase and 5-lipoxygenase metabolites of arachidonic acid by rat gastric mucosa and inflammatory tissue. Oral treatment with indomethacin dose-dependently inhibits ex vivo formation of both gastric mucosal PGE_2 and LTC_4 [18]. The inhibitory action is, however, more pronounced on formation of the cyclooxygenase (IC_{50} 3.4 mg/kg) than on the 5-lipoxygenase product (IC_{50} 16 mg/kg) resulting in a decreased quotient of gastric PGE_2/ LTC_4 (Table 1). Similar results were obtained after treatment of rats with diclofenac. This is in contrast to the effect of indomethacin on formation of arachidonic acid metabolites in inflammatory exudates induced by implantation of carrageenan-soaked sponges [18]. Thus, treatment with 5 mg/kg indomethacin simultaneously with sponge implantation decreased concentrations (ng/ml, mean ± SEM, $n = 6$) of PGE_2 in the inflammatory exudates from 9.3 ± 1.1 to 2.0 ± 0.5 ($P < 0.001$), but enhaced concentrations of LTC_4 from 3.0 ± 0.2 to 4.6 ± 0.5 ($P < 0.025$). These results show that blockade of the cyclooxygenase pathway of arachidonate metabolism may increase release of 5-lipoxygenase-derived products from some tissues, but not others. The more pronounced inhibitory action of nonsteroidal anti-inflammatory drugs on the gastric mucosal cyclooxygenase as compared to the 5-lipoxygenase pathway may alter the balance between protective and potentially ulcerogenic arachidonate metabolites, an effect that could contribute to the gastrointestinal irritancy caused by these drugs.

Effect of PGE_2 and Drugs that Activate the Endogenous Gastric Prostaglandin System

Gastroprotection is not always accompanied by inhibition of ethanol-induced stimulation of gastric LTC_4 formation. Thus, pretreatment of rats with PGE_2 (0.2 mg/kg)

reduced ethanol-induced mucosal injury by 78%, but did not affect gastric mucosal LTC_4 formation [17]. As reported previously [19, 20], pretreatment of rats with sucralfate (500 mg/kg) or the Al/Mg hydroxide-containing antacid Maalox 70 (1.5 ml/kg) prior to ethanol instillation stimulated gastric mucosal PGE_2 biosynthesis by 46% and 45%, respectively ($P < 0.05$ each) and simultaneously inhibited lesion production by 62% and 77%, respectively ($P < 0.001$ each). Similarly to PGE_2 neither drug prevented ethanol-induced stimulation of mucosal LTC_4 formation suggesting that their protective action is due rather to functional antagonism of LTC_4 effects. The finding that ethanol-induced stimulation of gastric mucosal LTC_4 synthesis occurs despite pronounced protection implies that the activation of the 5-lipoxygenase pathway of arachidonate metabolism is not a secondary phenomenon resulting from gastric mucosal injury.

Effect of a Leukotriene Receptor Antagonist

L-649,923 (sodium-4-(3-(4-acetyl-3-hydroxy-2-propylphenoxy)propylthio)-hydroxymethyl-benzene benzoate) inhibits binding of (^3H)LTD_4 and to a lesser extent (^3H)LTC_4 to guinea pig lung homogenates and antagonizes various effects of sulfidopeptide leukotrienes after oral administration in vivo (for details see [21] and Ford-Hutchinson, this volume). Oral pretreatment with L-649,923 significantly reduces mucosal damage caused by intragastric ethanol (Table 2). The protective action of L-649,923 is also found when indomethacin is used as a gastric irritant (Table 2, see also Ford-Hutchinson, this volume). In both experimental models pretreatment with L-649,923 did not affect mucosal LTC_4 release. Previous studies using high-pressure liquid chromatography analysis have revealed that during incubation of rat gastric mucosa in vitro, LTC_4 is by far the predominating 5-lipoxygenase product formed. If the same pattern of formation of sulfidopeptide leukotrienes also occurs in vivo, this

Table 2. Effect of the leukotriene receptor antagonist L-649,923 on gastric mucosal damage and LTC_4 formation in rats treated with indomethacin or ethanol

Treatment	Experiments (n)	Ulcer index	LTC_4 (ng/g/10 min)
Indomethacin	6	13 ± 4	7.2 ± 1.5
Indomethacin and L-649,923 (10 mg/kg)	6	7 ± 5	5.8 ± 2.2
Indomethacin and L-649,923 (50 mg/kg)	6	1 ± 1*	8.1 ± 3.0
Ethanol	9	50 ± 2	304 ± 40
Ethanol and L-649,923 (50 mg/kg)	6	21 ± 4**	388 ± 131

Rats were pretreated orally with L-649,923 30 min prior to oral administration of either indomethacin (20 mg/kg) or ethanol (1.5 ml). Rats were killed 4 h after indomethacin adminstration or 5 min after ethanol treatment. Gastric damage and mucosal LTC_4 release was determined as described elsewhere [7]. Results give the mean ± SEM. * $P < 0.025$, ** $P < 0.01$ as compared to rats receiving the noxius agent only (Student's *t* test)

could explain the relatively high doses of L-649,923 necessary to confer protection as the compound exhibits weaker antagonism against effects of LTC_4 compared to LTD_4. However, as discussed in this volume (see Ford-Hutchinson) further studies are necessary to clarify whether the gastroprotective action of L-649,923 is due to leukotriene receptor blockade or other effects of the compound. In this context it is of interest that FPL55712, another sulfidopeptide leukotriene receptor antagonist [22], has recently been found to protect against stress-induced gastric lesions in rats [23].

Conclusions

Activation of the 5-lipoxygenase pathway of arachidonate metabolism seems to be a crucial factor in acute mucosal damage caused by agents such as ethanol. Inhibition of gastric LTC_4 formation prevents ethanol-induced gastric injury and may underly or contribute to the mechanism of action of gastroprotective drugs such as lipoxygenase inhibitors, carbenoxolone, or agents modulating gastric mucosal sulfhydryl levels. Protection by prostaglandins and drugs stimulating the endogenous gastric prostaglandin system, on the other hand, is due rather to functional antagonism of leukotriene effects. Nonsteroidal anti-inflammatory drugs inhibit both the gastric cyclooxygenase and 5-lipoxygenase pathway of arachidonate metabolism. As the inhibitory action is more pronounced on formation of prostaglandins than of leukotrienes a shift in the balance of protective to potentially ulcerogenic arachidonate metabolites might contribute to the gastric irritancy caused by these drugs. Finally, the protective effect of the leukotriene receptor antagonist L-649,923 supports the hypothesis that sulfidopeptide leukotrienes are involved in gastric mucosal damage caused by ethanol or nonsteroidal anti-inflammatory compounds.

References

1. Whittle BJR, Oren-Wolman N, Guth PH (1985) Gastric vasoconstrictor actions of leukotriene C_4 $PGF_{2\alpha}$, and thromboxane mimetic U-46619 on rat submucosal microcirculation in vivo. Am J Physiol 248: G580–G586
2. Samuelsson B (1983) Leukotrienes: Mediators of immediate hypersensitivity reactions and inflammation. Science 220: 568–575
3. Hua XY, Dahlén SE, Lundberg S, Hammarström S, Hedqvist P (1985) Leukotrines C_4, D_4 and E_4 cause widespread and extensive plasma extravasation in the guinea-pig. Naunyn-Schmiedeberg's Arch Pharmacol 330: 136–141
4. Guth PH, Paulsen G, Nagata H (1984) Histologic and microcirculatory changes in alcohol-induced gastric lesions in the rat: Effect of prostaglandin cytoprotection. Gastroenterology 87: 1083–1090
5. Szabo S, Trier JS, Brown A, Schnoor J (1985) Early vascular injury and ioncreased vascular permeability in gastric mucosal injury caused by ethanol in the rat. Gastroenterology 88: 228–236
6. Pihan G, Majzoubi D, Haudenschild C, Trier JS, Szabo S (1986) Early microcirculatory stasis in acute gastric mucosal injury in the rat and prevention by 16,16-dimethyl-prostaglandin E_2 or sodium thiosulfate. Gastroenterology 91: 1415–1426
7. Peskar BM, Lange K, Hoppe U, Peskar BA (1986) Ethanol stimulates formation of leukotriene C_4 in rat gastric mucosa. Prostaglandins 31: 283–293
8. Whittle BJR, Kauffman GL, Moncada S (1981) Vasoconstriction with thromboxane A_2 induces ulceration of the gastric mucosa. Nature 292: 472–474

9. Wallace JL, Whittle BJR (1985) Role of prostanoids in the protective actions of BW755C on the gastric mucosa. Eur J Pharmacol 115: 45-52
10. Peskar BM, Holland A, Peskar BA (1976) Effect of carbenoxolone on prostaglandin synthesis and degradation. J Pharm Pharmac 28: 146-148
11. Peskar BM, Weiler H (1983) Carbenoxolone inhibits thromboxane B_2 synthesis by human gastric mucosa. Gut 24: A480
12. Rask-Madsen J, Bukhave K, Madsen PER, Bekker C (1983) Effect of carbenoxolone on gastric prostaglandin E_2 levels in patients with peptic ulcer disease following vagal and pentagastrin stimulation. Eur J Clin Invest 13: 351-356
13. Bennett A, Melhuish PB, Stamford IF (1985) Carbenoxolone and deglycyrrhized liquorice have little or no effect on prostanoid synthesis by rat gastric mucosa ex vivo. Br J Pharmac 86: 693-695
14. Dreyling KW, Lange K, Peskar BA, Peskar BM (1986) Release of leukotrienes by rat and human gastric mucosa and its pharmacological modification. Br J Pharmacol 88: 236P
15. Konturek SJ, Brzozowski T, Piastucki I, Radecki T, Szabo S (1983) Gastric cytoprotection by agents altering gastric mucosal sulfhydryl compounds: Role of endogenous prostaglandins. In: Advances in Prostaglandin, Thromboxane and Leukotriene Research, Vol 12 (B Samuelsson, R Paoletti and P. Ramwell eds), Raven Press, New York, pp 411-416
16. Robert A, Eberle D, Kaplowitz N (1984) Role of glutathione in gastric mucosal cytoprotection. Am J Physiol 247: G296-G340
17. Lange K, Peskar BA, Peskar BM (1987) Stimulation of rat gastric mucosal leukotriene C_4 formation by ethanol and effect of gastric protective drugs. In: Advances in Prostaglandin, Thromboxane and Leukotriene Research, Vol 17 (B Samuelsson, R Paoletti and PW Ramwell eds), Raven Press, New York, pp 299-302
18. Hoppe U, Peskar BA, Peskar BM (1987) Effect of indomethacin on prostaglandin and leukotriene formation in rat gastric mucosa and inflammatory exudate. Naunyn-Schmiedeberg's Arch Pharmacol, 335, Suppl: (R 41)
19. Hollander W, Tarnawski A, Gergeley H, Zipser RD (1984) Sucralfate protection of the gastric mucosa against ethanol-induced injury: a prostaglandin-mediated process? Scand J Gastroenterol 19 (Suppl) 101: 97-102
20. Szelenyi I, Postius S, Engler H (1983) Evidence for a functional cytoprotective effect produced by antacids in the rat stomach. Eur J Clin Pharmacol 88: 403-406
21. Jones TR, Young R, Champion E, Charette L, Denis D, Ford-Hutchinson AW, Frenette R, Gauthier JY, Guindon Y, Kakushima M, Masson P, McFarlane C, Piechuta H, Rokach J, Zamboni R (1986). L-649,923, sodium (−S*, γR*)-4-(3-(4-acetyl-3-hydroxy-2-propylphenoxy)-propylthio)-γ-hydroxy-β-methyl-benzene-butanoate, a selective orally active leukotriene receptor antagonist. Can J Physiol Pharmacol 64: 1068-1075
22. Augstein J, Farmer JR, Lee TB, Sheard P, Tattersall ML (1973) Selective inhibitor of slow-reacting substance of anaphylaxis. Nature, New Biol 245: 215-217
23. Ogle CW, Cho CH (1986) FPL55712, a leukotriene-receptor antagonist, protects against stress-induced gastric ulcers in rats. IRCS Med Sci 14: 114-115

Discussion Following the Report of Prof. Peskar

SZABO

I have two questions. One is related to the finding that LTC_4 generation is increased by ethanol, while LTD_4 release was not affected. Do you think this might be due to the fact that the changes observed are very rapid? LTC_4 is the first cysteinyl leukotriene synthesized with the entire glutathione being attached. LTD_4 is the next metabolite formed by shortening the amino acid side chain. Since the ethanol effect is so rapid, there might not be enough time for the generation of LTD_4.

PESKAR

I do not think that this explains the findings. Even when the tissue is incubated for up to 1 h, or incubation media are stored for 24 h prior to the HPLC analysis, no conversion of LTC_4 to LTD_4 or LTE_4 in rat gastric-mucosal incubates can be observed. This is in contrast to other tissues such as human gastric mucosa where conversion of LTC_4 to LTD_4 and LTE_4 occurs within minutes. Rat gastric mucosa contains high concentrations of glutathione which may be released from the chopped tissue, and this could possibly prevent the metabolism of LTC_4. Thus, we have been able to show that addition of gluthathione to incubation media of human gastric mucosa results in release of LTC_4 only obviously preventing formation of LTD_4 and LTE_4.

SZABO

My second question is: How do you explain that both diethyl maleate and cysteamine inhibit release of leukotrienes? Is it due to the decrease of glutathione which is needed for the complete synthesis of leukotrienes? We have measured dimished levels of glutathione in the gastric mucosa of rats given diethylmaleate.

PESKAR

We do not know the mechanism by which sulfhydryl-containing or-blocking agents inhibit gastric leukotriene formation. Depletion of glutathione could be one explanation. It is of interest that the two drugs differ in their effect on basal gastric leukotriene formation in rats not treated with ethanol. While diethyl maleate causes profound inhibition of LTC_4 release, cysteamine has no effect. Thus, cysteamine may prevent the stimulatory action of ethanol on leukotriene formation by a different mechanism, acting not primarily at the enzyme level.

WHITTLE

One of the most intriguing observations is the ability of nonsteroidal cyclooxygenase inhibitors apparently to prevent the formation of leukotriene C_4. This is in contrast to many of the studies on purified preparations of the 5-lipoxygenase enzyme. Do you think these compounds are directly interfering with the enzymic biosynthesis of the compounds, or is it some other unrelated effect, perhaps on the release of precursors?

PESKAR

We have not yet investigated this possibility. As I have mentioned in other organ systems, such as inflammatory tissue, inhibition of cyclooxygenase is paralleled by an increased release of leukotrienes. We do not know what mechanism is responsible for the difference in the action of nonsteroidal anti-inflammatory compounds on leukotriene release by gastric and inflammatory tissue, but an indirect mechanism and not effects on the 5-lipoxygenase enzyme seem to be a more likely explanation.

Effect of Prostaglandins on the Motility of the Digestive Tract

P. DEMOL

Introduction

A variety of synthetic analogues of prostaglandins (PGs) of the E-type (PGE) have been shown to be effective in treatment of ulcer disease [1–4]. PGEs also protect the gastroduodenal mucosa against several irritants as for example acetyl salicylic acid (ASA) and other nonsteroidal anti-inflammatory drugs (NSAIDs) [5–8]. The major side effect which has been observed during treatment with PGE is diarrhea (softening or increase in the number of stools or, more rarely, watery stools coupled with abdominal colics). This diarrhea has been classically explained by the enteropooling effect of these substances [9, 10].

However, animal studies have shown that PGEs influence gastric and intestinal smooth muscle activity [12, 13], and a recent work even suggests that changes of gastric contractility induced by PGE could play an important role in their cytoprotective activity [14]. This study reviews the in vitro and in vivo effects of PG on the gastrointestinal smooth muscle and considers the relevance of these effects in diarrhea and the protection of the gastric mucosa.

Synthesis of PG

Microsomes from mammalian circular and longitudinal muscles convert enzymatically arachidonic acid into (AA) a variety of prostanoid products [15]. The most abundant metabolic product is 6-keto PGF_1 (product of spontaneous breakdown of PGI_2). Other products are PGE_2, PGF_2, and thromboxane [15, 16].

As Sanders states in a review article [13], it seems paradoxical that different PGs with contradictory effects on the mechanical activity of the circular and longitudinal muscles are released together in these adjacent muscle layers. The explanation could be that the stimuli controlling AA liberation could be unique to each muscle layer [13].

Regulation of PG Synthesis

Various stimuli enhance PG synthesis by smooth muscle: strech [16], vagal nerve stimulation [17], and various drugs and toxins [18]. The most important level of PG synthesis appears to be the liberation of AA, a constituent of membrane phospholipids

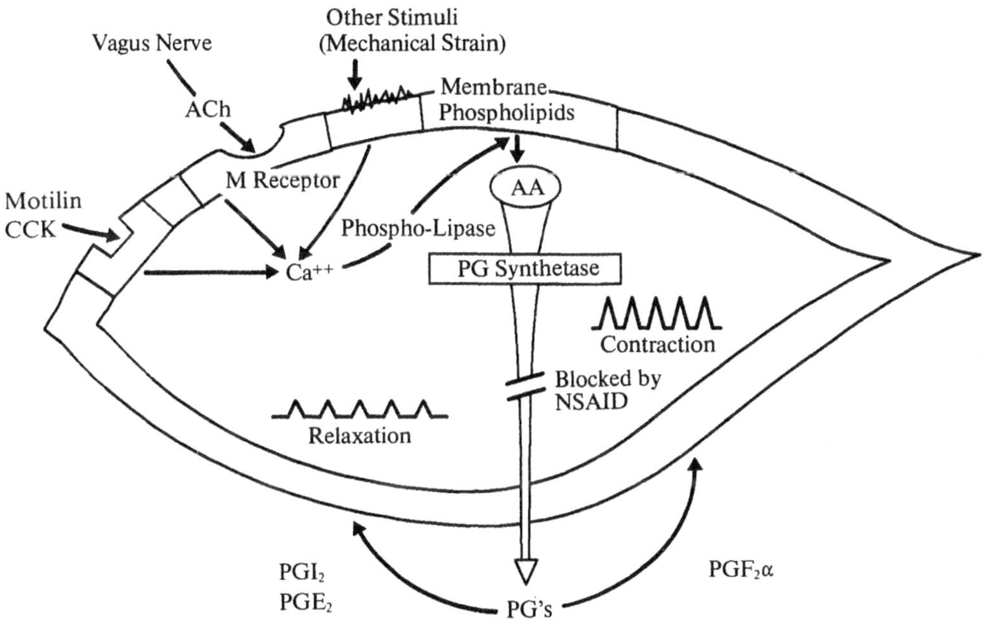

Fig. 1. Mechanisms of PG's from the gi muscle (Adapted from [52]). Activation of the menbrane receptors by different mechanisms (mechanical, neural or hormonal) induce the mobilisation of intracellular Ca** which activates the phospholipase. This enzyme produces arachidonic acid (AA) from the membrane phospholipids. The PG synthetase transforms AA in different PG's which are then released in the milieu and directly influence the electrical and mechanical activity of the adjacent muscle cells

[15]. The common messenger mediating PG synthesis to the stimuli could be the intracellular calcium. Its increase at the beginning of smooth muscle cell activation is supposed to stimulate the activity of phospholipase which then releases AA from the membranes (Fig. 1).

Effect of PG on Electrical and Mechanical Activity in the Gastrointestinal Tract

In Vitro Studies

Stomach

PGE_1 and PGE_2 contract the isolated longitudinal muscle of the human, guinea pig, and rat proximal stomach [13, 19]. This stimulation probably occurs by excitation of the intrinsic cholinergic nerves since it is blocked by tetrodotoxin and potentiated by cholinesterase inhibitors. More recently, PGE_2 has been shown to have an excitatory presynaptic influence on the release of acetylcholine from cholinergic nerve terminals through a specific receptor [20]. On the other hand, the circular muscle of the human, guinea pig, and rat antrum are inhibited by PGE_1 and PGE_2, apparently by a direct action on the muscle cells. Recent extensive in vitro studies by Sanders [13, 21] have analyzed the role of PG in the modulation of gastric motility. In these studies Sanders showed that indomethacin increases significantly the spontaneous electrical and mechanical activities of the isolated canine antral circular muscle, demonstrating that PG must have an inhibitory effect on the tonus. In fact, PGs have antagonistic effects: PGE_2 and PGI_2 have a dose-related inhibitory effect on the antral circular muscle contractions, while PGF_2 and PGD_2 stimulate these contractions (Fig. 2) [13].

The inhibitory effect of PGE_2 on mechanical activity is explained by a decrease in amplitude of basal electrical activity of the muscle cells (also called "slow waves"), probably due to an increased membrane conductance to potassium [13]. In summary, the local PGs seem to stimulate the proximal stomach responsible for emptying of liquids, and to reduce the force of the antral contractions which are responsible for the grinding up and emptying of solids.

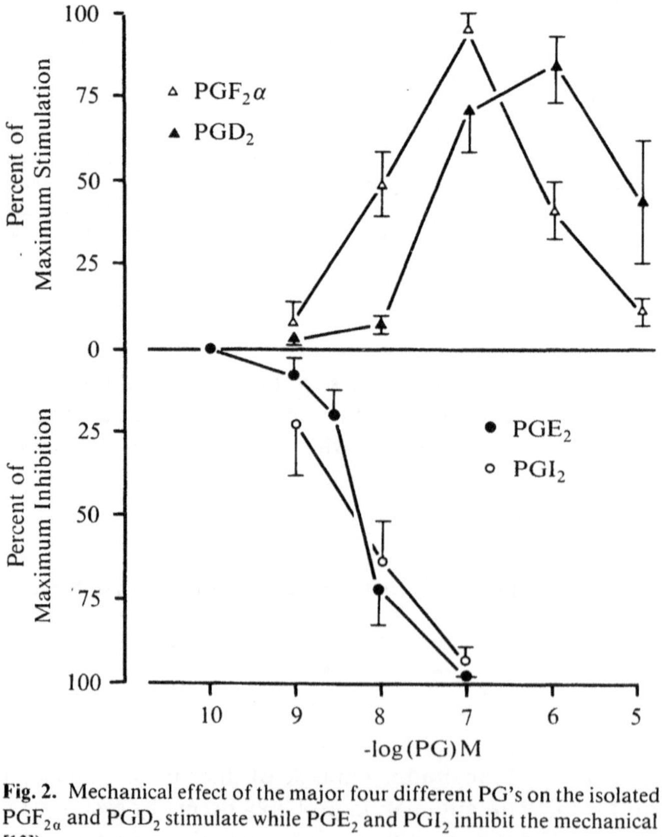

Fig. 2. Mechanical effect of the major four different PG's on the isolated canine antral circular muscle. $PGF_{2\alpha}$ and PGD_2 stimulate while PGE_2 and PGI_2 inhibit the mechanical activity of this muscle. (From [13])

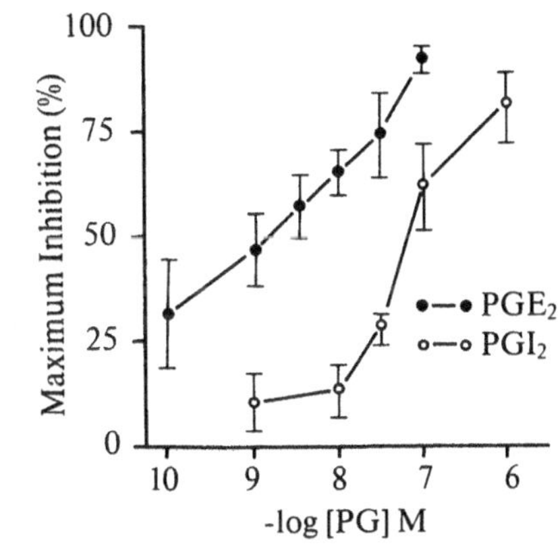

Fig. 3. PGE_2 and PGI_2 inhibit dose-dependantly the acetylcholine stimulated contractions of the isolated canine ileal circular muscle. (From [22])

Intestine

As for the antral circular muscle, Sanders [22] showed that PGE_2 and PGI_2 dose-dependently decreased the acetylcholine-stimulated phasic contractions of the canine ileal curcular muscle (Fig. 3).

Sanders showed further that PGI_2 totally inhibited the action potentials of ileal circular muscle recorded by intracellular recordings. As PGI_2 is the most abundant metabolite of AA in the circular ileal muscle [15], these data suggest that PGI_2 plays a major role in limiting the membrane excitability of ileal circular muscle. As depolarizing stimuli increase the PG concentration [18], and as PGE_2 and PGI_2 limit the degree of depolarization during slow waves, it can be assumed that these PGs function as a local negative feedback in regulating the electrical and contractile behavior of circular muscles (Fig. 1) [22].

In Vivo Studies

Experiments in dogs have shown that an i. v. injection of a methyl-PGE_1 abolishes the spike potentials and produces a profound inhibition of the nonstimulated and morphine-stimulated circular muscle contractions [23].

The interdigestive (fasting) period is characterized by the regular occurrence of short periods of intense motor activity, called "activity front" or "phase III", of the interdigestive motor complex (IMC). This motor activity is induced by the regular occurrence of short bursts of electrical spike activity superimposed on the continuous basal activity (called "slow waves").

Konturek et al. [24] showed that an i. v. infusion of PGE_2 (40 $\mu g\ kg^{-1}\ h^{-1}$) significantly delayed the appearance of the activity front while PGF_2 (80 $\mu g\ kg^{-1}\ h^{-1}$) in

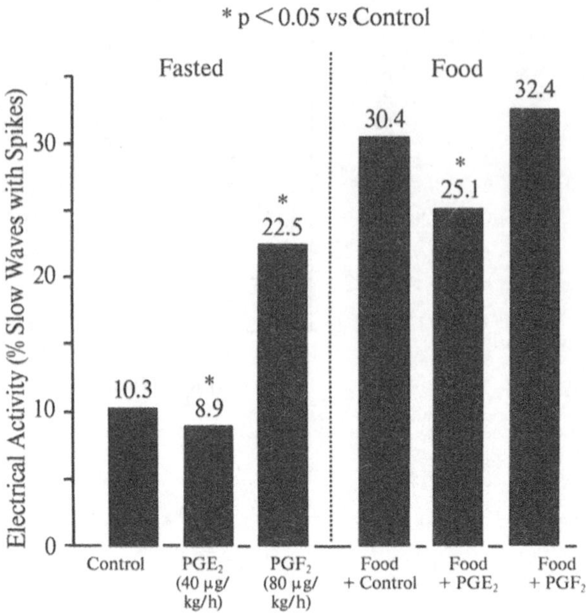

Fig. 4. Effect of i.v. PGE_2 and PGF_2 on the fasted and food stimulated electrical activity of the small intestinal of the dog. PGE_2 inhibit while PGF_2 stimulate both of these activities. (From [24])

creased the percentage of slow waves with spikes and the mechanical activity (Fig. 4). Likewise, PGE_2 decreased the food-induced activity while PGF_2 increased the electricalfood-induced activity.

In volunteers the oral administration of 100 μg of a synthetic derivative of a PGE_2 (15(R),15-methyl-PGE_2) was associated with a significant reduction in amplitude of antral and duodenal contractions during phase II of the interdigestive motor complex (IMC) [25]. Paradoxically, 650 mg aspirin had very similar effects. In a similar study Nylander and Andersson [26] observed that the oral administration of 140 μg of a 16,16-dimethyl-PGE_2 produced a significant decrease in the spontaneous motor activity in both the gastric antrum and duodenum.

Recent studies of Fargeas et al. [27] showed that PGE_2 could be the cerebral mediator of the actions of calcitonin and neurotensin on the gastrointestinal myoelectric activity in rats and dogs. When injected in microamounts in the cerebral ventricles these two peptides restored the fact pattern of the jejunal electrical activity, which was interrupted by a meal. This effect was blocked by indomethacin and restored by the intraventricular administration of very small amounts of PGE_2 (Fig. 5).

Effect of PGs on Gastric Emptying and Intestinal Transit

Gastric Emptying

Most studies have analyzed the effect of PGEs on the emptying of a liquid and not of a solid meal. In 1975 Nylander and Mattsson [28] observed that the oral administration

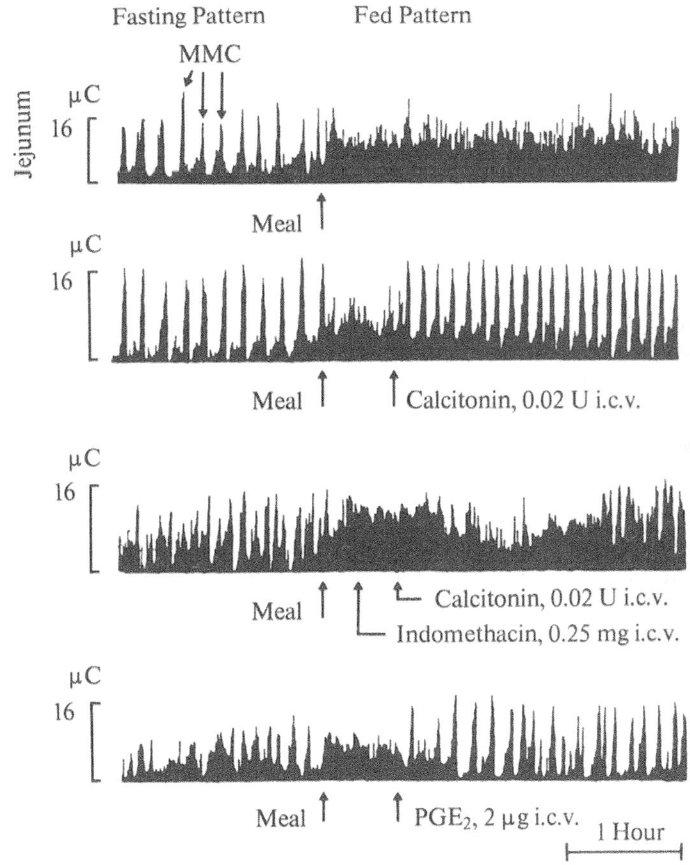

Fig. 5. Intracerebroventricular (i.c.v.) administration of calcitonin after a meal in the rat restores the fasting pattern. This effect is blocked by a preceding administration of indomethacin probably by blocking the local synthesis of PG's. PGE_2 i.c.v. administration has the same effect as calcitonin. (From [27])

of 140 μg 16,16-dimethyl-PGE_2 enhanced the gastric emptying (GE) of a barium liquid test meal in eight volunteers. This effect was explained by the reduction in duodenal pressure and thus the decrease of duodenal resistance toward the gastric outflow which had been observed in their previous work [26]. These results were confirmed by Johansson and Ekelund [29] with a more sophisticated technique (a multiple indicator dilution technique). The same dose of PGE_2 reduced the GE of a liquid meal by about 50% (Fig. 6).

In contrast, a recent work by Moore et al. [30] showed that oral administration of a therapeutic dose (200 μg) of a synthetic PGE_1 analogue (misoprostol) given four times a day decreased the rate of GE of a liquid meal when analyzed with an isotope method in patients with healed duodenal ulcer. In this work it was observed that misoprostol had no effect on the GE of a solid food meal. On the other hand, rioprostil, a compound similar to misoprostol, has been shown to increase the speed of GE of a liquid meal in normal volunteers when compared to ranitidine or a placebo [31]. However, the differences between the groups were small. These conflicting results could be explained by differences in the dosage of the PGE used and also by the differences in the population. The i.v. administration of a 15S-(15)-methyl-PGE_2 in

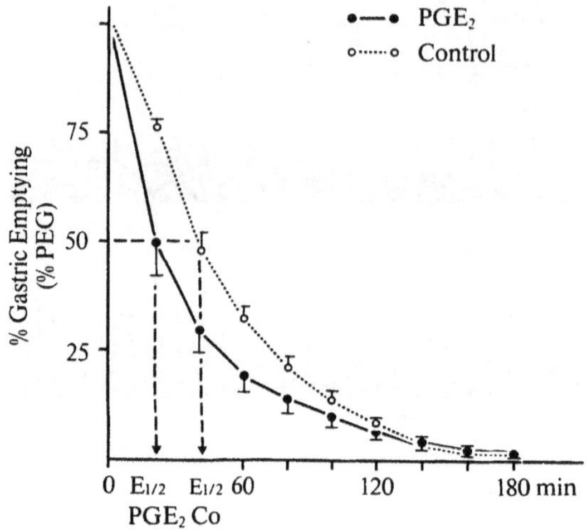

Fig. 6. In man the oral administration of 140 µg of a 16 dimethyl PGE_2 increases the rate of emptying of a liquid meal. The duration of emtying of half on the meal ($E_{1/2}$) is nearly the half after intake of the PGE_2. (From [21])

conscious rhesus monkeys induced a dose-dependent increase of the GE of a liquid and solid meal [32]. However, as indomethacin also increased the GE of both solid and liquid meals, the authors suggest that it is PGI_2 (which slows GE) that plays a physiologic role in modulating the GE.

We have recently observed that the oral administration of 600 µg rioprostil with digoxin followed by a breakfast reduced the maximal plasma level (C_{max}) of digoxin by 50% and delayed the t_{max} by around 30 min (Fig. 7) [33]. As it has been shown that there is an inverse correlation between GE and the C_{max} of paracetamol [34], our

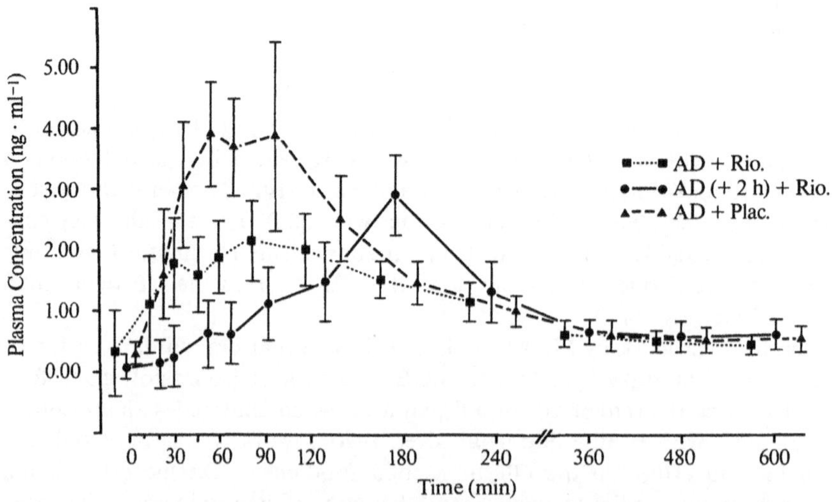

Fig. 7. In 9 volunteers the oral administration of a synthetic PGE_2 analogue, rioprostil, given concomitantly (AD Rio) or 2 h before (AD (+ 2 h) + Rio) the intake of acetyl-digoxin (AD) induce both a significant decrease of the maximal peak concentration and an increase of the time taken to reach this peak of concentration (t_{max} of digoxin in the plasma, when compared to the effect of a placebo given togehter with AD (AD + Rio). (From [33])

results suggest that rioprostil slows GE of a solid meal, possibly by an inhibition of the circular antral muscle activity as demonstrated in vitro by Sanders [21]. As the antrum is responsible for the emptying of solid meals [35], the inhibition of its activity would also explain the increase of t_{max}.

Intestinal Transit

In the first study analyzing the effect of PGs in humans, Misiewicz et al. [36] observed that a high dose of PGE_1 (2 mg) induced colic or the desire to defecate in the four volunteers and increased strikingly the propulsion of a telemetric capsule into the colon. This dose of PGE_1 also speeded the elimination of ingested radiopaque capsules, demonstrating that PGE_1 reduced the oro-anal transit time.

In a more recent X-ray study [37], i. v. administration of a synthetic 16,16-dimethyl-PGE_2 to volunteers increased the GE of radiopaque capsules; however, it slowed their small intestinal, transit afterward, which confirmed the observation by Johansson and Ekelund [29].

We have also recently observed that the oral application of rioprostil increases the transit time from mouth to caecum as analyzed by the H_2 breath test in volunteers (Fig. 8) [38]. The slowing of the small intestinal transit could be explained by a decrease of propulsive activity induced by PGE. This effect is also observed with PGI_2 [39]. On the other hand, 16,16-dimethyl-PGE_2 strongly increased the speed of the colonic transit in rats [40] (Fig. 9), by stimulation of the colonic transit, could play a major role in PGE-induced diarrhea according to Rush and Ruwart [40].

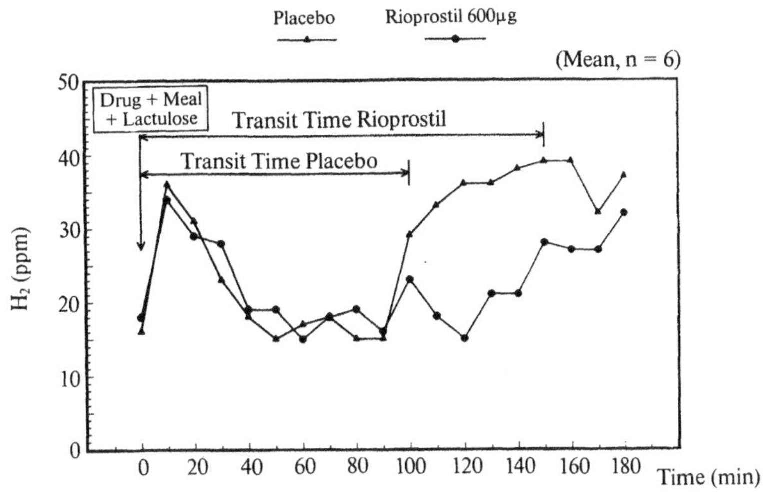

Fig. 8. Effect of the oral administration of rioprostil, a synthetic PGE_2 analogue, compared to a placebo on the H_2 breath concentrations after the intake of a liquid meal with lactulose in healthy volunteers. Rioprostil delayed by around 50 min the stable increase of H_2 in the breath. (From [38])

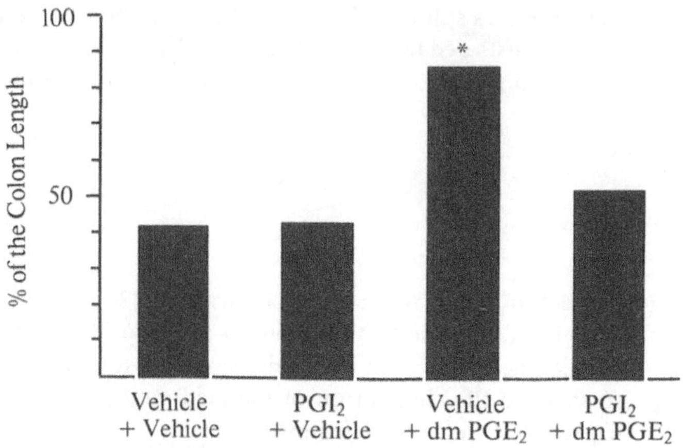

Fig. 9. Effect of PGI_2 or PGE_2 on the speed of colon transit in the rat. The administration of dm PGE_2 increases significantly the perceantage of the colon length which is transited by the marker after a predetermined time. This acceleration effect is prevented by the previous administration of PGI_2. (Adapted from [40])

Role of Prostanoids in Dysregulation of Gastrointestinal Motility

Gastroesophageal Reflux

PGE_1 and PGE_2 given i.v. or i.a. decrease the esophageal peristaltic amplitude and inhibit the tonus of the lower esophageal sphincter (LES) in several animals [41, 42] and in man [43]. However, a recent study in man showed that trimoprostil, a synthetic PGE_2 administered orally, had no lowering effect on the tonus of LES in man [44].

Studies with the radiation-induced esophagitis model in the opossum have shown that the local increase of PGE_2 could be a direct cause of inflammation in this model [45]. Within this study it was demonstrated that indomethacin decreased the intensity of inflammation and lesions, and that prostaglandin-pretreated animals showed more severe evidence of esophagitis than control animals. As it was suggested in an editorial by Goyal [46], these findings are contrary to what would be expected on the basis of the cytoprotective role of prostaglandins. However, the relevance of this model to the reflux esophagitis observed in humans is unclear.

Stomach

Kim et al. [47] have observed that intra-arterial injection of PGE_2 in the dog could induce electrical dysrhytmias (either retrograde tachygastrias or anterograde bradygastrias). These dysrhytmias could induce slowing of GE of solid meal and the alteration of the speed of absorption of certain drugs, which have been observed with PGEs [33]. These effects could be explained by the alteration of the basal electrical activity,

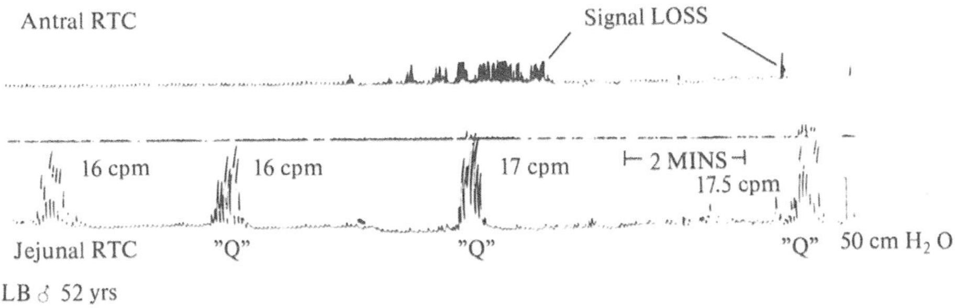

Fig. 10. Paroxysmal tachyrhythmia (Q Complexes) observed in the jejunum of patients with different gi diseases. These abnormal complexes are characterized by bursts of high pressure waves occuring at a frequency of 16–17.5 cycles per minute (cpm). Lower trace is a normal phase 3 of the interdigestive motor complex (Phase III MMC). (From [49])

which has been reported by Sanders [13]. Recently the same group [48] demonstrated that PGs could play a role in the regulation of the amplitude of antral contractions. Their role in the induction of abnormal electrical rhythms, however, remains uncertain.

Intestine

Acute administration of PGE can induce the following abnormalities of the interdigestive motility pattern presented according to the new classification proposed by Vantrappen et al. [49]:

1. Paroxysmal tachyrhythmia, also called "Q complex", which is characterized by discrete bursts of regular contraction waves of high amplitude (Fig. 10).
2. Abnormal migrating action potential complexes (MAPCs), also described as "peristalsic rushes", are observed in rabbits after administration of cholera enterotoxin [50] and in man after administration of PGF_2 [49]. Their incidence is increased in patients with secretory diarrhea and they could be a response of the intestine to eliminate the excess of fluid present in the lumen [49].

The pathogenetic role of PGs in the secretory diarrheas is reviewed in by Madsen in this volume.

Gastric Motility and Cytoprotection; Role of PGE

Several studies have reported that stress-induced lesions in rats are associated with an increase in amplitude and frequency of gastric contractions. Garrick et al. [51] studied the exact relation between motility and ulcer appearance in rats submitted to cold restraint. They observed that, compared to a meal, this sort of stress decreased the frequency but increased significantly the duration of high-amplitude gastric contractions

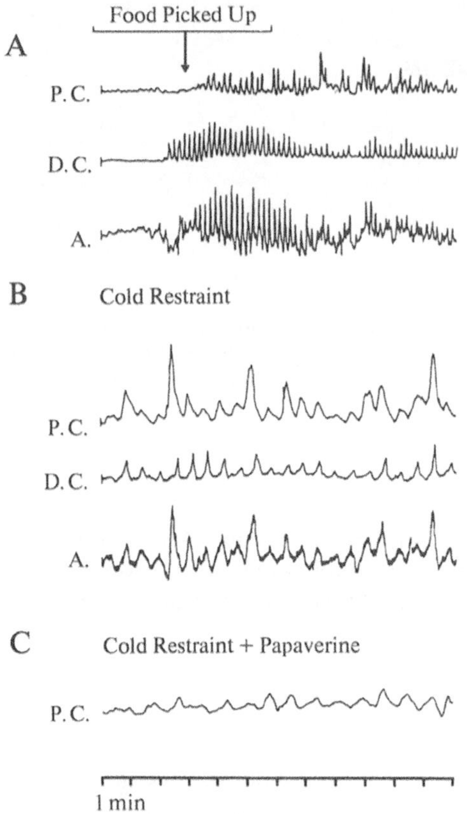

Fig. 11. Effect of cold restraint compared to a meal on the gastric motility in rats. Cold restraint (B) induce a significant increase in the duration of amplitude of contraction waves of the corpus and antrum when compared to the contraction waves induced by the intake of a meal (A). Papaverine administration blocks the appearance of these high amplitude contractans (C) and reduces the mucosal lesions induced by cold restraint. (From [51])

(Fig. 11) which correlated with the formation of gastric lesions and seemed to be the critical factor for the authors. Papaverine, 50 or 100 μg/kg, decreased significantly the number of high-amplitude contractions and the lesion surface area in this model, substantiating the causal relation between motility and mucosal damage in cold restraint.

Another work by Japanese authors [14] showed that instillation of absolute ethanol, 0.6 N HCl, 0.2 *M* NaOH, or 4 *M* NaCl produced streak lesions in the glandular stomach which were preceded by violent contractions (Fig. 12). Intragastric administration of 16-dimethyl-PGE_2 30 min before the necrotizing agents dose-dependently lessened the amplitude and number of contractions and prevented the lesions (Fig. 13). These studies suggest that inhibition of excessive gastric contractions may contribute to the protective action of PGEs in the prevention of gastric lesions in the rat. This interesting hypothesis has yet to be confirmed in humans.

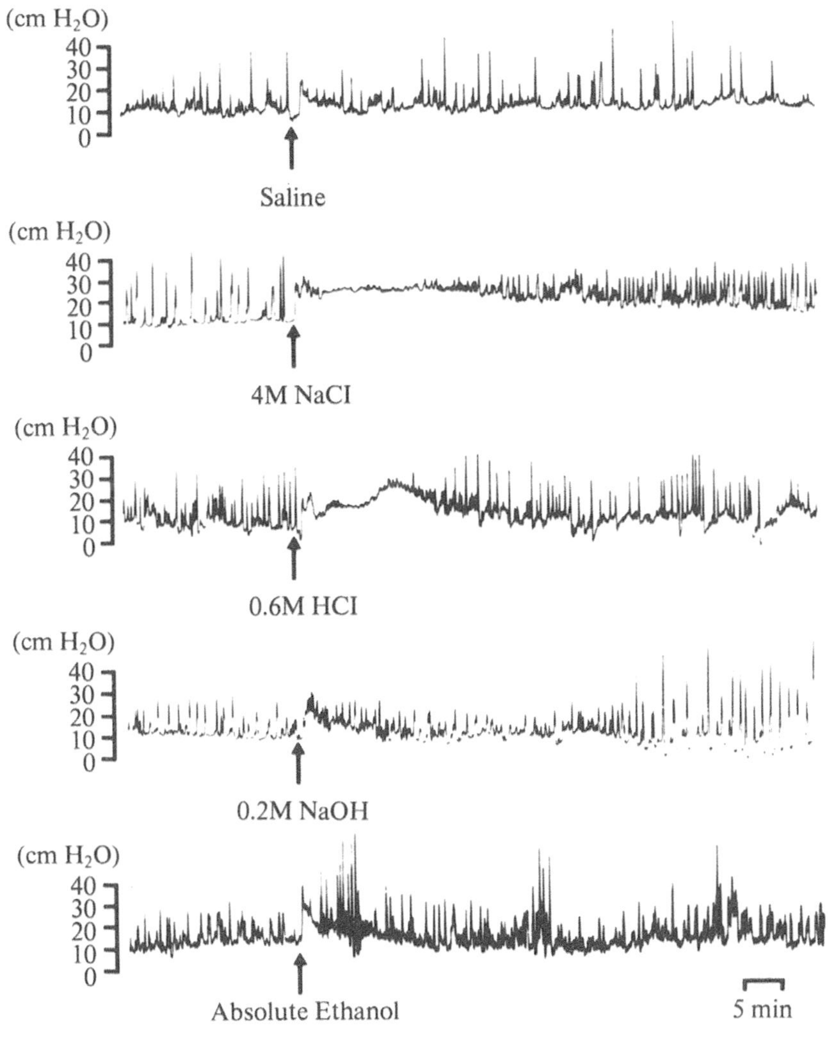

Fig. 12. Effect of different necrotizing agents (concentrated NaCL, HCl, NaOH or Ethanol) on the antral motility of the rat. All these agressors increase significantly the frequence of the antral contractions when compared to saline. (From [14])

Conclusions

1. Prostaglandins play an important modulatory role in the regulation of the digestive tract motility
2. Changes of the motility induced by exogenous administration of PGEs could play a role in the diarrhea which is sometimes observed in patients taking these substances as drugs
3. Inhibition of the antral motility could play an important role in the protection of the gastric mucosa against different aggressors.

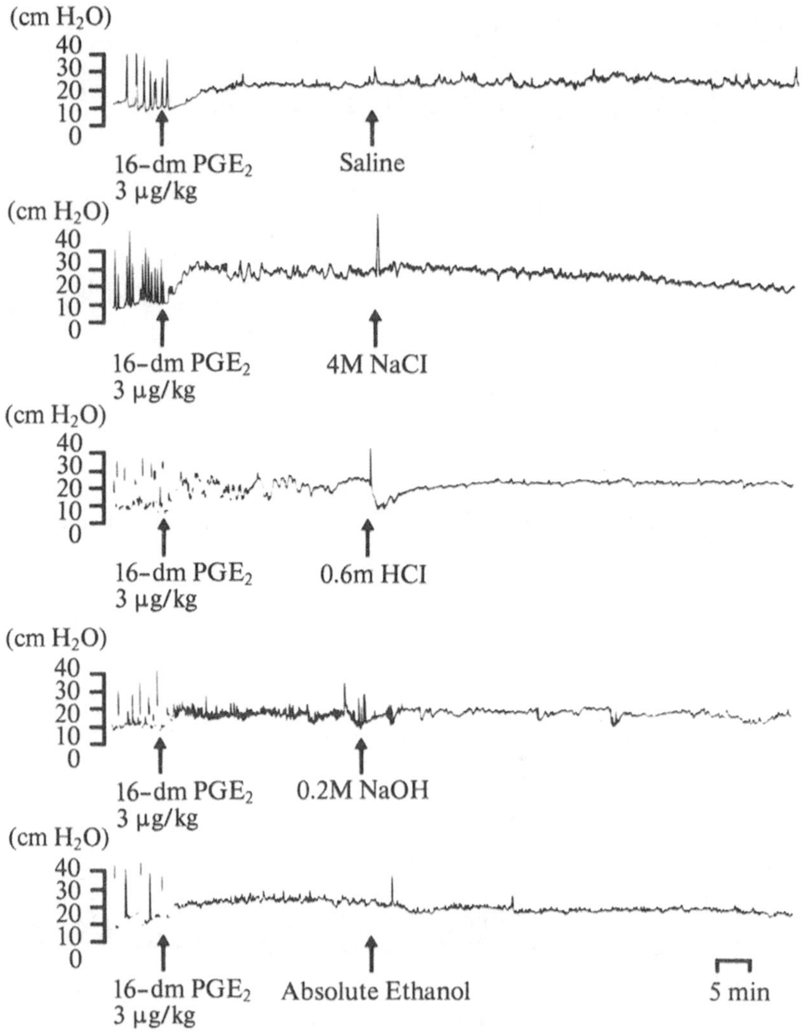

Fig. 13. The effect of intragastric administration of a 16-dm PGE_2 on antral motility in the rat. The PGE_2 induce an immediate and strong reduction of the amplitude of antral contractions in the contral situation (saline) and prevent totally the strong increase of the antral contraction observed in fig. 12 after administration of the necrotizing agents. (From [14])

References

1. Fung WP, Karim SMM, Tye CY (1974) Effect of 15 (R)-15-methyl-prostaglandin E_2-methyl-ester on healing of gastric ulcers. Lancet 2: 10–12
2. Rybicka J, Gibinski K (1978) Methyl-prostaglandin E_2 analogues for healing of gastroduodenal ulcers. Scand J Gastroenterol 13: 155–159
3. Vantrappen G, Popiela T, Tygat DNJ, Lambert R, Robert A (1980) A multicenter trial of 15(R)-15-methyl prostaglandin E_2 in duodenal ulcer. Gastroenterology 78: 1238 (Abst)

4. Dammann HG, Walter TA, Müller P, Simon B (1986) Rioprostil nocte: high duodenal ulcer healing rates, low incidence of side effects. Gastroenterology 90:1386 (Abst)
5. Hunt JN, Smith JL, Jian CL et al (1983) Effect of synthetic prostaglandin E_1 analog on aspirin-induced gastric bleeding and secretion. Dig Dis Sci 28: 897-902
6. Gilbert DA, Surawicz CM, Silverstein FE et al (1984) Prevention of acute aspirin-induced gastric mucosal injury by 15-R-15-methyl-prostaglandin E_2: An endoscopic study. Gastroenterology 86: 339-345
7. Detweiler DK, Harrison CA, Rollins DE et al (1984) Effect of rioprostil on aspirin-induced gastrointestinal mucosal changes in normal volunteers. Gastroenterology 86:1062 (Abst)
8. Demol P, Schmitz HD, Weihrauch TR, Kuhlmann J (1986) Prevention of acetylsalicylic acid-induced changes of gastric potential difference by the new synthetic prostaglandin E_1 analogue Mioprostil. Arzneim.-Forsch./Drug Res. 36 (II): 1406-1408
9. Robert A, Nezamis JE, Lancaster C, Hanchar AJ, Klepper MS (1976) Enteropooling assay: a test for diarrhea produced by prostaglandins. Prostaglandins 11: 809-828
10. Robert A (1981) Prostaglandins and the gastrointestinal tract in: Physiology of the Gastrointestinal Tract, edited by Johnson LR, Raven Press, New York
12. Bennett A, Hensby CN, Sanger GJ, Stamford IF (1981) Metabolites of arachidonic acid formed by human gastrointestinal tissues and their actions on the muscle layers. Br J Pharmacol 74: 435-444
13. Sanders KM (1984) Role of prostaglandins in regulating gastric motility. Am J Physiol 247: G117-G126
14. Takeuchi K, Nobuhara Y (1985) Inhibition of gastric motor activity by 16,16-dimethyl prostaglandin E_2. A possible explanation of cytoprotection. Dig Dis Sc 30: 1181-1188
15. Sanders KM, Northrup TE (1983) Prostaglandin synthesis by microsomes of circular and longitudinal gastrointestinal muscles. Am J Physiol 244: G442-G-448
16. Bennett A, Friedman CA, Vane JR (1967) Release of prostaglandins E_1 from the rat stomach. Nature 216: 873-876
17. Radmonovic B (1968) Prostaglandins in perfusates of the rat intestine after vagal stimulation. Jugoslov Physiol Pharm Acta 4: 123-124
18. Sanders KM (1978) Endogenous prostaglandin E and contractile activity of isolated ileal smooth muscle. Am J Physiol 234: E209-E212
19. Bennett AK, Fleschler B (1970) Prostaglandins and the gastrointestinal tract. Gastroenterology 59: 590-800
20. Das M, Ganguly DK (1984) Effect of prostaglandin E_2 on the acetylcholine release from some peripheral cholinergic nerve terminals. Europ J: Pharmacol 100: 41-46
21. Sanders KM, Szurszewski J (1980) Does endogenous prostaglandin affect gastric antral motility? Am Physiol 241:G191-G195
22. Sanders KM (1984) Evidence that prostaglandins are local regulatory agents in canine ileal circular muscle. Am J Physiol 246: G361-G371
23. Dajani EZ, Roge EAW, Bertermann RE (1975) Effects of E prostaglandins, diphenoxylate and morphine on intestinal motility in vivo. European J Pharmacol 34: 105-113
24. Konturek SJ, Thor P, Pawlik W et al (1982) Role of prostaglandins in the myoelectric motor and metabolic activity of the small intestine in the dog in: Motility of the digestive tract, Ed M Wienbeck, Raven Press, NY: 437-444
25. Dooley CP, Mello WO, Valenzuela JE (1985) Effects of aspirin and prostaglandin E_2 on interdigestive motility complex and duodenogastric reflux in man. Dig Dis Sc 30: 513-521
26. Nylander B, Andersson S (1975) Effect of two methylated prostaglandin E_2 analogs on gastroduodenal pressure in man. Scand J Gastroenterol 10: 91-95
27. Fargeas MJ, Fioramomti J, Bueno L (1984) Prostaglandin E_2: a central neuromodulator of intestinal motility involved in the effects of calcitonin in rats. Gastroenterology 179 (A)
28. Nylander B, Mattson O (1975) Effect of 16,16-dimethyl-PGE_2 on gastric emptying of barium food test meal in man. Scand J Gastroenterol 10: 289-292
29. Johansson C, Ekelund K (1977) Effect of 16,16-dimethyl prostaglandin E_2 on the integrated response to a meal. In: HL Duthie (Ed). Gastrointestinal Motility in Health and Disease, University Park Press, Baltimore: 195-204
30. Moore JG, Alazraki N, Clay GD (1986) Effect of synthetic prostaglandin E_1 analog on gastric emptying of meals in man. Dig Dis Sc 31: 16-20

31. Penston JG, Johnston DA, Wormsley KG (1986) The effects of rioprostil on gastric emptying and intragastric acidity. Hepatogastroenterol 33, in press
32. Dubois A, C'Connell L, Bailey H, Conklin JJ (1986) Prostaglandins and gastric emptying. 6th International Conference on Prostaglandins and related compounds, Florenz, 495 (Abst)
33. Demol P, Wingender W, Weihrauch TR, Kuhlmann J (1986) Effect of rioprostil, a synthetic prostaglandin E_1 on the bioavailability of digoxin. Gastroenterology 92: 1368 (Abst)
34. Heading RC, Nimmo J, Presscott LF, Tothill P (1973) The dependance of paracetamol absorption on the rate of gastric emptying. Brit J Pharmacol 47: 415-421
35. Kelly KA (1980) Gastric emptying of liquids and solids: roles of the proximal and distal stomach. Am J Phys 239: G71-G76
36. Misiewicz JJ, Waller SL, Kiley N, Horton EW (1969) Effect of oral prostaglandin E_1 on intestinal transit in man. Lancet I: 648-651
37. Reele SB, Ruwart MJ, Noah ML (1982) Gastrointestinal propulsion measurement with radiopaque capsules during 16,16-methyl-PGE_2. Prostagl Leukot Medic 9: 629-640
38. Demol P, Wingender W, Weihrauch TR, Kuhlmann J (1986) Effect of Rioprostil, a 16-hydroxy-16-methyl-PGE_1, on the mouth to caecum transit time and gastrin release in volunteers. 6th Int Conf Prostagl Florenz, 213 (Abst.)
39. Ruwart MJ, Klepper MS, Rush BD (1980) PGI_2 inhibitors gastric emptying and small intestinal transit. Gastroenterology 78: 1248
40. Rush BD, Ruwart MJ (1984) The role of acceledrated colonic transit in prostaglandin-induced diarrhoea and its inhibition by prostacyclin. Br J Pharmac 83: 157-159
41. Goyal RK, Rattan S (1974) Mechanism of the lower esophageal sphincter relaxation. Action of prostaglandin E_1 and theophylline. J Clin Invest 52: 337-341
42. Sinar DR, Fletcher JR, Castell DO (1981) Prostaglandin E_1 effects on resting and cholinergically-stimulated lower esophageal sphincter pressure in cats. Prostaglandins 21 (4): 581-590
43. Mukhopadhyay A, Rattan A, Goyal RK (1975) Effect of prostaglandin E_2 on esophageal motility in man. J Appl Physiol 39: 479-481
44. Schwartz GJ, Levine RA, Sondheimer JM et al (1985) Effect of trimoprostil, a PGE_2 analog, on esophageal motility in man. Gastroenterology 88: 1577 (Abstract)
45. Northway MG, Libshitz HI, Osborne BM, Feldman MS, Mamel JJ, West JH, Szwarc IA (1980) Radiation esophagitis in the opossum: Radioprotection with indomethacin. Gastroenterology 78: 883-892
46. Goyal RK (1980) Deleterious effect of prostaglandins on esophageal mucosa. Gastroenterology 78: 1085-1087
47. Kim CH, Azpiroz F, Malagelada JR (1986) Characteristics of spontaneous and drug-induced gastric dysrhythmias in a chronic canine model. Gastroenterology 90: 421-427
48. Kim CH, Hanson R, Abell T, Malagelada JR (1986) The role of prostaglandins in the regulation of human gastric electromechanical activity. Gastroenterology 91: 4 (Abstract)
49. Vantrappen G, Janssens J, Coremans G, Jian R (1986) Gastrointestinal motility disorders. Dig Dis Sc 31, 9 (Suppl): 5S-25S
50. Mathias JR, Carlson GM, Bertiger G, Martin JL, Cohen S (1977) Migrating action potential complex of cholera: a possible prostaglandin-induced response. Am J Physiol 235: E529-E534
51. Garrick T, Buack S, Bass P (1986) Gastric motility is a major factor in cold restraint-induced lesion formation in rats. Am J Physiol 250: G191-G199
52. Konturek SJ, Pawlik W (1986) Physiology and pharmacology of prostaglandins. Dig Dis Sc 31:6S-19S
53. Konturek SJ, Thor P, Pawlik W, GustawP, Dembinski A (1982) Role of prostaglandins in the myoelectric, motor, and metabolic activity of the small intestine in the dog. In: Motility of the digestive tract. Wienbeck M (ed), Raven Press, New York: 437-444
54. Fargeas MJ, Fioramonti J, Bueno L (1984) Prostaglandin E_2: a neuromodulator in the central control of gastrointestinal motility and feeding behaviour by calcitonin. Science 225: 1050-1052
55. Foster GE, Arden-Jones JR, Evans DF, Beahie A, Hardcastle JD (1982) Abnormal jejunal motility in gastrointestinal disease: the Q complex. In: Motility of the digestive tract. Wienbeck M (ed), Raven Press, New York: 427-432

Discussion Following the Report of Dr. Demol

SZABO

Just a comment on your last point concerning hypermotility and cytoprotection. I think it is very likely that hypermotility plays a role in the development in both gastric and even duodenal lesions. We have recent studies showing that even the cysteamine-induced duodenal ulcer is preceded by hypermotility. In this context Takeuchi's studies should be mentioned. The trouble is that he looked at hypermotility only in the antrum, while most of the lesions after necrotizing agents develop in the acid-secreting part of the mucosa. Do you have any information from your own studies that hypermotility possibly also occurs in the rest of the stomach and not only in the antrum?

DEMOL

We have not done any study in animals. It is possible that motility could also play a role in the ulcer disease in humans as it has recently been shown by Malagelada. At least some patients with gastric ulcer have a lower motility index in the antrum. In contrast, he has shown previously that duodenal ulcer patients had a faster emptying of acid. However, the role of motility in ulcer pathogenesis in humans is still very controversial.

HOLTERMÜLLER

Slow-release drugs are now widely used in clinical medicine. Has the rioprostil-induced delay of gastric emptying been examined on the bioavailability of these drugs?

DEMOL

I do not think that there is a major problem. The only effect is a delayed gastric transport of the drug. All in all, the bioavailability remains unchanged. For example rioprostil does not modify the steady state of digoxin. We have to perform studies such as this to analyze whether absorption of any of these drugs is affected.

DAMMANN

Dr. DEMOL, you have showed us studies which observe the postprandial antral motility. Have data been collected under fasting conditions?

DEMOL

The works of Takeuchi were done in fasted rats. In humans Valenzuela analyzed the effect of PGE_2 on interdigestive motility. His data are difficult to interpret because he showed that prostaglandins *and* aspirin modify interdigestive motility.

DAMMANN

Is human enteromotility also decreased under fasting conditions?

DEMOL

There is a study by Nylander from Sweden showing that a single dose of PGE_2 inhibits antrum motility and decreases the amplitude of contractions of basal motility in fasting volunteers.

Addendum: VANTRAPPEN has recently shown that Rioprostil decreased the phase II activity of the IMC.

DAMMANN

Do you think that these results favor a protective activity of prostaglandin analogues?

DEMOL

This is difficult to prove. It would surely be interesting to look for it in humans but, in fact, I do not recall any data on this subject.

WEIHRAUCH

Two comments. I remember a short communication on trimoprostil and its effects on the lower esophagus sphincter. After the application of prostaglandins the radiologically induced esophagitis increased in the opossum. It may be different in man. This certainly has to be looked into also for other prostaglandins. The second point concerns motility and gastric ulcer: there are placebo-controlled studies with metoclopramide as well as with domperidon which clearly show that there is acceleration of gastric ulcer healing, even though, admittedly, the number of patients is small.

COHEN

How can we be sure that the changes in contractility that you are showing us are not the result of mucosal injury rather than the cause of it? And if hypercontractility is the cause of damage, how does this explain the relative sparing of the antrum compared to the fundus in most animal species and also the focal nature of the lesions as a result of injurious agents, rather than more symmetrical or linear lesions which one would expect to find if contractility was important?

DEMOL

Based on studies in rats, Takeuchi speculated that hypercontractility contributes largely to the finding of streak lesions.

BONMELEAR

Have other drugs, known to inhibit gastric motility, been shown to have any cytoprotective effects?

DEMOL

No, I do not know of any.

BONMELEAR

It has been claimed for atropin by Dr. Guth, but atropin is also an antisecretory.

Gastroduodenal Bicarbonate Secretion in Mucosal Protection *

G. FLEMSTRÖM

Introduction

It was proposed by Pavlov already in 1898 [26] that "alkaline mucus" lining the gastric mucosa neutralized luminal acid and that it had a protective role. Many years later, Hollander postulated the occurrence of gastric secretion of an alkaline (non-parietal fluid) and that this fluid was produced at a constant rate [15]. He also demonstrated the occurrence of bicarbonate in the secretion from gastric fundic pouches in dogs after inhibition of the acid secretion by vagotomy and antrectomy. During the last ten years it has been found in all species tested that gastric antral and fundic mucosa secretes bicarbonate to the lumen and that this secretion can be stimulated and inhibited by a variety of means. The secretion most probably originates from the surface epithelial cells. Furthermore, the surface epithelium in duodenal segments devoid of Brunner's glands possesses a similarly metabolism dependent secretion of bicarbonate. The rates of secretion (per unit surface area) are higher in the duodenum than in the stomach and higher in proximal than in more distal segments of the duodenum. In addition, there are distinct differences between the duodenum and the stomach with respect to both the processes of transport of bicarbonate and pathways for stimulation of the secretion [8, 9].

The secretion of bicarbonate together with the mucus gel adherent to the gastric and the duodenal surface is most probably important in the protection of these epithelia against acid and pepsin. The use of pH-sensitive microelectrodes inserted into the gel has permitted experimental demonstration in animals and in man [3, 7, 20, 27, 29] that the pH within the gel is near neutral in spite of high acidities in the gastric lumen (pH 2–3). A surface pH gradient is maintained in the duodenum even at luminal pH 1.5. At higher luminal acidities in the stomach (pH <2–3), the surface gel is acidified and other mechanisms for protection and repair (restitution) of the epithelium should be important. In the duodenum, however, pH in the lumen seldomly falls below 2 even in ulcer patients. Mucosal secretion of bicarbonate is therefore most probably a main mechanism in the protection of this mucosa. This is further supported by the recent demonstration that duodenal intraluminal pH in healthy subjects and patiens with exocrine pancreatic insufficiency is very similar [25]. For both gastric and duodenal mucosa, it has been demonstrated that ulcerogenic agents such as aspirin, in-

* This work was supported by the Swedish Medical Research Council: grant 04X-3515.

domethacin, ethanol and acetazolamide inhibit the alkaline secretion. Furthermore, prostaglandins with ulceroprotective action stimulate the secretion of bicarbonate and mucus in both stomach and duodenum.

Physiological control of gastroduodenal bicarbonate secretion.

Three ways in which mucosal protection by bicarbonate against local acid could be enhanced are:

a) neural stimulation of gastroduodenal bicarbonate secretion simultaneously with gastric acid secretion,
b) local mucosal linkage between the process of parietal cell hydrogen ion secretion and that of secretion of bicarbonate by the surface epithelial cell, and
c) stimulation of the gastric and duodenal bicarbonate secretion by acid present in the lumen. Recent studies have provided evidence that all three mechanisms do operate.

Sham-feeding has been shown to stimulate gastric bicarbonate secretion in humans [6, 10] and to stimulate duodenal mucosal bicarbonate secretion in conscious dogs [22]. These findings indicate that the secretions like gastric secretion of acid are under extrinsic neural control. Fundic distension increases the alkaline secretion in the human stomach [11]. The thus induced rise in secretion was very similar in healthy volunteers and in vagotomized patients, suggesting that the secretion is also under control of the enteric nervous system. Electrical stimulation of the vagal nerves increases both gastric and duodenal bicarbonate secretion in animals [18, 24]. This response is inhibited by alpha$_2$-adrenergic agonists and is enhanced by splanchnicotomy and/or adrenal ligation [18]. The antimuscarinic (M_1) antagonist pirenzepine stimulates duodenal mucosal secretion in rats. This drug binds to ganglia and to some areas in the brain and the stimulation by pirenzepine is abolished by vagotomy suggesting that the effect is exerted centrally and mediated by the vagal nerves. Diazepam has a similar but smaller stimulatory effect [28].

Stimulation of parietal cell acid secretion enhances the ability of the stomach to resist instilled hydrochloric acid and potent inhibition of the acid secretory process decreases this ability. Parenteral infusion of bicarbonate but not other buffer species has a similar protective effect [19]. Furthermore, recent work by Gannon and collaborators [12] has indicated the presence of fenestrated capillaries in the rat and human gastric mucosa which may facilitate vascular transport of bicarbonate, released interstitially from the parietal cell during acid secretion, to the surface epithelial cells. Increased availability of bicarbonate to the surface epithelial cells together with stimulation of their secretion by neural and other influences may all contribute to mucosal protection (Fig. 1).

Presence of acid in the lumen is a stimulant of the alkaline secretion and both the stomach and duodenum. This was first demonstrated in dogs with vagally denervated pouches [13]. Instillation of hydrochloric acid (10–100 mM) into the gastric remnant thus increased the alkaline secretion of the pouch. Strong evidence for humoral mediation of responce to acid has been obtained in in vitro experiments where two isolated mucosae were mounted in parallel facing a common buffered solution [14]. Exposure of the luminal side of fundus to pH 2 or duodenum to pH 4 stimulated the secretion

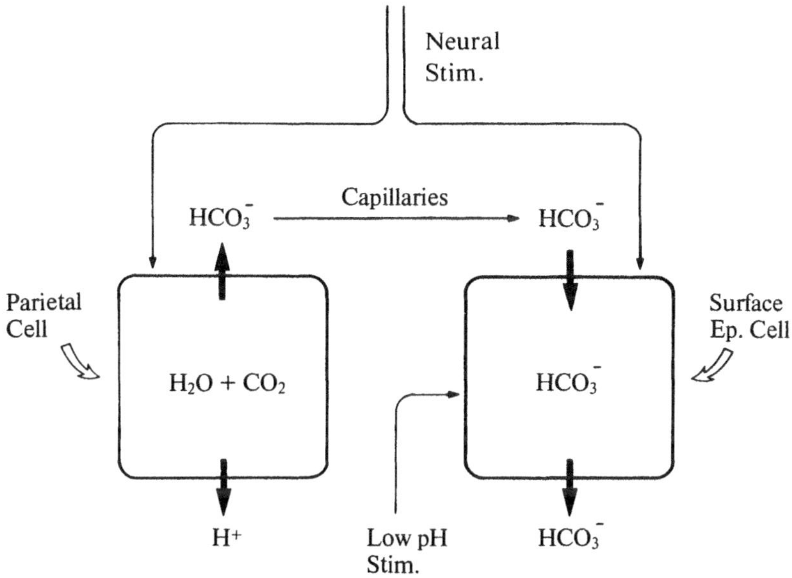

Fig. 1. Model for protection of gastric mucosa. Stimulation of the H^+ secretion by the parietal cells may increase the amount of HCO_3^- available for secretion by the surface epithelial cells. Stimulation of the HCO_3^- secretory process per se, simultaneously with H^+ secretion by neural stimuli, and subsequently by the low intraluminal pH created by the H^+ secretion should further increase protection

by the parallel non-acid exposed tissue. Neural mechanisms are also important in mediating the rise in mucosal alkaline secretion in response to local acid. The stimulation of alkaline secretion by luminal acid in rat duodenum is thus greatly inhibited by pretreatment with the anti-muscarinic agent atropine or the ganglionic blocking agent hexamethonium. Pretreatment with cyclooxygenase inhibitors such as aspirin or indomethacin similarly depresses the ability of the duodenal mucosa to respond to local acid with a rise in bicarbonate secretion. This has been demonstrated in several species, including man, and is strong evidence for a role for mucosal production of prostaglandins in mediating the response (Fig. 2). Furthermore, it has been shown in both animals and man that the rise in alkaline secretion is associated with increased release of E-type prostaglandins to the duodenal lumen. The rise in prostaglandin release after acid exposure has been observed also in the stomach in humans [1]. Finally it should be noted that stimulation of duodenal mucosal alkaline secretion by the prostaglandin precursor arachidonic acid is inhibited by indomethacin [21].

Fig. 2. Pathway for mediating the rise in duodenal mucosal alkaline secretion in response to luminal acid

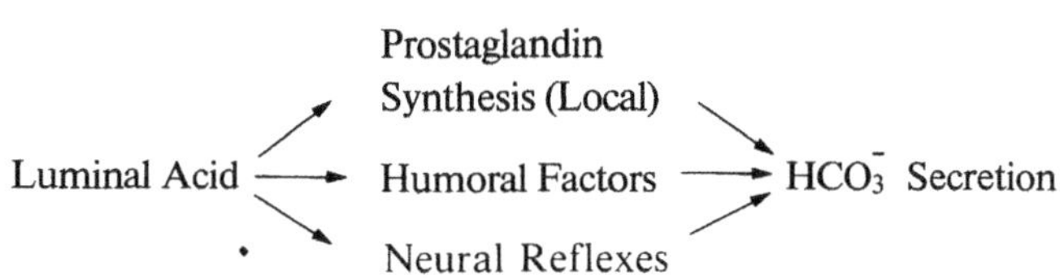

Stimulation by some exogenous prostaglandins.

Stimulation by gastric mucosal alkaline secretion by prostaglandins was first observed in dogs with the analog 16,16-dimethyl PGE_2 [4]. It has later been demonstrated in both stomach and duodenum in a variety of species in vitro and in vivo [2]. Many studies have been performed in vitro and in conscious dogs with denervated pouches but E-type prostaglandins are also effective stimulants of the alkaline secretion in stomach and duodenum of human volunteers [5, 16, 17]. Failure of 16,16-dimethyl PGE_2 to stimulate gastric alkaline secretion has been reported in bullfrog fundus in vitro and the cat stomach in vivo is relatively insensitive to this compound. This may possibly reflect high concentrations of endogenous prostaglandin in these preparations, making exogenous prostaglandins apparently without effect. Luminal administration of the prostaglandin generally results in greater maximal responses than those obtained after parenteral injection. Finally, a possible link between prostaglandin and cholinergic stimulation of gastric alkaline secretion has been observed in the dog [23]. The stimulation by 16,16-dimethyl prostaglandin E_2 was thus blocked by atropine and also by the neural blocking agent tetrodotoxin. Further studies of the interrelation between local prostaglandins and neural influences in the control of gastroduodenal mucosal alkaline secretion and ulceroprotection seem of considerable interest.

References

1. Aly A, Green K Johansson C (1985) Acid instillation increases gastric luminal prostaglandin E_2 output in man. Acta Med Scand 218: 505–510
2. Aly, A Flemström G (1988) Alkaline secretion by the stomach and intestine: Effects of eicosanoids and anti-inflammatory drugs. In: Eicosanoids and the Gastrointestinal Tract. K Hillier, Ed MTP Press, Lancaster
3. Bahari HMM, Ross IN, Turnberg LA (1982) Demonstration of a pH gradient across the mucus layer on the surface of human gastric mucosa in vitro. Gut 23: 513–516
4. Bolton JP, Cohen MM (1978) Stimulation of non-parietal cell secretion in canine Heidenhain pouches by 16,16-dimethyl prostaglandin E_2. Digestion 17: 291–299
5. Feldman M, Barnett CC (1983) Gastric bicarbonate secretion in humans. Effects of pentagastrin, bethanechol, and 11,16,16-trimethyl prostaglandin E_2. J Clin Invest 72: 295–303
6. Feldman M (1985) Gastric H^+ and HCO_3^- secretion in response to sham feeding in humans. Am J Physiol 248: G188–G191
7. Flemström G, Kivilaakso E (1983) Demonstration of a pH gradient at the luminal surface of rat duodenum in vivo and its dependence on mucosal alkaline secretion. Gastroenterology 84: 787–794
8. Flemström G, Turnberg LA (1984) Gastroduodenal defence mechanisms. Clin Gastroenterol 13: 327–354
9. Flemström G (1987) Gastric and duodenal mucosal bicarbonate secretion In: Physiology of the Gastrointestinal Tract, Second Edition. LR Johnson et al., Eds Raven Press, New York pp. 1011–1029
10. Forssell H, Stenquist B, Olbe L (1985) Vagal stimulation of human gastric bicarbonate secretion. Gastroenterology 89: 581–586
11. Forssell H, Olbe L (1987) Effects of fundic distension on gastric bicarbonate secretion in man. Scand J Gastroenterol 22: 627–633
12. Gannon B, Browning J, O'Brien P, Rogers P (1984) Mucosal microvascular architecture of the fundus and body of human stomach. Gastroenterology 86: 866–875
13. Garner A, Hurst BC (1981) Alkaline secretion by the canine Heidenhain pouch in response to exogenous acid, some gastrointestinal hormones and prostaglandin. Adv Physiol Sci 12: 215–219

14. Heylings JR, Garner A, Flemström, G (1984) Regulation of gastroduodenal HCO_3^- transport by luminal acid in the frog in vitro. Am J Physiol 246: G235-G242
15. Hollander F (1963) The electrolyte pattern of gastric mucinous secretions: its implication for cystic fibrosis. Ann NY Acad Sci 106: 757-766
16. Isenberg JI, Hogan DL, Koss MA, Selling JA (1986) Human duodenal mucosal bicarbonate secretion. Evidence for basal secretion and stimulation by hydrochloric acid and a synthetic prostaglandin E_1 analog. Gastroenterolgy 91: 370-378
17. Johansson C, Aly A, Nilsson E, Flemström G (1983) Stimulation of gastric bicarbonate secretion by E_2 prostaglandins in man. Adv Prostaglandin Thromboxane Leukotriene Res 12: 395-401
18. Jönsson C, Nylander O, Flemström G, Fändriks L (1986) Vagal stimulation of duodenal HCO_3^- secretion in anesthetized rats. Acta Physiol Scand 128: 65-70
19. Kivilaakso E (1981) High plasma HCO_3^- protects gastric mucosa against acute ulceration in the rat. Gastroenterology 81: 921-927
20. Kivilaakso E, Flemström G (1984) Surface pH gradient in gastroduodenal mucosa. Scand J Gastroenterol 19 (suppl 105): 50-52
21. Konturek SJ, Tasler J, Bilski J, Kania J (1983) Prostaglandins and alkaline secretion from oxyntic, antral, and duodenal mucosa of the dog. Am J Physiol 245: G539-G546
22. Konturek SJ, Thor P, Tasler J, Bilski J (1986) Cyclic changes in duodenal alkaline secretion and motility patterns in dogs. Role of vagus and prostaglandins (abstr). Proc Internat Union Physiol Sci 16: 105
23. Miller TA, Henagan JM, Watkins LA, Loy TM (1983) Prostaglandin induced bicarbonate secretion in the canine stomach: Characteristics and evidence for a cholinergic mechanism. J Surg Res 35: 105-112
24. Nylander O, Flemström G, Delbro D, Fändriks L (1987) Vagal influence on gastroduodenal HCO_3^- secretion in the cat in vivo. Am J Physiol 252: G522-G528
25. Ovesen I, Bendtsen F, Tage-Jensen U, Pedersen NT, Gram BR, Rune SJ (1986) Intraluminal pH in the stomach, duodenum, and proximal jejunum in normal subjects and patients with exocrine pancreatic insufficiency. Gastroenterology 90: 958-962
26. Pavlov JP (1898) Die Arbeit der Verdauungsdrüsen. Wiesbaden: JF Bergman Verlag, 30-56
27. Quigley EMM, Turnberg LA (1987) pH of the micro-climate lining luman gastric and duodenal mucosa in vivo. Studies in control subjects and in duodenal ulcer patients. Gastroenterology 92: 1876-1884
28. Säfsten B, Flemström G (1986) Stimulatory effect of pirenzepine on mucosal bicarbonate secretion in rat duodenum in vivo. Acta Physiol Scand 127: 267-268
29. Takeuchi K, Magee D, Critchlow J, Matthews J, Silen W (1983) Studies of the pH gradient and thickness of frog gastric mucus gel. Gastroenterology 84: 331-340

Discussion Following the Report of Dr. Flemström

REES

This is very interesting work. We have used a slightly different technique to come up with essentially the same outcome. Based on Ken Hubel's technique, we have applied electrical field stimulation to in vitro mucosa-amphibian gastric and duodenal mucosa. With field stimulation we found a very similar response to that which you have found, with marked stimulation of alkaline secretion, which is almost completely abolished by pretreatment with atropine. Also, we have found after pretreatment with atropine some sort of inhibitory mechanism as well, so it perhaps is a complex effect. Coming back to your luminal acidification experiments my question is: If we accept that prostaglandins possibly may be important, and may be neural factors, and if we accept that there is a pH gradient across mucus gel, how do you think that altering luminal pH triggers the sequence of events, giving some sort of autoregulation of bicarbonate? What is the surface event that triggers the alkali response?

FLEMSTRÖM

It was demonstrated some 15 years ago (Quart J Physiol *56*: 221, 1971) that there are neural receptors in the stomach and duodenum, which respond to local acid. There is also quite strong evidence for an alkaline layer at the surface of these epithelia. Perhaps receptor filaments penetrate into the surface layer, as suggested for the gastric gastrin cells.

REES

May I just come back and ask: How does it get across the gradient? Do you think that the concentrations of acid you are applying to the luminal surface lower the pH at the cell surface, despite the pH gradient? Perhaps you can overwhelm the gradient, but that usually occurs with higher concentrations of acid.

FLEMSTRÖM

Luminal acid may move a zone of neutralization closer to the endothelial surface, exposing pH receptors. There may also be a generation of carbon dioxide closer to the surface, and carbon dioxide sensitive receptors are well known.

SOLL

I was just wondering whether tetrodotoxin would inhibit the bicarbonate response to acid? These findings might provide evidence for a neutral component in this response.

FLEMSTRÖM

This is a very good suggestion but the experiment has not been done. May I just add one note of caution: We are talking about mediation of the response to local acid via both local nerves and prostaglandins. Cutting away one mediation may just result in the other taking over.

Prostaglandins and Cellular Restitution – Physiological and Pathological Implications

T. MIYAKE, M. MURAKAMI, and Y. KOBAYASHI

Introduction

Gastric mucosa is known to heal rapidly after injury induced by various agents such as luminal acid, bile salts, and ethanol. Recent studies suggest that endogenous and exogenous prostaglandins (PGs) play an important role in the protection of the gastric mucosa against the deleterious effects of these agents. Cytoprotection of PGs appears to be mediated by the stimulation of defensive mechanisms such as bicarbonate mucus barriers and maintenance of gastric microcirculation. We evaluated the effects of PGs on restitution of epithelial cells after damage of the gastric mucosa induced by ethanol in terms of gastric potential difference (PD), gastric mucosal blood flow, and autoradiography of the gastric mucosa.

Materials and Methods

Male Sprague-Dawley rats, weighing 180–220 g, were used after 24-h fasting. Gastric mucosal blood flow (GMBF) was measured by laser Doppler velocimetry (Periflux) and gastric transmucosal PD was measured using agar gel electrodes containing 3 *M* KCl in urethane-anesthesized rats. The probe was introduced into the stomach through an incision of the forestomach. Ethanol (intragastric administration) was used as a necrotizing agent or mild irritant. Controls were pretreated with water. Cell proliferation was assessed by autoradiography of H^3-thymidine incorporation in ICR-mice weighing 25–30 g. Detailed morphological changes of the mucosal surface of mice were observed under a scanning electron microscope (JSM-U3, Hitachi Co., Japan).

Results

Effects of 20% Ethanol and 16,16-Dimethyl-PGE_2 on the Gastric Blood Flow and PD in Ethanol-Induced Gastric Mucosal Lesions

After administration of 20% ethanol, a significant increase of blood flow and drop of PD were observed. Absolute ethanol produced marked decreases of blood flow and PD, and there was no recovery of blood flow and PD during the period studied.

Pretreatment with 20% ethanol significantly inhibited the decrease of blood flow and also attentuated the drop of PD 1 h after absolute ethanol administration.

When dimethyl-PGE_2 (10 μg/kg, intragastric administration) was given 15 min before administration of absolute ethanol (1 ml), the decrease of blood flow was significantly inhibited compared with the control group (distilled water pretreatment). Pretreatment with dimethyl-PGE_2 did not prevent the drop of PD immediately after ethanol administration, but significantly promoted recovery of PD.

Effects of 16,16-dimethyl-PGE_2 on the Mitotic Activity Rates and Scanning-Electron-Microscopical Findings in Ethanol-Induced Mucosal Lesions

In mice given absolute ethanol, the mucosal mitotic activity was significantly depressed after 1 h. Mitotic activity was significantly increased in animals exposed to 40% ethanol after 1 h and further increased by pretreatment with dimethyl-PGE_2 (10 μg/kg). In control rats, deep craters in completely denuded lamina propria were observed 1 h after absolute ethanol administration (Fig. 1), whereas in dimethyl-PGE_2-pretreated animals, numerous cells emerging from the gastric pits migrated to cover the denuded lamins (Fig. 2).

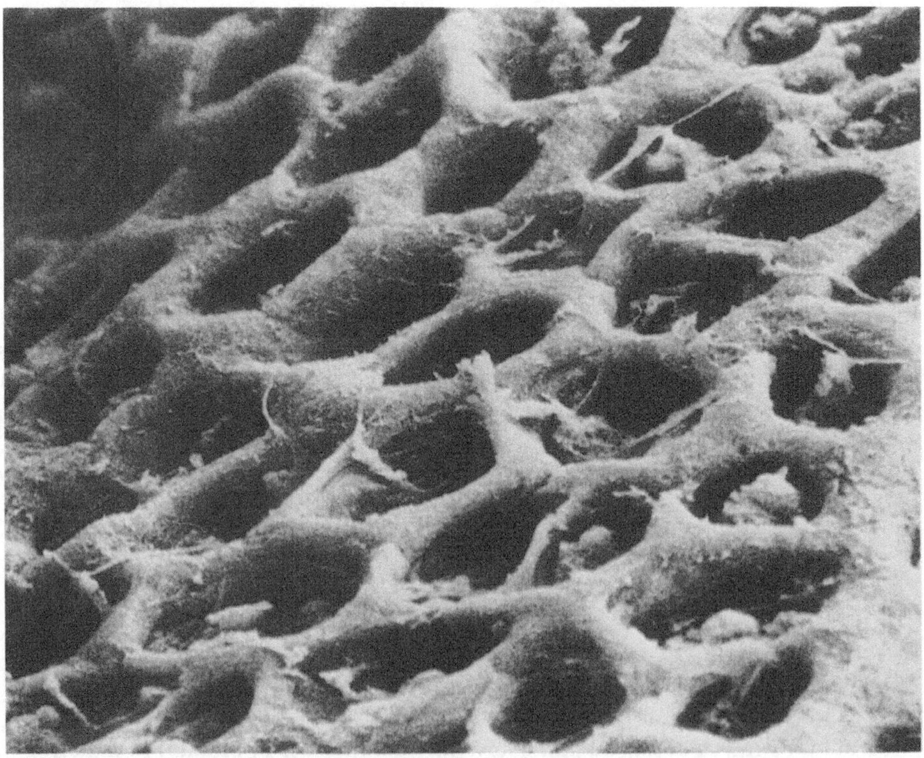

Fig. 1. Control mice. Deep craters in completely denuded lamina propria 1 h after assolute ethanol administration.

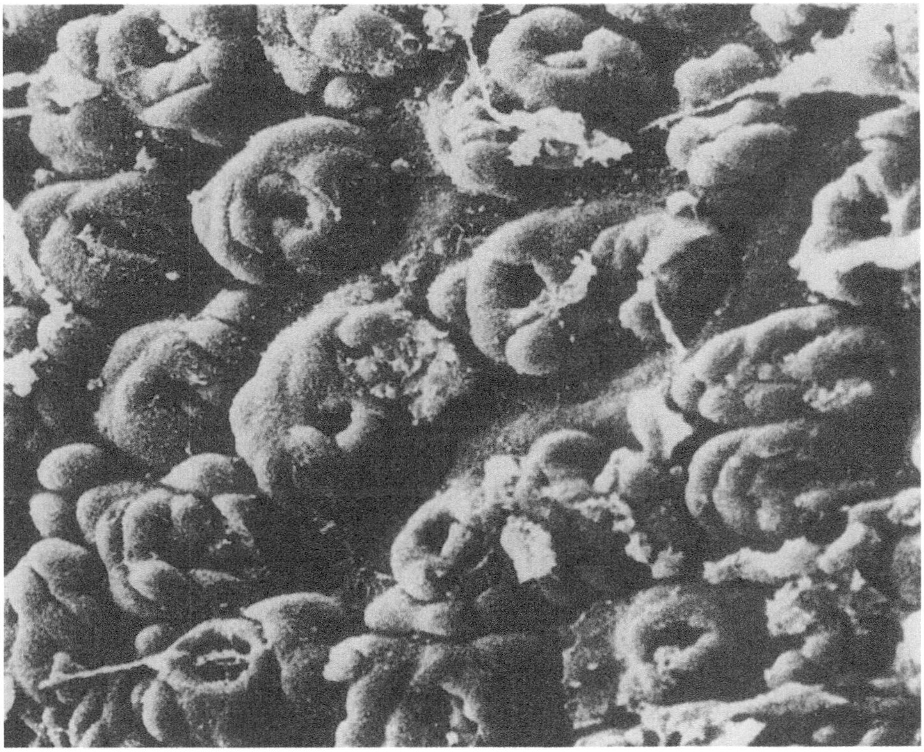

Fig. 2. Dimethyl-PGE_2-pretreated mice. Numerous cells emerging from the gastric pits migrated to cover the denuded lamins.

Discussion

PGs protect ethanol-induced gastric lesions in gross macroscopic appearance from deep mucosal necrosis but do not prevent the initial morphological disruption of the surface epithelium [1, 2]. It was reported that PGs prevent the development of deep mucosal necrosis and cells that will restore the superficial epithelium by migration from the proliferative zone [3]. It has also been demonstrated that the process of early restitution does not require cell proliferation. A histological study by Lacy and Ito demonstrated that PGs have no effect on the rate or extent of restitution when only the surface epithelium is damaged [2]. In an in vitro study using frog gastric mucosa (without blood supply), PGs had no effect on the sequence of electrophysiological changes that accompany the recovery process [4]. Tarnawski et al. reported that the feature of prostaglandin protection of the deep gastric mucosa against ethanol-induced injury is protection of the mucosal proliferative zone, which enables prompt morphological and functional restoration of mucosal integrity [3]. Black et al. reported the importance of blood flow as the mechanism by which deep gastric mucosa is protected and indicated that at the site where epithelial destruction coincides with impairment of the microvasulature, luminal acid can enter the lamina propria without significant neutralization by bicarbonate and destroy the basal lamina, impairing the short-term repair mechanisms [5]. The critical feature that governs whether or not recovery is successful is thought to be the integrity of the mucosal microvasculature [6]. We reported that mild irritants increased gastric blood flow, decreased PD, but that pretreatment with mild irritants promoted the recovery of the decreased PD induced by strong irritants [7, 8].

In contrast, strong irritants decreased gastric blood flow and PD, and no recovery of PD was observed during 1 h of observation [7]. This decrease of blood flow and PD was attentuated by pretreatment with exogenous 16,16-dimethyl-PGE_2. No decrease of blood flow was observed for 10 min after administration of ethanol in the 16,16-dimethyl-PGE_2 pretreatment group [8]. In the present experiment with mice, the number of labeled cells was significantly increased in the mice treated with 16,16-dimethyl-PGE_2 before exposure to 40% ethanol but decreased in mice administered absolute ethanol. The activity of cell proliferation paralleled the protection of the proliferative zone. Our results suggest that endogenous and exogenous PGs prevent the development of deep mucosal necrosis protecting the mucosal microvasculature, and that the rate of restitution is affected by the integrity of mucosal microvasculature and direct response of blood flow to released mediators such as PGs.

References

1. Robert A, Nezamis JE, Lancaster C et al (1979) Cytoprotection by prostaglandins in rats. Prevention of gastric necrosis produced by alcohol, HCl, NaOH, and thermal injury. Gastroenterology 77: 433–443
2. Lacy ER, Ito S (1984) Ethanol-induced insult to the superficial rat gastric epithelium: A study of damage and rapid repair. In: Allen A, et al. eds. Mechanisms of mucosal protection in the upper gastrointestinal tract. New York, Raven 49–56
3. Tarnawski A, Hollander D, Stachura J, Krause WJ, Gergely H (1985) Prostaglandin protection of the gastric mucosa against alcohol injury – A dynamic time-related process. Role of the mucosal proliferative zone. Gastroenterology 88: 334–352
4. Svanes K, Critchlow J, Takeuchi K, Magee D, Ito S, Silen W (1984) Factors influencing reconstitution of frog gastric mucosa: Role of prostaglandins. In: Allen A, et al., eds. Mechanisms of mucosal protection in the upper gastrointestinal tract. New York, Raven 33–39
5. Black BA, Morris GP, Wallace JL (1985) Effect of acid on the basal lamina of the rat stomach and duodenum. Virchows Arch (Cell Pathol) 50: 109–118
6. Morris GP (1986) Prostaglandins and cellular restitution in the gastric mucosa. AM J Med 81: 23–29
7. Murakami M, Mizuno M, Saita H et al (1985) Effect of mild irritants on the gastric mucosal blood flow and potential difference in the rat. Gastroenterology (abstr.) 88: 1512
8. Murakami M, Mizuno, Ashida Y et al (1985) Role of microcirculation in the adaptive cytoprotection by diluted ethanol against ethanol-induced gastric lesions in the rat. Dig Dis Sci (abstr.) 30: 390

Discussion Following the Report of Prof. Miyake

WHITTLE

I have a comment which is related to the terminology regarding restitution and the protection of the proliferative zone. The process of restitution can occur, as you have pointed out, within 10–30 min – very rapidly, far more rapidly than cells can actually turn over. These cells do not necessarily come from the proliferative zone. Rapid restitution is not cell proliferation; it is cell migration.

MIYAKE

The proliferative zone or generative zone is situated at the glandular neck in the fundic area. In the proliferative zone a high synthesis rate of DNA can be observed as an indicator of high mitotic activity. The epithelial cells normally migrate to the mucosal surface. Mild or strong mucosal irritants lead to a massive exfoliation, and thus a defect occurs. In the migration of the regenerating epithelial cells to the mucosal defect the role of basement membrane becomes very important. Since regenerating epithelial cells creep up from the gastric pit along this basement membrane, they do, in fact, migrate within a short time to the damaged area.

WHITTLE

May I just say that I completely agree with this; all I am saying is that the process of epithelial restitution does not require new cells to be formed. It simply requires the existing cells to migrate.

MIYAKE

I agree, but when the mucosal damage is so deep that it includes both the proliferative zone and the basement membrane, the migration of epithelial cells from the proliferative zone is impossible. The protective effect of prostaglandins could maintain a normal microcirculation which in turn preserves the physiological role of the proliferative zone and the basement membrane in the restitution process.

SZABO

I would like to support the comment of Dr. Whittle about the meaning of restitution. In fact, we should be more specific about this term because the proliferative zone does not simply imply dividing cells but also migrating cells, which are most essential for restitution. We should differentiate strictly between dividing cells and migrating cells.

Prostanoid Inhibition of Acid Secretion – Cellular Mechanisms in Canine Fundic Mucosa*

A. H. SOLL

Introduction

Prostaglandins (PGs) have antisecretory actions in several species including man, dog and rat. This review will provide an overview of current information relating to the cellular mechanisms underlying the antisecretory actions of prostaglandins. Discussion of the cellular mechanisms by which either inhibitory or stimulatory chemotransmitters modulate acid secretion is complicated by the fact that several interrelated pathways regulate acid secretion. Three pathways deliver chemical messengers that regulate acid secretion: neural (transmitters released from postganglionic nerves in the stomach wall); endocrine (hormones, such as gastrin, delivered by blood), and paracrine (transmitters released from local storage sites move across the intercellualar space to their local target cell). In vivo the parietal cell (PG) is exposed to many potential chemical transmitters that modulate its function and therefore it has been difficult in vivo to sort out the direct and indirect regulators of secretion. An additional factor complicating the physiology of acid secretion is an interdependency that exists between the pathways regulating acid secretion. This interdependency is clearly evident in the apparent non-specificity displayed by H_2 and muscarinic receptor blockers. These drugs not only respectively inhibit the response to histamine and cholinergic stimulation, but they also block the response to gastrin, food, and vagal stimulation. Prostaglandins in vivo also inhibit all forms of acid secretion: basal secretion as well as the secretory response to food, histamine, gastrin, and cholinergic agents. As a result of these considerations, in vivo studies cannot discern whether the receptors mediating the response to the various chemostransmitters reside on the PC itself, or on other cell types, such as the fundic cells storing histamine or somatostatin.

In recent years a good deal of information regarding the cellular mechanisms regulating acid secretion have come from studies in which cells or gastric glands have been dispersed from fundic mucosa using enzymes, and techniques developed for studying function [1, 2]. This brief summary will focus largely upon our studies of prostaglandin action on canine fundic mucosal cells. Because of the cellular heterogeneity of the stomach mucosa, cell separation is necessary in order to evaluate the potential role of various cell types; both size (velocity) and density separation have been useful. In this review prostaglandin action on parietal cells will first be considered; subse-

* Supported by NIAMDD grants AM-17328, AM-19984, and by the Medical Research Service of the Veterans Administration.

quently attention will be turned to possible prostaglandin action on other cells, including histamine cells and antral gastrin cells. Since isolated parietal cells lose their polar orientation in the mucosa, acid secretion cannot be used as an index of cell function; acid secreted at the apical surface is neutralized by bicarbonate secreted from the basal surface. Therefore, PC function is monitored indirectly using techniques such as the intracellular accumulation by pH partition of the weak base aminopyrine (AP) or the consumption of oxygen or glucose [1, 2]

PC Responses and Receptors

Regardless of the index monitored, canine PC respond to histamine, acetylcholine, and gastrin. Specific receptor antagonists have allowed characterization of the receptors involved [1–3]. H_2-receptor antagonists selectively inhibit histamine stimulation of PC function, with dissociation constants similar to those found in other H_2-receptor systems. The interaction of H_2 antagonists with receptors on isolated PCs appears to provide an excellent model for the site and mechanism of the antisecretory action of these agents. The response to cholinergic agents is blocked by muscarinic antagonists, such as atropine, producing a result indicative of competitive inhibition. Although both H_2 blockers and antimuscarinic agents display an apparent non-specificity in vivo, these drugs are respectively specific against histamine and cholinergic stimulation of the isolated PC. Studying canine PC, gastrin caused a small stimulation of function that was not inhibited by muscarinic or H_2-receptor antagonists, suggesting that gastrin was acting at a separate receptor site. The existence of specific receptors for gastrin has been confirmed using a gastrin analogue labelled with radioactive iodine, ^{125}I-[Leu^{15}]-gastrin [4]. Receptors for this biologically active tracer were localized to PC in studies that produced highly enriched parietal cells using sequential velocity and density cell separation techniques. Gastrin inhibition of tracer binding and stimulation of PC function were correlated over the gastrin dose response curve and both gastrin binding and action were proportionately inhibited by proglumide, a selective antagonist of the family of the gastrin/cholecystokinin receptors. Therefore, current data indicate that the parietal cell has specific receptors for histamine, acetylcholine and gastrin.

Potentiating Interactions Amplify PC Responses

Potentiating interactions between histamine and both gastrin and acetylcholine are evident in studies of PC function [2]. Although muscarinic and H_2 receptor antagonists are specific in their site of action, when PC are treated with combinations of agents, cimetidine and atropine display an apparent lack of specificity, reminiscent of that found in vivo and probably reflecting blockade of the histamine and cholinergic components of the amplification process. At present, it appears that potentiating interactions at the PC are only one of several components of the interactions that occur between the pathways regulating acid secretion.

Prostaglandin Effects on Parietal Cell Function

Evidence has been accumulated that prostaglandins of the E and I groups in nanomolar concentrations directly inhibit PC function [5–10]. Prostanoids inhibit AP accumulation stimulated by histamine and the phosphodiesterase inhibitior isobutyl methyl xanthine (IBMX), alone and in combination. Inhibition was dose dependent over PGE_2 concentrations from 0.1 nM to 1 $^{-}$M; the ID_{50} values (dose producing 50% inhibition of the response) were between 1 and 10 nM against these stimuli. Maximal inhibition by PGE_2 or analogs such as enprostil or misoprostil are produced at doses between 10 and 100 nM and generally ranged from 65 to 95% of the initial response over basal to histamine or IBMX. The inhibition of histamine by PGs is only partly surmounted at higher doses of histamine and therefore was not indicative of competitive inhibition. The presence or absence of the phosphodiesterase inhibitor IBMX did not alter the inhibitory actions of PGs.

Forskolin, a diterpene that appears to directly activate the catalytic subunit of adenylate cyclase [11], stimulates PC function. Stimulation of canine PC AP accumulation by 10 $^{-}$M forskol is inhibited by both enprostil and PGE_2. However, interpretation of these data required controlling for the interactions between histamine and forskolin, since the response to forskolin is inhibited by the H_2 antagonist cimetidine. Therefore, studies of forskolin inhibition by enprostil were performed in the presence of 10 $^{-}$M cimetidine; under these conditions forskolin stimulation of AP accumulation was also markedly inhibited by nanomolar concentrations of enprostil and PGE_2 (10). PG was not found to inhibit forskolin stimulation of rat PC [12]; the reason for these divergent findings is not clear, but there may be some differences in PG action among species, as considered below.

Prostanoid inhibition of canine PC function is specific for histamine; PGs of the E and I groups do not inhibit stimulation of AP accumulation by the cholinergic agonist carbachol or by the dibutyryl analog of cyclic AMP (dbcAMP). These prostanoids also failed to significantly inhibit the response to heptadecapeptide gastrin (G17). However, when gastrin action is potentiated by histamine or IBMX (presumably acting by enhancing the action of endogenous histamine), PGs caused marked inhibition. In contrast, when gastrin response was enhanced by interaction with dbcAMP, no PG inhibition was produced.

Mechanisms of PG inhibition

Once agonists bind to receptors secondary changes take place that transduce the signal, thereby activating cell function. These activation mechanisms fall into two categories, those related to the generation of cyclic adenosine monophosphate (AMP) and those related to increases in calcium concentration in the cell. Stimulation of PC function by histamine, but not by cholinergic or gastrin, is closely linked to enhanced formation of cyclic AMP. Histamine presumably stimulates parietal cell function by increasing cyclic AMP production and thus activating specific cyclic AMP-dependent protein kinases. Since histamine action on PC function appears specific for histamine, a direct effect of PGs on histamine – stimulated cyclic AMP generation was a reasonable first hypothesis to test.

Histamine and PG Stimulated of Cyclic AMP Production

Previous studies have indicated that histamine stimulation of cyclic AMP production is accounted for by the parietal cell content of the elutriator-separated fractions [13]. We have confirmed this result by examining further subjecting elutriator – enriched parietal cell fractions to subsequent density gradient separation, producing fractions respectively enriched to greater than 90% parietal or chief cells. In these fractions histamine stimulation of cyclic AMP production correlated closely with the parietal cell content. Consistent with previous findings with elutriator enriched fractions (13), secretin only stimulated cyclic AMP production in chief cell-, but not PC-enriched fractions.

PGE_2 also stimulates cyclic AMP production in fundic mucosa and previous studies indicated this effect was more pronounced in non-parietal cells [13, 14]. This stimulatory action of PGE_2 is generally found at higher concentration (0.1 to 100 ¯M) than those inhibiting histamine-stimulated parietal cell function. In step gradient enriched fractions of canine parietal and chief cells, PGE_2 (1 ¯M) stimulated cyclic AMP production in chief cells, but not in the parietal cell enriched fractions. Stimulation of cyclic AMP production is not a property shared by all PGE analogues. Previous studies found that the 16-phenoxy analog of $PGE_{1\delta}$, inhibited histamine-stimulated PC function with a potency equal to PGE_2, but failed to increase cyclic AMP production at any concentration tested. Enprostil, another PGE analog substituted at the 16 position, also failed to increase cyclic AMP production in any of the canine fundic mucosal cell fractions studied [10].

PG Inhibition of Histamine-stimulated Cyclic AMP Production

PGs of the E and I group have been found to inhibit histamine-stimulated cyclic AMP production over the same nanomolar concentration range of prostaglandins in which inhibition of histamine-stimulated aminopyrine accumulation occurs [5, 6, 7, 10, 12, 14, 15]. As noted above, histamine, but not cholinergic agents nor gastrin, activates cyclic AMP production in parietal cells, and this difference in cell activation mechanisms probably accounts for the specificity of PGs against histamine. In canine parietal cells the proportionate inhibition by PGs of histamine stimulated function and cyclic generation are comparable, suggesting a causal association. Enprostil inhibition of histamine-stimulated parietal cell function and cyclic AMP production were studied with a background of 10 ¯M IBMX; enprostil produced about 70% inhibition of maximal histamine stimulation of both AP accumulation and cyclic AMP production. Interpretation of PG inhibition of histamine-stimulated cyclic AMP production can be complicated by the independent action of PG stimulating cyclic AMP production, especially when the fractions studied include a significant number of non-parietal cells.

To confirm that PG inhibition of histamine-stimulated parietal cell function was a direct action on parietal cells, PG inhibition was studied in fractions highly enriched in parietal cells by sequential elutriation and step density gradient separation. In these fractions cyclic AMP formation stimulated by 10 ¯M histamine plus 10 ¯M IBMX, was dose dependently inhibited by enprostil. These studies therefore support the view that PG inhibition is a direct action on parietal cells.

Mechanism of PG Inhibition of Histamine-stimulation of Adenylate Cyclase

Increasing knowledge has indicated that adenylate cyclase is composed of both stimulatory and inhibitory components. Stimulatory hormone receptors, such as the H_2 receptor, activate a stimulatory guanine nucleotide binding protein, G_s, that in turn induces the catalytic subunit to convert ATP to cyclic AMP [16]. A mirror image of G_s exists that serves to inhibit, rather than stimulate, the catalytic subunit. This inhibitory G protein is termed G_i or N_i. Inhibitory receptors act via G_i to reduce cyclic AMP generation [16, 17]. An important tool for dissecting these mechanisms is provided by the toxin produced by *Bordetella pertussis.* Pertussis toxin, originally recognized for its ability to activate islets, inducing the secretion of insulin [18]. This "islet activating protein" was found to interact with G_i, rendering this GTP binding protein incapable of inhibiting the catalytic subunit [19]. This inactivation resulted from the transfer of an ADP-ribose group to the 41K δ-subunit of G_i. Several agents, such as opioids, δ_2-adrenergic agents, and muscarinic agents, have an inhibitory action on cell function mediated by this inhibitory GTP-binding protein of adenylate cyclase [16, 17, 20]. Pertussis toxin treatment of PC has been used to evaluate the involvement of the inhibitory GTP-binding protein, G_i, in prostanoid inhibition of parietal cell function [12, 21].

Pertussis Toxin Effects on PC Function and Cyclic AMP Production

To study the effects of PT, PC were cultured overnight in the presence and absence of PT. A similar pattern of histamine, carbachol, and dbcAMP stimulation and prostanoid inhibition of histamine stimulation was found after this culture period. In parietal cells treated overnight with PT, enprostil inhibition of histamine-stimulated AP accumulation was markedly attenuated. PGE_2 inhibition of histamine-stimulated AP accumulation was also attenuated in pertussis toxin-treated cells. PG inhibition of forskolin-stimulated AP accumulation was also markedly attenuated in PT-treated cells compared to control cells after a similar culture period.

In these PC after overnight culture, enprostil dose-dependently inhibited histamine stimulated cyclic AMP production [21]. In PT-treated cells, histamine was at least as effective in stimulating cyclic AMP production, but in parallel with the patterns found with functional studies, enprostil inhibition of histamine-stimulated cyclic AMP production was markedly attentuated. Forskolin stimulation of cyclic AMP production was inhibited by enprostil treatment in control, but not PT-treated cells.

Prostaglandin Actions on other Fundic Mucosal Cells

Prostaglandin actions on physiological functions are frequently complex. For example, although the hypotensive action of prostanoids is associated with direct relaxation of vascular smooth muscle, several other mechanisms also contribute, such as modifying smooth muscle responsiveness to norepinephrine or neuronal release of norepinephrine. Prostanoid inhibition of acid secretion may also reflect multiple actions, only one of which is inhibition of histamine-stimulated PC function. Prostanoid action in the fundic mucosa has already been noted to reflect two actions: inhibition of histamine-stimulated cyclic AMP production, an effect probably reflecting interaction with inhibitory receptors linked to the inhibitory GTP binding protein of adenylate cyclase. In addition, prostanoids also stimulate cyclic AMP production, probably primarily in non-parietal cells. Two other actions of prostanoids in fundic mucosa have thus far been found, as discussed below; there are probably several others that remain to be recognized.

PG Modulation of Histamine Release

Histamine in the canine fundic mucosa is stored in mast cells [22]. In contrast to the rat and probably the rabbit fundic mucosa, current evidence indicates that no major stores of histamine are present in endocrine – like cells. Evidence supporting this view comes from studies with isolated fundic mucosal cells in which sequential velocity and density gradient separation have revealed a close correlation between histamine content and mast cell number [22]. To study histamine release, canine fundic mast cells were placed in overnight suspension culture. Using this culture system, histamine release has been stimulated by the lectin Conçonavalin A. Histamine release was found to be inhibited by adrenergic agents acting at a beta-adrenergic receptor. PGE_2, but not enprostil, also inhibited histamine release (A. H. Soll, M. Toomey, M. Beaven, manuscript in preparation). This effect of PGE_2 was only observed at concentrations of PGE_2 ranging from 0.1 to 100 ~M. This concentration range is considerably higher than that producing inhibition of parietal cell function and corresponds to the concentration range in which PGE_2 stimulates adenylate cyclase. Although the role of cyclic AMP in mast cell function is controversal, previous studies have indicated that agents that stimulate cyclic AMP, such as adrenergic agents, inhibit mast cell histamine release. The failure of enprostil to inhibit mast cell histamine release may relate to finding that enprostil does not stimulate cyclic AMP production.

Prostaglandin action in rabbit gastric glands appears to differ in one major aspect from the findings reviewed for canine fundic cells. In rabbit glands PGs stimulate, rather than inhibit, histamine release [9]. The reason for this difference probably relates to histamine being stored in an endocrine-like cell in the fundic mucosa of some species, including rabbit and rat. This difference in the nature of cells storing histamine may explain the differences observed in prostaglandin action on histamine release between studies on dog cells and rabbit gastric glands.

Prostanoid Modulation of Gastrin Release

Selected prostanoid analogs, including 16,16-dimethyl PGE_2 and enprostil, appear to inhibit release of gastrin in vivo [23, 24]. Recently in vitro systems have been developed to allow dispersion and culture of canine antral gastrin cells [25]. Using this system, enprostil, but not PGE_2, inhibits bombesin stimulated gastrin release [26]. Somatostatin also inhibits gastrin release in this system [25], but since there is a very low content of somatostatin cells in this culture system, it is unlikely that prostanoid action is mediated via release of somatostatin. Thus prostanoid analogs appear to inhibit gastrin release by direct actions on antral G cells; the cellular mechanisms underlying this action of enprostil remain to be established.

A Family of Prostaglandin Receptors

The receptors that mediate prostanoid action in the fundic mucosa appear to comprise a complex family of related receptor subtypes. Present data suggest that canine fundic mucosa possesses at least three receptors that can functionally discriminate subtle structural differences between E- and I-type prostanoids. Inhibition of parietal cell function is mediated by a receptor that interacts with prostanoid analogs of the PGE or PGI groups; PGE_2, PGI_2, and related analogs inhibit parietal cell function with roughly comparable potency and efficacy. Thus, the structural modifications of analogs such as enprostil, misoprostil, and 5,9-epoxy-16-phenoxy-PGF_1 do not alter interaction at the parietal cell receptor linked to inhibition via the inhibitory GTP binding protein of adenylate cyclase. However, PGE_2, but not enprostil or 5,9-epoxy-16-phenoxy-PGF_1, stimulates cyclic AMP production; thus modifications affecting the 16 position of the prostanoid structure may impair interaction with the PG receptor that mediates stimulation of adenylate cyclase. This group of prostanoids would thus not be expected to share the ability of PGE_2 to inhibit mast cell histamine release, an effect that appears to reflect stimulation of adenylate cyclase. A third possible PG receptor "subtype" may mediate PG actions on the antral gastrin cell, a view supported by the finding that enprostil, but not PGE_2, inhibits bombesin-stimulated gastrin release. Receptors mediating prostanoid inhibition of parietal cell function, antral G cell secretion, and histamine release display subtle differences in specificity. These differences in receptor specificity may markedly influence the spectrum of prostaglandin action and thus shape the therapeutic actions and potential side effects of these compounds. These distinctions between receptors are tentatively presented since they are based upon functional differences in specifity and potency of agonists; differentiation of receptor subtypes generally requires selective receptor antagonists and direct radioligand studies. Other factors such as differences in degradation or access (delivery to a receptor) can alter the apparent spectrum of action of an agonist.

The Role of Endogenously Produced Prostaglandins

Endogenously produced prostanoids may be an important modulator of parietal cell function under certain conditions and may account for a relative impairment in the response to stimulation both in vivo and in vitro. When dog gastric glands were prepared in the presence of indomethacin, the histamine response was increased 3-fold compared to control, whereas the gastrin and acetylcholine responses were unchanged [27]. Furthermore, in vivo studies found that indomethacin enhanced acid secretion in vivo [28, 29]. Although indomethacin may have actions other than inhibition of cyclooxygenase, and thus prostaglandin production, these data suggest an inhibitory role for endogenous prostaglandins. Understanding the role of endogenous prostanoids will be greatly advanced by elucidating the cell types responsible for prostanoid production and the factors regulating this production. Obviously a great deal of knowledge needs to be gained before the role of endogenous prostanoids can be sorted out.

The present review has considered three possible mechanisms of the antisecretory actions of prostanoids. In ex vivo and in vivo systems prostaglandins have also been shown to have other actions, such as stimulation of somatostatin secretion and modulation of neurotransmitter release. It is possible that additional mechanisms to the ones presently considered also contribute to the antisecretory actions of PGs. Also considered has focused upon PGs only acting by either stimulating or inhibiting adenylate cyclase. It is also possible that prostanoids have other mechanisms of actions, such as modulating the calcium-protein kinase C pathways for cell activation.

References

1. Berglindh, T (1984) The mammalian gastric parietal cell in vitro. Ann Rev Physiol 46: 377-392
2. Soll AH, Berglindh T (1985) Physiology of isolated gastric glands and cells: Receptora and effectors regulating secretion. Physiology of Gastrointestinal Tract, Raven Press, LR Johnson, Ed., in press.
3. Soll AH (1980) Secretagogue stimulation of ^{14}C-aminopyrine accumulation by isolated canine parietal cells. Am J Physiol 238: G366-G375
4. Soll AH, Amirian DA, Thomas LP, Reedy TJ, Elashoff JD (1984) Gastrin receptors on isolated canine parietal cells. J Clin Invest 73: 1434-1447
5. Soll AH (1978) Specific inhibition by prostaglandins E_2 and I_2 of histamine-stimulated [^{14}C]aminopyrine accumulation and cyclic adenosine monophosphate generation by isolated canine parietal cells. J Clin Invest 65: 1222-1229
6. Schepp W, Heim H-K, Ruoff H-J (1983) Comparison of the effect of PGE_2 and somatostatin on histamine stimulated ^{14}C-aminopyrine uptake and cyclic AMP formation in isolated rat gastric mucosal cells. Agents and Actions, 13(2/3): 200-206
7. Levine RA, Kohen KR, Schwartzel EH Jr, Ramsay, CE (1982) Prostaglandin E_2-histamine interactions on cAMP, cGMP, and acid production in isolated fundic glands. Am. J Physiol. 242 (Gastrointest Liver Physiol 5): G21-G26
8. Skoglund ML, Nies AS, Gerber JG (1982) Inhibition of acid secretion in isolated canine parietal cells by prostaglandins. J Pharm Exper Ther 220: 371-374
9. Nylander O, Berglindh T, Obrink KJ (1986) Prostaglandin interaction with histamine release and parietal cell activity in isolated gastric glands. Am J Physiol 250 (Gastrointest Liver Physiol 13): G607-G616
10. Soll AH, Chen M-CY, Amirian DA, Toomey M, Sanders MJ Prostanoid inhibition of canine parietal cells: Mediation by the inhibitory GTP-binding protein of adenylate cyclase. Submitted, Am J Med
11. Barovsky K, Pedone C, Brooker, G (1984) Distinct Mechanisms of forskolin-stimulated cyclic AMP accumulation and forskolin-potentiated hormone responses in C6-2B cells. Mol Pharm 25: 256-260
12. Rosenfeld G (1986) Prostaglandin E_2 Inhibition of Secretagogue-Stimulated [^{14}C]amonopyrine Accumulation in Rat Parietal Cells: A Model for its Mechanism of Action. J Pharm Exp Therp 237(2): 513-518
13. Wollin A, Soll AH, Samloff IM (1979) Actions of histamine, secretin, and PGE_2 on cyclic AMP production by isolated canine fundic mucosal cells. Am J Physiol 237: E437-E443
14. Major JS, Scholes P (1978) The localization of a histamine H_2-receptor adenylate cyclase system in canine parietal cells and its inhibition by prostaglandins. Agents and Actions 8: 324-31
15. Becker M, Ruoff H-J (1982) Inhibition by prostaglandin E_2, somatostatin and secretin of histamine-sensitive adenylate cyclase in human gastric mucosa. Digestion 23: 194-200
16. Spiegel AM, Gierschik P, Levine MA, Downs, RW Jr (1985) Clinical implications of guanine nucleotide-binding proteins as receptor-effector couplers. N Engl J Med 312(1): 26-33
17. Moss J, Burns DL, Hsia JA, Hewlett EL, Guerrant RL, Vaughan M (1984) Cyclic nucleotides: Mediators of bacterial toxin action in disease. Ann Int Med 101: 653-666

18. Katada T, Ui M (1981) Islet-activating protein: a modifier of receptor-mediated regulation of rat islet adenylate cyclease. J Biol Chem 256: 8310–17
19. Murayama T, Ui M (1983) Loss of the inhibitory function of the guanine nucleotide regulatory component of adenylate cyclase due to its ADP ribosylation by islet-activating protein, pertussis toxin, in adipocyte membranes. J Biol Chem 258(5): 3319–3326
20. Ui M (1984) Islet-activating protein, pertussis toxin: probe for functions of the inhibitory guanine nucleotide regulatory component of adenylate cyclase. Trnds Pharm Sci 5: 277–299
21. Soll AH, Chen M, Amirian DA, Toomey M, Sanders MJ Enprostil and PGE_2 inhibition of canine parietal cells: mediation by the inhibitory GTP binding protein of adenylate cyclase. Gastroenterology, abstract, 90(5): 1642.
22. Soll AH, Lewin K, Beaven MA (1979) Isolation of histamine containing cells from canine fundic mucosa. Gastroenterology. 77: 1283–1290
23. Mahachai V, Walker K, Sevelius H, Thomson ABR (1985) Antisecretory and serum gastrin lowering effect of enprostil in patients with diodenal ulcer disease. Gastroenterology 89: 555–61
24. Ippoliti AF, Isenberg JI, Hagie L (1981) Effect of oral and intravenous 16,16-dimethyl prostaglandin E_2 in duodenal ulcer and zollinger-ellison syndrome patients Gastroenterology, 80: 55–59
25. Giraud A, Soll AH, Cuttita F, Walsh J (1986) Bombesin stimulation of gastrin release by isolated canine cells in short term culture. In press Amer J Phys
26. Giraud AS, Walsh JH, Soll AH (1986) Prostanoids of the PGE_2 series diffentially affect gastrin (G) release from canine G-cells in short term culture. Gastroenterology, 90(5): 1428
27. Berglindh T, Hansen D (1984) Characterization of isolated gastric glands from the dog Fed Proc 43: 996
28. Feldman M, Colturi TJ (1984) Effect of indomethacin on gastric acid and bicarbonate secretion in humans. Gastroenterology 87: 1339–1343
29. Levine RA, Schwartzel EH (1984) Effect of indomethacin on basal and histamine – stimulated human gastric acid secretion. Gut. 25: 718–722

Discussion Following the Report of Dr. Soll

DAMMANN

Dr. Soll, do you think that it might be clinically relevant to combine prostaglandin analogues with other antisecretory drugs, firstly with respect to their gastrin-lowering properties and secondly with respect to their gastrin acid inhibitory effect?

SOLL

Since potent antisecretory agents can enhance gastrin secretion, adding a prostaglandin analogue that would reduce gastric release might be a very nice compliment to a highly potent antisecretory therapy, which leads to achlorhydria and consequently to hypergastrinemia. The degree to which such a combination will reduce gastrin levels has not been studied in man. A gastrin-receptor antagonist might be another alternative to use in this setting. To answer your second question, the potential benefits of combining two anti-secretory agents that act by different mechanisms have not been carefully studied. I doubt either antisecretory or ulcer-healing effects will justify the use of two drugs, especially when one of the drugs is either a very potent, long-acting H_2 blocker or omeprazole.

HALTER

I would like to comment. We have tested the effect of the combination omeprazole with enprostil on serum gastrin in the rat. Our data so far available suggest that the prostaglandin analogue, enprostil, has no influence on the hypergastrinemia induced by omeprazole. We cannot exclude, however, that this may be a specific phenomenon in the rat. I am interested in another problem: Have you tested omeprazole with your isolated G-cell model? What happens with gastrin release in this model?

SOLL

We have yet to do that study. But I would anticipate that omeprazole will have no direct effect on antral G cells.

DAMANN

Dr. Halter, could you tell us something about the doses of omeprazole and enprostil which have been used in your experiments?

HALTER

We have not finished our investigations yet, so I cannot tell you whether enprostil has already been used in an optimal dose.

SZABO

The quality of your pictures is impressive. The study design you have used affords a 10-min exposure of the tissue to ethanol. Also the casting takes time to get fixed, and so on. During the course of time a reduction of capillaries can be seen. Do you think that this is due to acute necrosis, since a 10-min alcohol exposure leads to quite an extensive damage of the mucosa, or is the casting material unable to reach all capillaries because of the stasis in the microcirculation, or something else?

O'Brien

I personally assume that the cast does not include all vessels present. But I do not think that there was any occlusion of the vessels which were filled, such as arteriols, capillaries, or venules. Therefore we place it at the capillary network or the submucosal arterioles. I note the data from yourself and Paul Guth which do not support the view that the arterioles are closed, but Brendan Whittle has provided us with a somewhat alternative view. From our casting experiments I can only suspect that a block has occurred at the capillary level.

Rees

Did your technique give you any insight into whether regional variations occur in the normal rat gastric mucosa? For example, did you find any areas where the microvasculature differed substantially, and if so, could this account for the predisposition of certain areas to develop peptic ulceration? Furthermore, did you look at any other mucosa-damaging agents, such as bile acids or NSAIDs, to see if they produce a similar type of response?

O'Brien

I agree that certain areas are more vulnerable. We have not yet studied this phenomenon, which would be most interesting, particularly in the antral mucosa and also in the antral fundic junction. All our studies have been in fundic mucosa. Concerning your second question, I have no data on the damaging agents you mentioned. We are in the process of looking at aspirin.

The Protective Effects of Prostaglandins on the Gastric Microvasculature

P. E. O'Brien

Introduction

The process of cytoprotection is a drug-induced enhancement of gastric mucosal resistance to various exogenous irritants [1]. The mechanisms of cytoprotection are still unclear. A number of observations point to a central role for the microcirculation of the stomach in the process [2].

In this study we have investigated the influence of prostaglandin E_2 (PGE_2) on the effects of topical ethanol (EtOH) on the gastric microvasculature. We have examined the structure of the microvessels using microvascular casting techniques, and have examined the permeability of the microvessels to macro molecules using fluorescein isothiocyanate labelled albumin (FITC albumin) as a probe.

Methods

We have utilized the basic rat model of cytoprotection as developed by Robert et al [1]. Adult male Porton rats (180–300 g), fasted for 24 hours, were given a pretreatment of either PGE_2 (100 μg/kg) in 1 ml of normal saline or 1 ml normal saline (control group) via an orogastric tube. Fifteen minutes later, 1 ml of either EtOH or normal saline was instilled into the stomach via the orogastric tube. The rat was sacrificed 15 minutes after this instillation.

Microvascular Casting

At 10 minutes after instillation of EtOH each animal was anaesthetized, the thoracic aorta was exposed and cannulated and the animal perfused with casting medium according to the technique previously described [3]. The casting medium contained methyl-methacrylate monomer, 5ml (Polysciences, U. S. A.), Mercox CL-2R-5, 15 ml (Vilene Hospital Ink and Chemical Co., Tokyo), and Mercox MA catalyst 1 g. After setting of the cast, the stomach was removed, the tissue corroded away, and the cast examined by scanning electron microscopy (Siemens-E. T. E. C. Autoscan). At least 10 casts were examined for each experimental group.

Capillary Macromolecular Permeability

This was assessed by examining the fluorescence within the interstitium of the gastric mucosa after intravenous infusion of FITC albumin. For these experiments, FITC albumin (250 mg/kg) was given intravenously 30 minutes prior to the pretreatment and treatment protocol. At 15 minutes after EtOH treatment the animal was sacrificed and the stomach was fixed in neutral phosphate-buffered 10% formalin, embedded in paraffin, sectioned at 5 μm and examined by fluorescence microscopy.

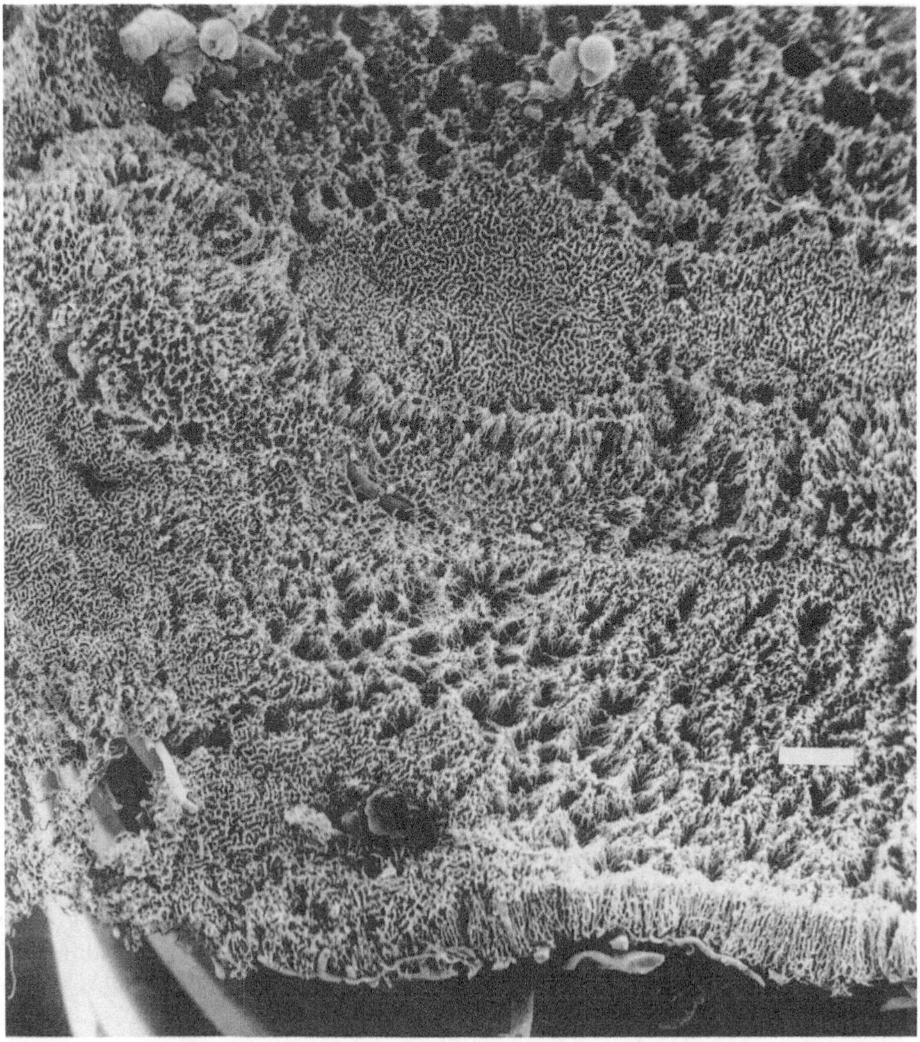

Fig. 1. An overview of the luminal aspect of a cast after EtOH damage. There is gross disturbance of the normal architecture with almost full thickness loss and visible submucosal vessels in the midzone. Calibration bar = 400 μ

Results

The normal microvascular architecture consists of capillaries which arise from the submucosal arterioles and pass upwards between the gastric glands towards the gastric lumen to form a network of linked capillaries around the neck of the glands immediately deep to the surface epithelium. These vessels then drain into infrequent venules which pass directly to the mucosa, without further tributaries to the submucosal veins [3]. This structure is best seen in Fig. 6 and 7. After FITC albumin, fluorescence microscopy of normal gastric mucosa shows the fluorescent label to be confined to the mucosal microvessels alone (Fig. 4).

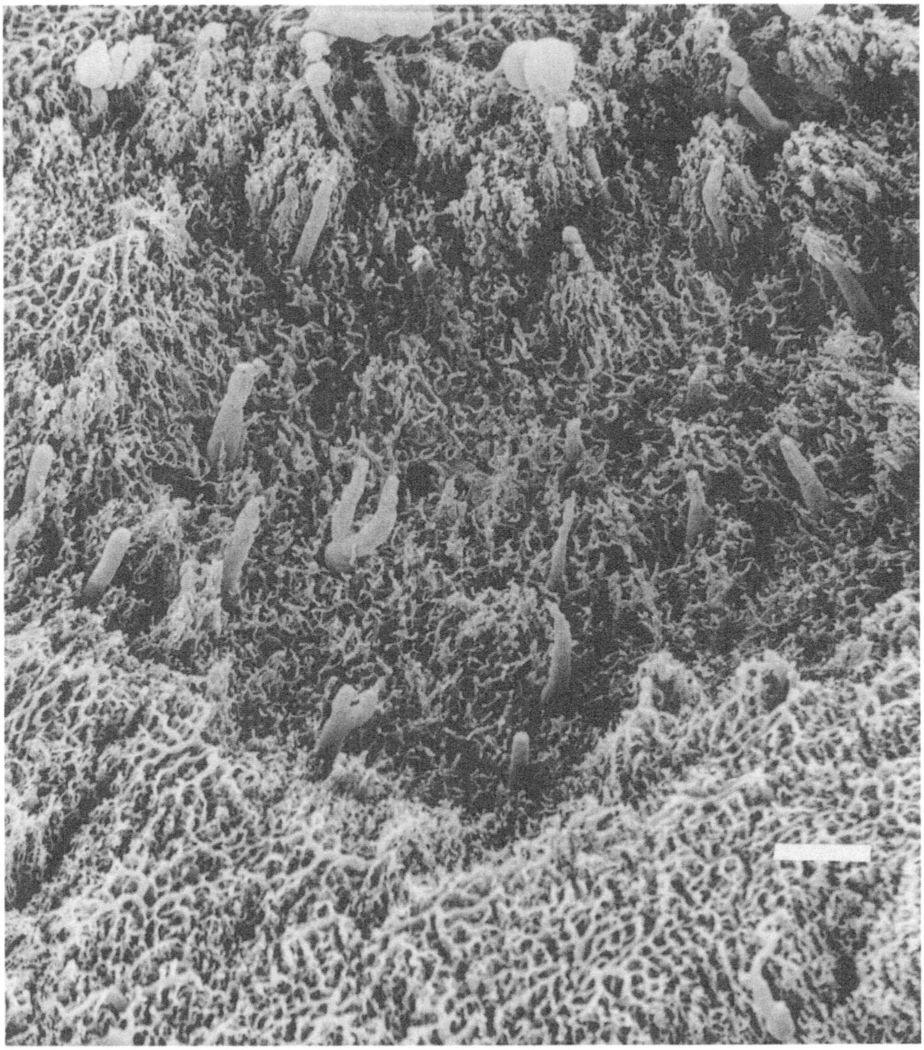

Fig. 2. A closer view of deep damage after EtOH exposure with complete loss of patency of the mucosal capillaries. Residual venules only are seen. Calibration bar = 250 μ

Ethanol Damage to the Microvasculature

EtOH damage to the microvasculature is characterized by the presence of areas in which the normal cast network of capillaries is absent, there is exudation of casting medium into the mucosal interstitium and onto the surface of the cast and increased interstitial fluorescence is seen throughout the thickness of the mucosa.

Figure 1 is an overview showing extensive damage to most areas of the cast, with absence of filling of capillaries and exudation of the casting medium. Closer examina-

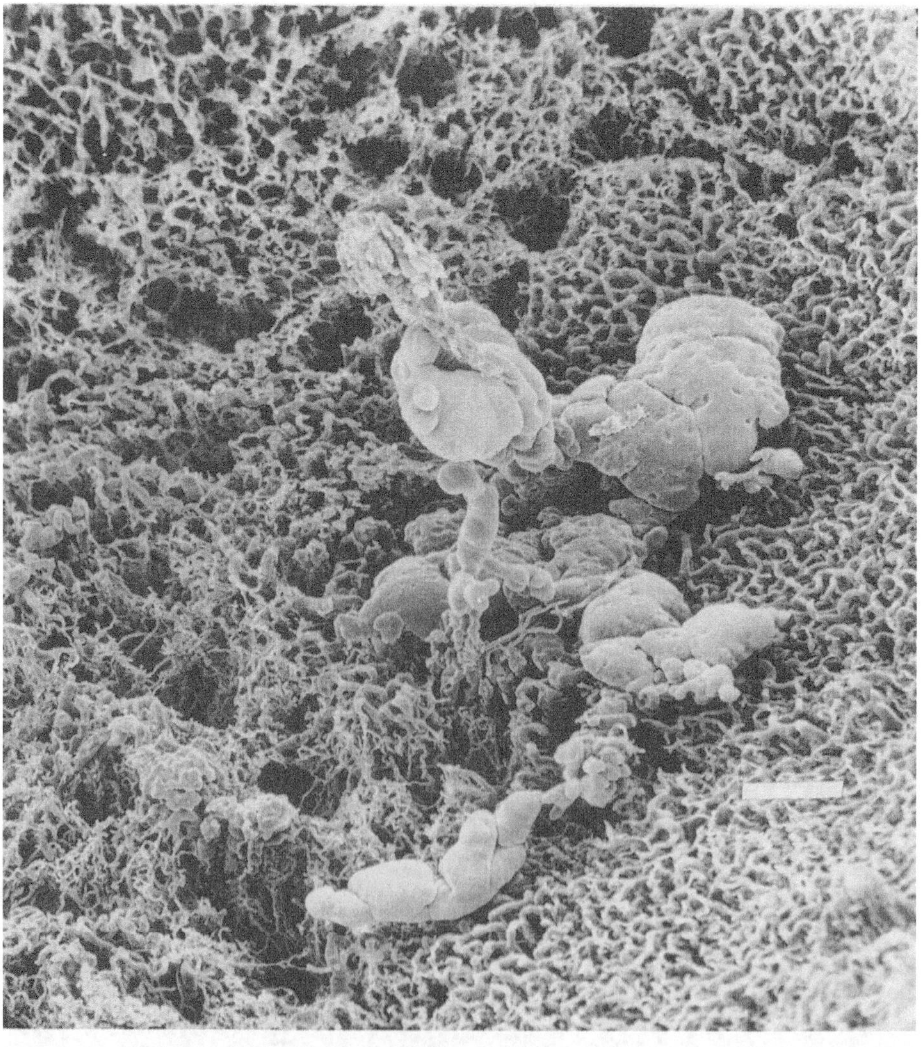

Fig. 3. EtOH damage. Exudates of casting medium onto the surface of the cast. Note the irregularity and pitting of the surface exudates suggesting the presence of an overlying intact epithelium at the time of casting. Calibration bar = 250 μ

tion of an area of "erosion" (Fig. 2) shows almost full thickness loss of the capillary network with residual filling of the venules, presumably by retrograde flow from adjacent submucosal vessels. The exudates onto the cast surface were characteristically large and multilobular with surface pitting (Fig. 3), and were frequently seen to be arising from within the cast. Intra-mucosal exudates were globular, encasing the capillaries down to the level of the submucosa (Fig. 4). Extensive leakage of FITC albumin occurred throughout the full thickness of the mucosa (Fig. 5).

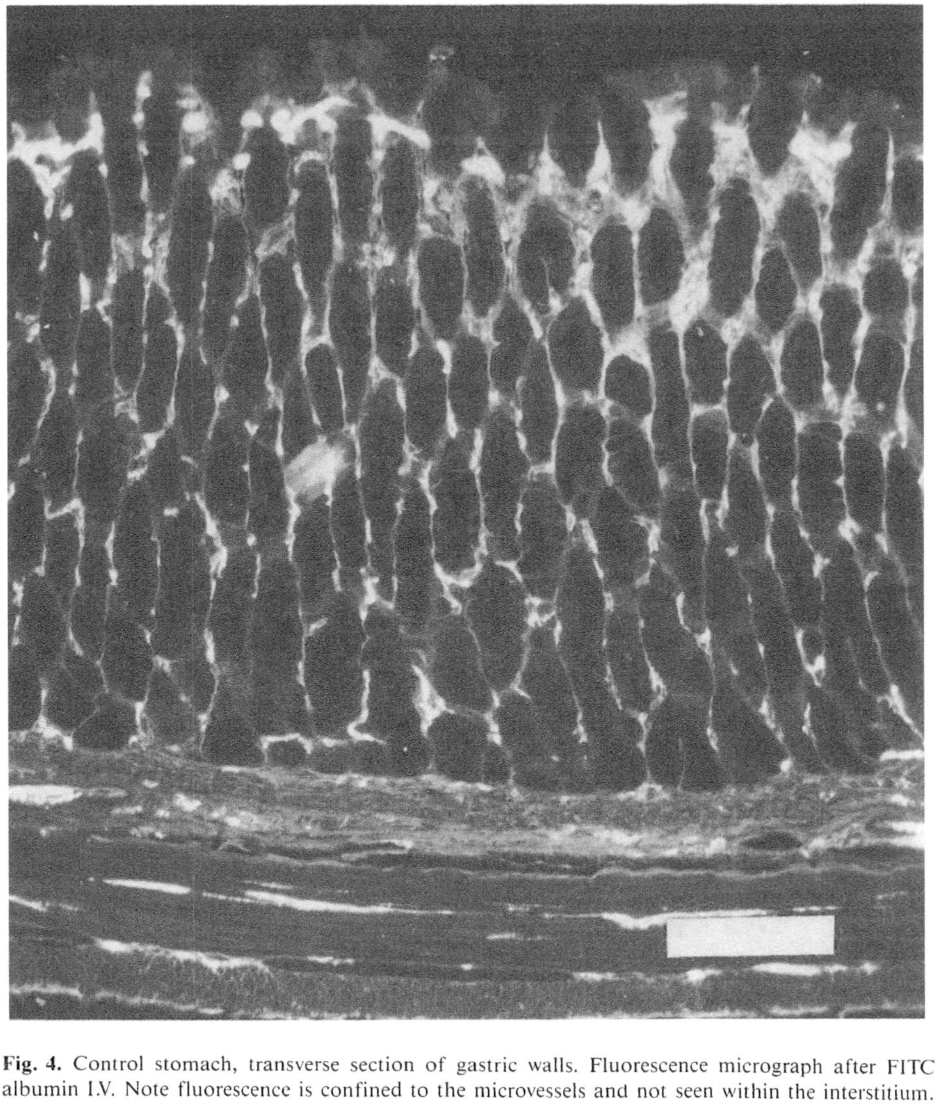

Fig. 4. Control stomach, transverse section of gastric walls. Fluorescence micrograph after FITC albumin I.V. Note fluorescence is confined to the microvessels and not seen within the interstitium. Calibration bar = 100 μ

The Effects of PGE_2 on EtOH Damage

The principal differences after pretreatment by PGE_2 are the virtual absence of areas of deep damage to the capillary network and the presence of small spherical surface exudates only. An overview of a microvascular cast after pretreatment by PGE_2

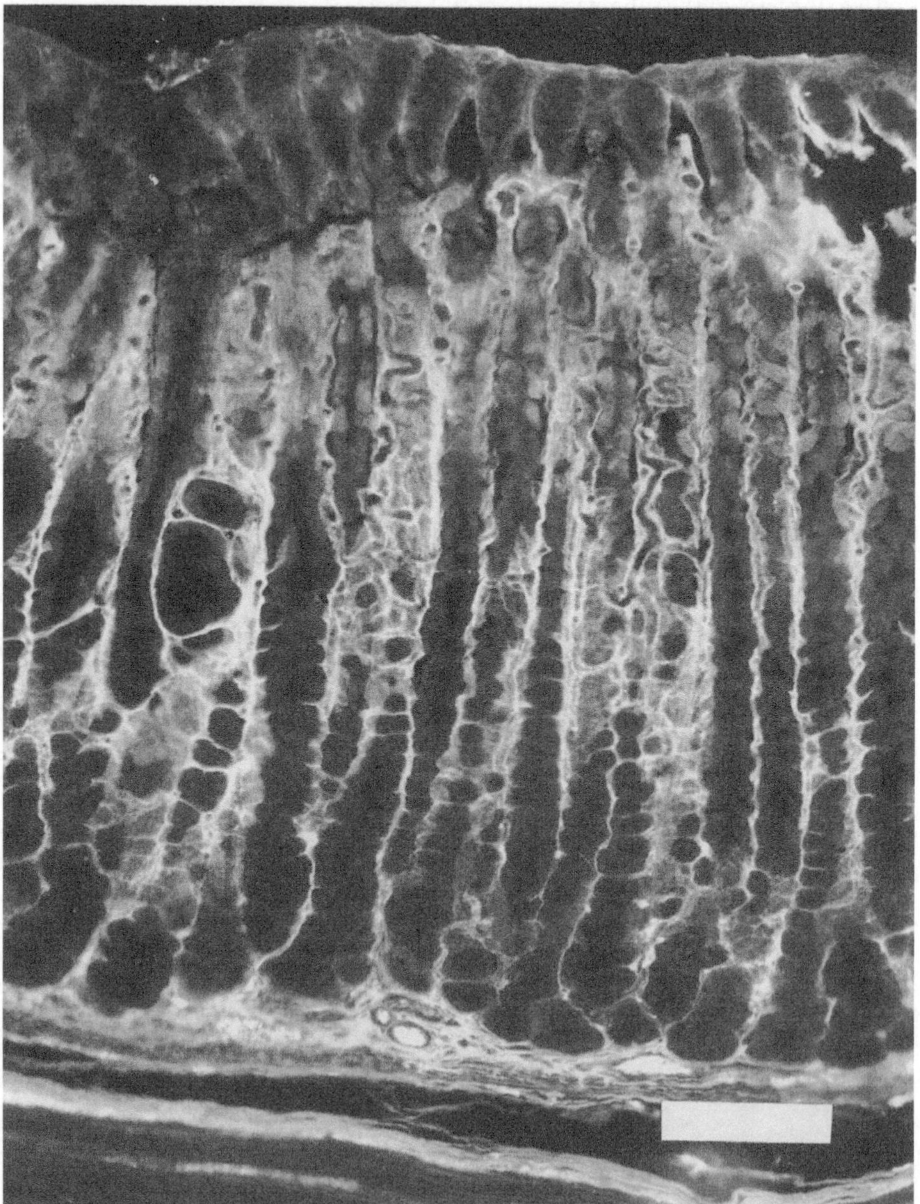

Fig. 5. EtOH damage. A fluorescence micrograph showing an area of intact epithelium with gross fluorescence of the interstitium extending deep to the submucosa. Calibration bar = 100 μ

followed by exposure to EtOH (Fig. 6) shows the relative uniformity of intact capillary networks. On lateral view (Fig. 7) the full thickness of the capillary network is seen to be preserved. Closer examination, however, shows some areas of incomplete casting of the most superficial capillary loops and exposure of the tips of the draining venules. Exudation of the casting material from the microvessels appeared to occur only at the surface of the cast and was of a characteristic smooth spherical shape, suggesting extravasation into the gastric lumen, rather than into the mucosa (Fig. 7). Leakage of FITC albumin into the interstitium was seen to occur only at the more superficial levels of the mucosa with virtually no areas of interstitial fluorescence deep in the mucosa (Fig. 8).

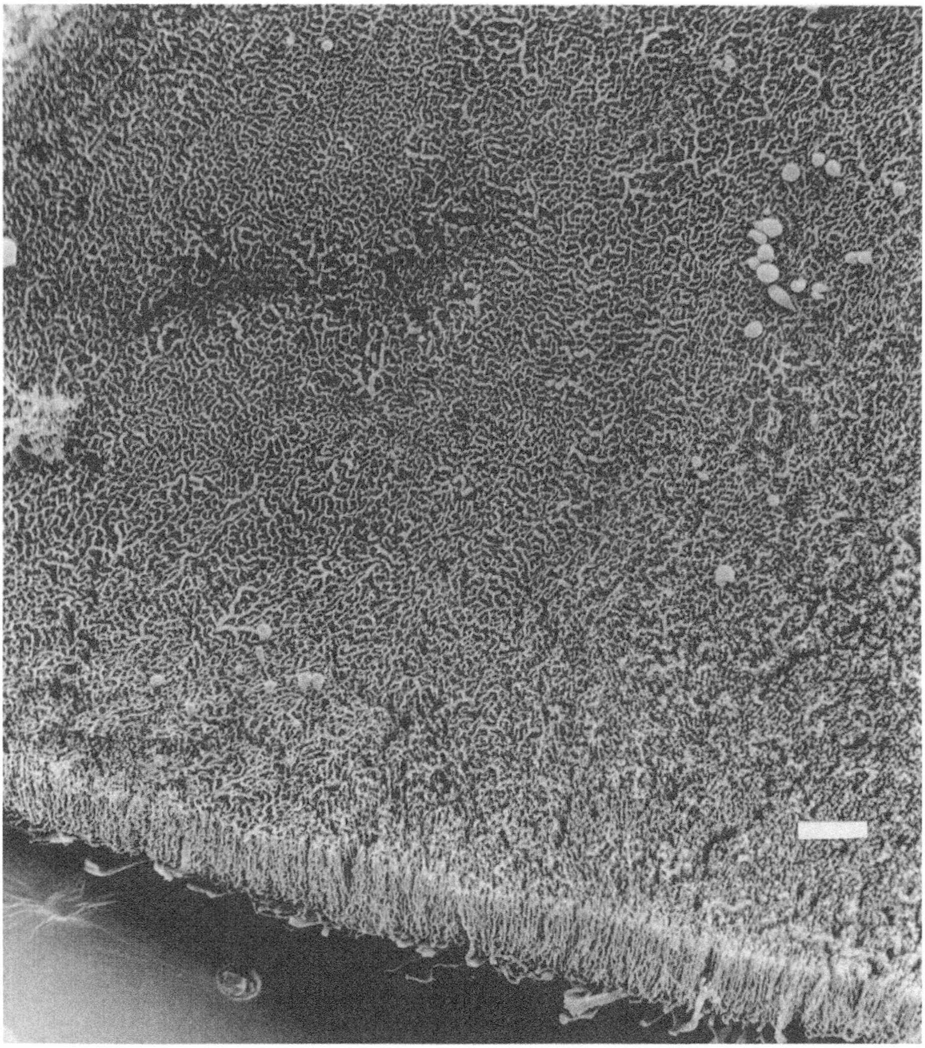

Fig. 6. PG-EtOH. This overview shows a generally intact cast. There are patch areas of incomplete filling of the most superficial capillary loops and some small spherical exudates. Calibration bar = 400 μ

Discussion

Microvascular casting techniques and fluorescence microscopy after FITC albumin reveal major damage to the microvasculature of the mucosa after exposure to EtOH (Fig. 9). These changes involve the full thickness of the microvasculature and from the appearance of pitting on the surface exudates of casting medium and the presence of interstitial fluorescence beneath an intact gastric epithelium indicates that damage to the microvessels has occurred prior to loss of epithelium. These findings suggest that EtOH damage to the gastric mucosa is initiated, at least in part, via the effects on the microcirculation of the stomach.

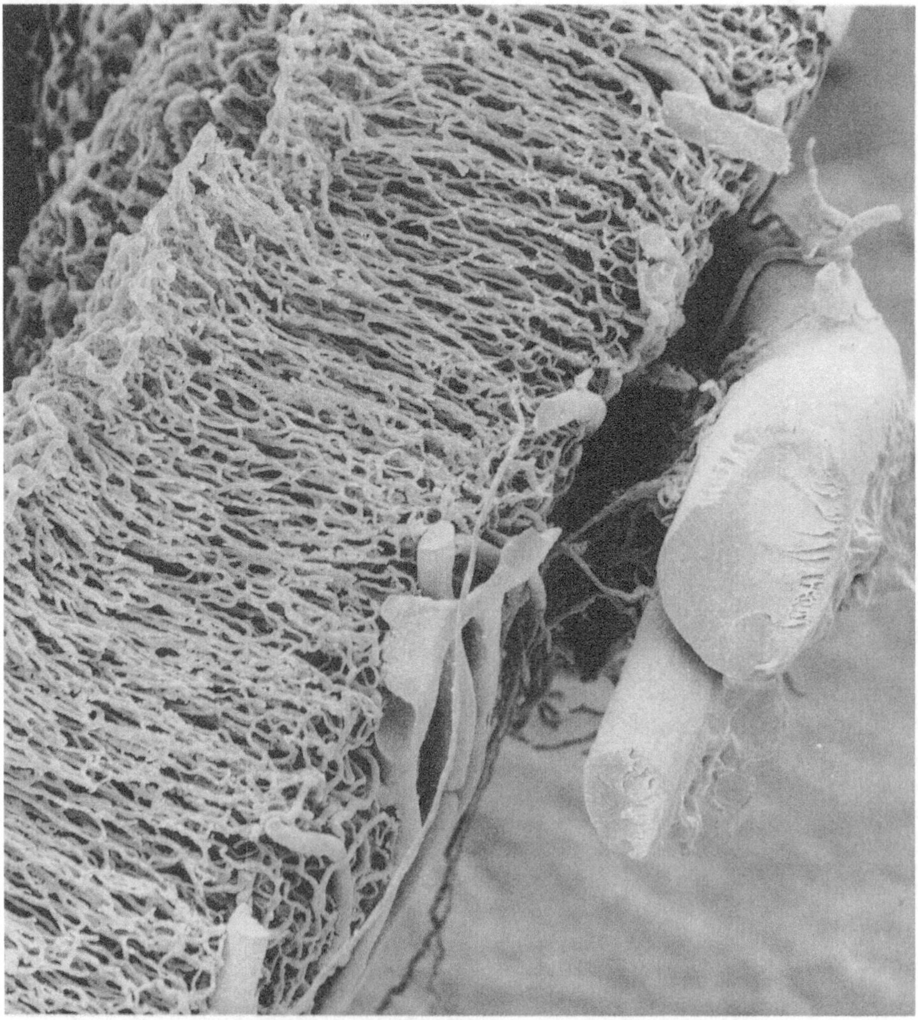

Fig. 7. PG-EtOH. View of the edge of a cast showing intact capillary network extending from the submucosa (right side of photo) to the lumen (left side of photo). Calibration bar = 100 μ

Pretreatment by PGE_2 has resulted in a clear protection of the microvasculature against EtOH damage. The damage is confined to the more superficial levels of the microvasculature and is less extensive. Intramucosal exudates which might be considered equivalent to the intramucosal haemorrhages, seen as red streaks on macroscopic examination, are common after EtOH alone. The virtual absence of intramucosal exudates in casts after pretreatment by PG correlates with the absence of red streaks on visual examination [1].

The absence of microvessels in the casts at the site of apparent damage may indicate loss of these vessels in association with adjacent tissue loss, closure of these vessels due to thrombosis, compression of the vessels by surrounding tissue or fluid, or constric-

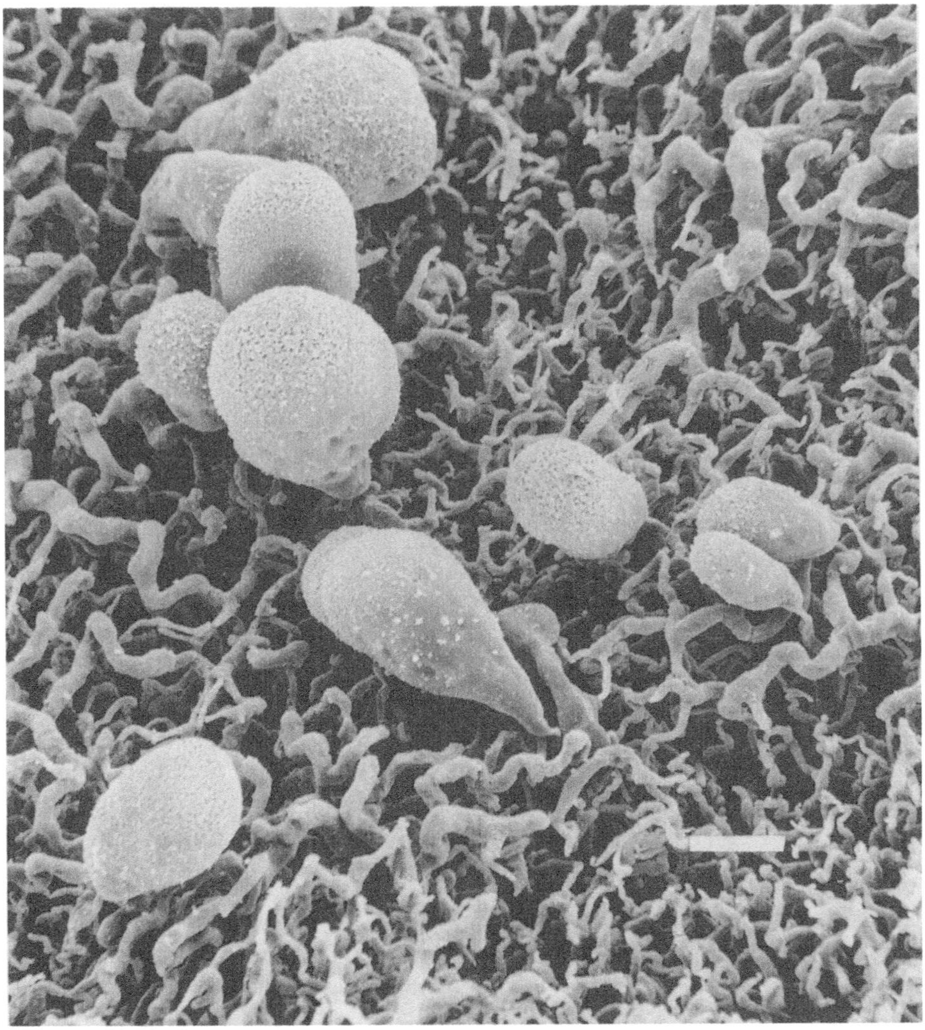

Fig. 8. PG-EtOH. A closer view of small exudates onto the surface of the cast. Note the smooth spherical shape and the apparent origin of the exudate from a surface capillary. Calibration bar = 50 μ

tion of the supplying vessels at the level of the submucosa with consequent failure of filling areas of the cast. By our current techniques we have not been able to identify the relative importance of these possible mechanisms. However, in the intact animal any of these changes would be associated with ischaemia of the adjacent areas of gastric mucosa and would thus be expected to reduce the capacity of this area of mucosa to tolerate exposure to an injurious agent.

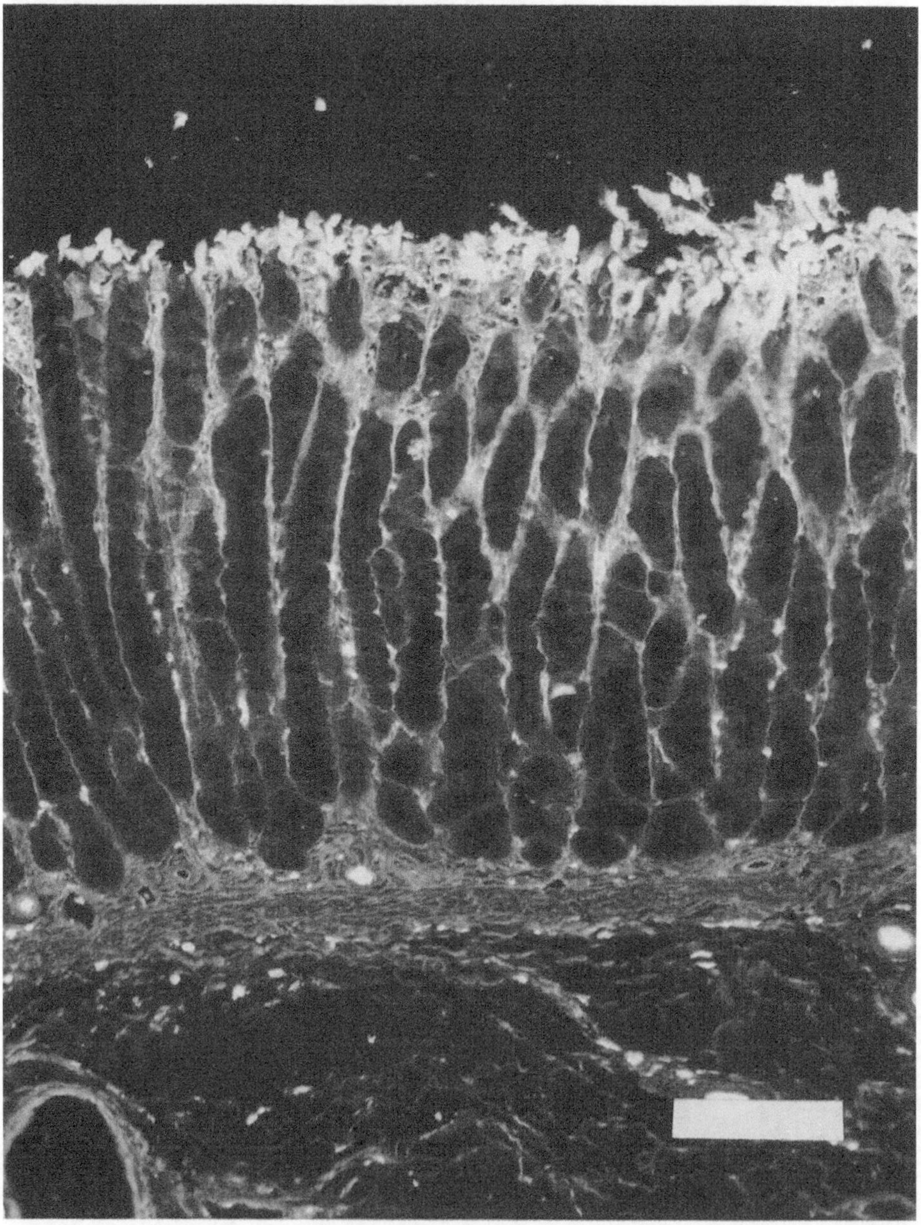

Fig. 9. PG-EtOH. A fluorescence micrograph after FITC albumin showing that fluorescence in the interstitium is confined to the most superficial layers of the mucosa only. Calibration bar = 100 μ

References

1. Robert A, Nezamis JE, Lancaster C, Hanchar AJ (1979) Cytoprotection by prostaglandins in rats: prevention of gastric necrosis produced by alcohol, HCL, NaOH, hypertonic NaCL, and thermal in jury. Gastroenterology 77: 433-443
2. Miller TA (1983) Protective effects of prostaglandins against gastric mucosal damage: Current knowledge and proposed mechanisms. Am J Physiol 245 (Gastrointest Liver Physiol. 8): G601-G623
3. Gannon BJ, Browning J, O'Brien P (1982) The microvascular achitecture of the glandular mucosa of the rat stomach. J Anat 135: 667-683

Non-steroidal Anti-inflammatory Drugs and Peptic Ulcer

M. J. S. LANGMAN

Introduction

Clinical suspicion, or prejudice, that non-steroidal anti-inflammatory drugs (NSAID) commonly cause dyspepsia and are liable to cause ulcer perforation and bleeding has been largely unsupported until recently, although NSAIDs have been marketed and widely used for over 20 years. That clinical opinion has been unsupported for so long, could arise for two reasons. Firstly, any claim of causal assocation could be false, and secondly, methodological difficulties could make it well-nigh impossible to demonstrate any association even if really present [1].

Peptic ulceration occurs in about 10% of men and 5% of women at some time in their lives. Therefore coincidental occurrence of ulceration with other diseases is to be expected. In these circumstances detecting association, which is more than coincidental, is difficult. Problems are compounded because associations between one disease and another may simply reflect a tendency to occur within the same social class or a common association with smoking. In addition, the patient with rheumatoid arthritis may be inherently liable to peptic ulceration. Methodological problems may also arise: thus Berkson's bias, which describes in essence the liability of individuals with one disease to have another detected more easily, makes the description of false association possible and likely.

Approaches to the problem can be by animal experimentation, by the quantification of noxious responses to treatment in healthy people or deseases individuals, and by epidemiological studies of disease occurence in association with NSAID treatment.

Animal Experiments

A very large number of experimental models of human peptic ulceration exists. Most involve measuring the number and size of ulcers or erosions induced by procedures such as cold stress or restraint, and their relevance to ordinary chronic human peptic ulcers is doubtful. Such models may serve well in screening for ulcer treatment, but even then their value in examining the virtues, or otherwise, of unconventional treatments is unclear. They may have no relevance as models of natural ulcer disease in man and therefore the ability or lack of ability to demonstrate NSAID – associated ulcers in experimental animals may be quite unimportant.

Human Experiments

Short-term exposure to NSAIDs can be followed by the occurence of submucosal haemorrhages or gastric erosions. Extrapolation to the conclusion that drugs which cause intragastric haemorrhage are those which can cause classical peptic ulcers or complications may be correct, but must be justified by more direct evidence. The use of young healthy individuals in experimental studies may lead to unwarranted conclusions about the liability or resistance of older people to peptic ulceration.

Studies in Deseased Individuals

Theoretically it should be easy to plan a programme in which elderly people who are prescribed NSAIDs have changes in ulcer frequency measured. However, it is almost impossible to study people requiring treatment before their first NSAID exposure. Even if such studies were possible, the size demanded would probably be prohibitive. Thus, although peptic ulceration might indeed occur at some time in their lives, in 10% of men the incidence rate over a defined period of say one month would be vanishingly small. Therefore a doubling or quadrupling of expectation, though important, would be quite undetectable in a group of 50 or 100 people.

If intensive investigation is impracticable, then surveillance of the outcome in a large sample of takers of NSAIDs might provide an acceptable alternative. However, it has to be remembered that takers are not a random, sample of the ordinary population and that base ulcer frequency rate calculations may be difficult. Conventionally, comparisons are made between periods "on" and "off" drug, but these are based upon untested assumptions about the likely duration of drug effects and on the fact that events occuring "off" treatment will be reported as assiduously as those occurring "on" treatment.

Retrospective Epidemiological Investigations

Provided a working hypothesis exists, it is possible to devise a retrospective study in which the antecedent experience of disease subjects and of controls is compared. The value of such comparisons will depend on a number of factors and these include the extent to which any control group can be regarded as the same as the ordinary population, and the extent to which the selected disease group is representative of the totality of the disease group. Assuming that both samples are representative, their responses will only be generalizable to the world at large if information about antecedent factors is uniformly and accurately collected. Thus the occurrence of disease may in itself influence responses to questioning and invalidate the information obtained. Retrospective epidemiological studies may nevertheless be the best means and even the only means of determining what happens in the ordinary world. We have therefore used classical case-control studies to try and determine whether NSAID treatment is associated with serious gastrointestinal hazards.

Methods

Case-control studies must be based upon comparisons which allow generalizable conclusions and this means that data collected in cases can be regarded as likely to be obtainable from the general run of patients with similar problems in the community. Likewise, the control groups chosen must be likely to be representative of the population at large. We therefore attempted to collect data from a coherent group of ulcer patients, all those with gastric or duodenal ulcer aged 60 or over, who exhibited haematemesis or melaena [2] within the study period. Where patients could not be questioned directly, we obtained information by consulting hospital or practitioner records. Two control groups were collected, one consisting of patients admitted on the same medical intake as the cases but suffering from conditions other than gastrointestinal bleeding, and the other was obtained from the ordinary population by taking the next individual matched for age and sex off the alphabetically ordered file of the general practitioner responsible for the index individual. Since all people register for medical care with a general medical practitioner, this gave us a general population sample to compare with our sick medical emergency control.

Questioning was of necessity unblinded as to whether cases or controls were under consideration and therefore bias cannot be excluded. We sought to minimize this by using standard questionnaires and methods of interrogation.

Since the two Nottingham hospitals are the only district general hospitals available to serve the local population, provided adequate numbers of patients and controls responded and the controls were appropriately chosen the answers obtained should have measured any real differences or lack of differences.

Results

Table 1 shows details of the patients and controls considered and questioned. During a two-year period 903 patients were admitted to the two Nottingham hospitals with haematemesis and melaena, of whom 406 had gastric or duodenal ulcers, and 290 were aged 60 and over. 230 of these were questioned. Cases were between two and four times as likely to be takers of NSAIDs, other than aspirin, as controls, but parallel differences were not noted for other drugs (Table 2). Histories of NSAID intake obtained by note review in the 60 patients with bleeding, whom we were unable to question, yielded no material differences from the data obtained in those who were questioned. Although 95% confidence limits varied quite widely, they did not overlap, and the bottom end of the scale indicated that takers of NSAID were at least twice as likely to suffer from upper gastrointestinal bleeding as non-takers and could have been up to six times as likely.

Similar differences were not seen for other varieties of drugs, though as might be expected, the inpatient controls tended to be more frequent takers of cardiovascular drugs and diuretics. Increases in risk of ulcer in assocation with NSAID intake seemed to vary little in men and women, and for gastric and diodenal ulcer, though confidence limits tended to be widely due to the small numbers in individual subgroups.

Table 1. Details of cases and controls questioned

CASES			
All haematemesis and melaena		903	
Diagnosed ulcer, gastric or duodenal		406	
	60 yrs and over		Under 60
	290		116
	Questioned	Not questioned	
	230	60	
CONTROLS			
	In-patients	Community	
	230	230	
Questioned	230	207	

Table 2. Drug use amongst cases and controls

	Cases with bleeding Questioned	(Not questioned)	In-patient Controls	Population Controls
No	230	(60)	230	207
NSAID	80	(20)	33	34
users %	35	(33)	14	16
Matched rel risk	(for those questioned compared with cases)		3.8	2.7
95% confidence limits			2.2–6.4	1.7–4.4
% using				
All drugs regularly	86		84	75
Diuretics	32		44	22
CVS drugs	23		39	26

Generalizability of the Data

The Nottingham hospitals serve a population of some 800,000 and there is no other substantial institution serving the same people. National figures suggest that some 24 million prescriptions are issued annually for NSAIDs half to individuals aged less than 60. If prescribing rates in Nottingham generally parallel those in the country as a whole, then we would expect some 300,000 prescriptions to be issued each year or about 600,000 during the period of study, half to older and half to younger people. In the elderly these 300,000 prescriptions were associated with 100 episodes of bleeding – not all caused – or one for every 3,000. Calculations of attributable risk by standard methods would indicate that about 20 to 25% of all ulcer bleeding is in fact caused by treatment and, generalized to the United Kingdom, the figures would be about 2,000 cases a year.

Indications that these conclusions and calculations do not over estimate include the common association of NSAID intake with ulcer bleeding and perforation in other case series, with suggestions using hospital controls only, that low proportions of people are ordinarily found to be takers [3–6].

Whether NSAID intake leads to bleeding or perforation of established lesions or to the development of new ulcers, is unclear. However, clinical endoscopic studies suggest that treatment is associated with the development of new lesions [7] and case control study in an endoscopy unit including the elderly is in conformity with this view [8, 9]. The failure of surveillance studies in the United Kingdom [10] to detect a risk may be attributable to two causes. Firstly, the size of patient samples, approximately 5,000 to 10,000, has been rather too small. At first sight this is surprising but it is the very magnitude of prescribing of NSAID which has brought the clinical problem to attention. Secondly, the risk may be concentrated in the elderly where as surveillance has been, very properly, conducted in individuals of all ages.

Whether the same phenomenon is detectable elsewhere, is unclear. Case control study in Australia [9] suggests a risk for gastric but not duodenal ulcer, although the rather younger population could conceivably explain the difference. In the United States a general parallelism between national cigarette consumption and ulcer mortality has suggested a dominant role for smoking [11] and surveillance studies comparing periods "on" and "off" NSAIDs have indicated no material risk[12]. However, interpretation could be affected by the lengths of periods defined as "on" or "off".

At least, so far as the United Kingdom is concerned, the data suggest a risk for elderly women, probably the elderly in general, of bleeding, perforated, and probably all ulcer diseases, whether gastric or duodenal. Evidence that NSAIDs inhibit prostaglandin E_2 release in the stomach and duodenum, thus reducing the effect of a potential protective mechanism, supplies a rational basis [13]. If this is true, then the prostaglandins should provide natural protective agents, although it should be noted that protection in the absence of single acid inhibition has yet to be demonstrated unequivocally.

References

1. Kurata JH, Elashoff JD, Grossman MI (1982) Inadequacy of the literature on the relationship between drugs, ulcers and gastrointestinal bleeding. Gastroenterology 82: 273–286
2. Somerville K, Faulkner G, Langman MJS (1986) Non-steroidal anti-inflammatory drugs and bleeding peptic ulcer. Lancet i, 462–4
3. Collier D St J, Pain JA (1985) Non-steroidal anti-inflammatory drugs and peptic ulcer perforation. Gut 26: 359–63
4. O'Brien JD, Burnham WR (1985) Bleeding from peptic ulcers and use of non-steroidal anti-inflammatory drugs in the Romford area. Br Med J 291: 1609–10
5. Armstrong CP, Blower AL (1986) Peptic ulcer complications and non-steroidal anti-inflammatory drugs. Gut 27: A609

6. Emmanuel JH, Montgomery RD (1971) Gastric ulcer and anti-arthritic drugs. Post grad Med J 47: 227–232
7. Caruso D, Porro GB (1980) Gastroscopic evaluation of anti-inflammatory drugs. Br Med J 1: 75–8
8. Clinch D, Banerjee AK, Ostick G, Levy DW (1983) Non steroidal anti-inflammatory drugs and gastro-intestinal adverse effects. JR Coll Physicians, Lond. 17: 228–230
9. Duggan JM, Dobson AJ, Johnson H, Fahey P (1986) Peptic ulcer and non steroidal anti-inflammatory agents. Gut 27: 929–933
10. Inman WHW (1984) Non-steroidal anti-inflammatory drugs. PEM News 2: 4–10
11. Kurata JH, Elashoff JD, Nogawa AN, Haile BM Sex and smoking differences in duodenal ulcer mortality. Amer J Publ Health, 76, 700–702
12. Jick H, Feld AD, Perera DR (1985) Certain non-steroidal anti-inflammatory drugs and hospitalization for upper gastrointestinal bleeding. Pharmacotherapy 289–294
13. Aly A, Selling JA, Hogan DL, Isenberg JI, Koss MA, Johansson C (1985) Gastric and duodenal prostaglandin E_2 (PGE_2) in humans: effect of luminal acidification (H^+) and indomethacin (I). Gastroenterology 88: A1305

Discussion Following the Report of Prof. Langman

GRAHAM

Could you give an estimate of how many of a thousand patients regularly taking NSAIDs including aspirin will bleed per year?

LANGMAN

I have not done the calculation on people over 60 years old for aspirin, but I can give you an estimation for the other nonsteroidals. In broad terms the rate in patients over 60 is about one in 3000 prescriptions. For those under 60 it may be in the order of one in 20000–30000 prescriptions. Thus, the bleeding incidence of NSAID users seems to be much higher in the elderly.

PESKAR

It has been suggested recently that the newer nonsteroidal anti-inflammatory drugs cause more intestinal lesions than the older ones due to extensive enterohepatic recirculation. Does your personal experience support this hypothesis?

LANGMAN

We have performed one study, in which we tried to get a more precise insight into the incidence of NSAID-induced bleeding admitted to the surgeons. In this investigation we looked at all cases of colonic and small-intestinal bleeding and perforation. In our investigation we entered all patients with these bowel emergencies except those who presented with ulcerative colitis, Crohn's disease, or cancer. There was about a two-fold increase in risk for nonsteroidal intake. It was not possible to separate the varieties of different NSAIDs.

WALAN

I wonder whether mortality is similar in patients who bled during NSAID intake in comparison to non-NSAID users with complications due to peptic ulcer?

LANGMAN

We are doing logistic analysis of the last 2500 cases of bleeding, where we have reasonable documentation of who was taking nonstero idals and who was not. There is no evidence from the data that nonsteroidals were particularly associated with death.

WEIHRAUCH

Could you make a comment on one of your papers in which you differentiated between the heavy ASA users which, so far as I can recall, were defined as those who took a certain amount of ASA grams at least 4 times a week and the occasional users on self-medication? The rate of complications depends very much on the ASA formulation. The Levy study showed us that there was not one single bleeding in 630 patients with gastrointestinal problems.

LANGMAN

The Boston collaborative study published by Levy in the New England Journal in 1974 suggested that there is no significant risk with occasional use, but that the risk doubles with continued use. Our data suggest that there is, in fact, a risk associated both with occasional and with continued use. It is difficult to explain the difference in the outcome of the two studies. One possible explanation may be that it is quite a complex question to work out to what extent ASA intake causes GI lesions or to what extent ASA is taken by patients with preexisting lesions. It is well known in England that aspirin is commonly taken to relieve the pain of dyspepsia despite information on the packets against doing so.

Mechanism of Injury to Gastric Mucosa by Non-Steroidal Anti-Inflammatory Drugs and the Protective Role of Prostaglandins

M. M. COHEN

Introduction

Non-steroidal anti-inflammatory drugs (NSAIDs) cause gastric mucosal injury primarily by interfering with the fundamental defensive properties of the mucosa and its underlying blood supply. They do not cause damage by increasing luminal acid or pepsin: indeed, the effect of NSAIDs on active transport is to reduce secretion. This inhibition of secretory activity may be harmful.

The gastric mucosa possesses an array of defensive mechanisms and NSAIDs have a deleterious effect on most of them. This results in a mucosa less able to cope with even a reduced acid load. The presence of acid appears to be a *sine qua non* for NSAIDs injury. Acid not only injures the mucosa by back diffusing from the lumen to cause tissue acidosis but also serves to increase drug absorption.

All of the NSAIDs are capable of causing mucosal damage but most of the experimental work has been done using salicylates. This brief review will therefore depend heavily on the data derived from work with salicylates.

Passive Ion Transport

The gastric mucosa permits the passive movement of hydrogen ion from lumen into mucosa. This is referred to as "back-diffusion" and considering the concentration gradient across the apical membrane of the surface epithelial cells, it is clear that in health the mucosa is not particularly permeable. This "barrier" to acid permeation of the mucosa can be readily damaged by the topical application of NSAIDs and especially by aspirin. However, an increase in permeability does not inevitably result in visible damage. This depends on the absolute amount of H^+ entering the mucosa and the ability of the mucosa to buffer it. It is of considerable interest that, whereas luminal salicylate in the presence of a moderate amount of acid (pH 3.5) causes both increased permeability and visible erosions, intravenous salicylate (at the same luminal pH) causes neither increased acid diffusion nor visible damage. However, at a luminal pH of 1.0 erosions appear even without any change in intramural pH [1].

The chemical structure of most NSAIDs displays an exposed carboxyl group and this is the likely cause of the increased permeability with luminal application or indeed oral ingestion (the usual route for NSAID therapy) [2]. As the undissociated molecule is absorbed more readily (depending upon its actual pKa), the greater the concentration of luminal acid, the greater will be the drug absorption and the more acid will diffuse into the mucosa as a result.

Active Ion Transport

In addition to their effects on permeability, the salicylates also inhibit oxidative phosphorylation. This results in a reduction of acid secretion. This apparent benefit is probably more than countered by the increased susceptibility to injury of a mucosa in which active transport is inhibited [3]. This may be due in part to reduced active bicarbonate secretion and thus a lessened buffering capacity. This is a clinically important concept as it suggests that a drug which inhibits acid secretion (eg.H_2-receptor antagonist) may not be the most appropriate prophylaxis or treatment of drug or stress-induced gastric injury.

Salicylate also inhibits active Cl^- transport. While exchange of Cl^- and HCO_3^- may be important in buffering H^+ diffusing into cells, the relative importance of chloride transport is not yet fully understood. Salicylate undoubtedly has other effects on active transport by the gastric mucosa which may be potentially damaging. It is also evident that the metabolic effects of salicylate, including inhibition of cyclooxygenase, are not alone sufficient to cause mucosal erosions.

Blood Flow

Recent experiments using the technique of hydrogen gas clearance have demonstrated that luminal aspirin causes a marked redistribution of mucosa blood flow. There is reduction in flow at the site of erosions and an augmentation of flow elsewhere, with an overall increase in total gastric blood flow [4]. This probably explains the previous failure to demonstrate mucosa ischemia in response to NSAIDs.

Both ethanol and NSAIDs cause intense focal constriction of submucosal venules. This may be mediated by products of the arachidonic acid cascade e.g. thromboxane. Indeed, the endogenous phospholipid platelet activating factor (PAF) has been shown to be an extremely potent damaging agent and this is probably due to intense venular constriction and capillary stasis [5]. It is not known whether NSAIDs can cause this local release of PAF.

The ability of the mucosal blood flow to provide bicarbonate, and to buffer and sweep away acid that has diffused into the mucosa, may be just as important as blood supply *per se*. Tissue bicarbonate availability is reduced by the administration NSAIDs.

Mucus

Adherent mucus gel provides a stable unstirred layer within which bicarbonate, secreted into the lumen, gets trapped. This mucus-bicarbonate barrier may slow the absorption of NSAIDs by increasing the concentration of the dissociated form of the molecule. The mucus itself is readily permeated by NSAIDs which have no major effect on the thickness of the mucus gel layer. Although there is absence of adherent mucus at the site of focal lesions, this cannot be attributed to an effect of the NSAID on mucus.

Nonetheless, NSAIDs do inhibit mucus secretion and aspirin reduces the pH gradient across the mucus layer [6]. It is not clear whether this latter effect is due to a reduced amount of mucus, an alteration in mucus structure, or due indirectly to mucosal damage. Any damaging agent, including NSAIDs, will increase the amount of soluble mucus present in the lumen probably by a process of washout of surface glycoprotein by the mucosal exudate [7].

Cellular Restitution

This is the process of rapid migration of viable surface epithelial cells to reepithelialize denuded areas of the gastric mucosa [8]. This restitution occurs within minutes of injury (presumably any injury, although it has been most studied in response to ethanol and aspirin) and is independent of cell division and regeneration, or the process of wound contraction. The factors which control cellular restitution are unknown. This process is capable of re-epithelializing only superficial damage. Repair of deep injury requires cell proliferation and takes several days.

While NSAIDs usually cause the kind of damage that can be readily repaired by cellular restitution, it is not known if the administration of NSAIDs or inhibition of cyclooxygenase can actually interfere with the ability of the mucosa to resurface itself in this remarkable manner.

Role of Prostaglandins

NSAIDs cause gastric mucosal injury and generally inhibit cyclooxygenase. It has been widely assumed that mucosal damage must be the result of inhibition of prostaglandin synthesis. There are, however, major problems with this theory.

For example, sodium salicylate which does not inhibit the cyclooxygenase system causes the same changes in ionic permeability and mucosa erosions as does aspirin [9]. The converse is also true. Complete inhibition of prostaglandin synthesis by aspirin does not cause mucosal lesions in either experimental animals or man unless the aspirin is given topically or the luminal pH is very low. It is likely that NSAID-induced inhibition of prostaglandin synthesis does not cause damage *per se* but produces a mucosa more susceptible to injury by acid, and agents such as bile salts or ethanol.

This raises the question of whether the endogeneous prostaglandins play any role in normal mucosa defense. While this is an attractive hypothesis, it remains unproven. Prostaglandins have been shown to have profound effects on the various defensive functions of the gastric mucosa. Thus, prostaglandins are capable of stimulating bicarbonate and mucus secretion, of augmenting mucosa blood flow, and preventing microvascular stasis [10]. Prostaglandins do not reduce the normal permeability of undamaged mucosa and have no major effect on the process of cellular restitution.

The experimental evidence with exogenous prostaglandins show convincingly that several prostanoids have a remarkable ability to protect the mucosa from acute injury by a variety of agents [11]. This protection is not complete. The surface cells cannot be totally preserved and there is always some microscopic damage. While it is clear that this protection of the deeper layer of the mucosa is independent of acid inhibition, its precise mechanism remains unclear. Until the mechanism of prostaglandin protection is fully understood, it will be difficult, if not impossible, to assess the protective function of endogenous mucosal prostaglandins [12].

Finally, the fact that NSAIDs and prostaglandins have opposite effects on many mucosal defensive functions makes it logical to test the efficacy of prostaglandins in the prevention and treatment of NSAID injury.

References

1. Fromm D, Kolis M (1982) Effects of sodium salicylate and acetylsalicylic acid on intramural pH and ulceration of rabbit antral mucosa. Surgery 91: 438-447
2. Rainsford KD (1978) Structure-activity relationship of non-steroidal anti-inflammatory drugs. I. Gastric ulcerogenic activity. Agents Actions 8: 587-605
3. Kivilaakso E, Fromm D, Silen W (1978) Effect of the acid secretory state on intramural pH of rabbit gastric mucosal. Gastroenterology 75: 641-648
4. Ashley SW, Sonnenschein LA, Cheung LY (1985) Focal gastric mucosa blood flow at the site of aspirin-induced ulceration. Amer J Surg 149: 53-59
5. Rosam A-C, Wallace JL, Whittle BJR (1986) Potent ulcerogenic actions of platelet-activating factor on the stomach. Nature 319: 54-56
6. Turner NC, Martin GP, Marriott C (1985) The influence of native procine gastric mucus gel on hydrogen ion diffusion: the effect of potentially ulcerogenic agents. J Pharm Pharmacol 37: 776-780
7. McQueen S, Hutton D, Allen A, Garner A (1983) Gastric and duodenal surface mucus gel thickness in rat: effects of prostaglandins and damaging agents. Amer J Physiol 245: G388-G393
8. Morris GP, Wallace JL (1981) The roles of ethanol and of acid in the production of gastric mucosal erosions in rats. Virchow's Arch 38: 23-38
9. Ligumsky M, Grossman MI, Kauffman GL Jr (1982) Endogenous gastric mucosa prostaglandins: their role in mucosal integrity. Amer J Physiol 242: G337-G341
10. Leung FW, Robert A, Guth PH (1985) Gastric mucosal blood flow in rats after administration of 16,16-dimethyl prostaglandin E_2 at a cytoprotective dose. Gastroenterology 88: 1948-1953
11. Cohen MM, McCready DR, Clark L, Sevelius H (1985) Protection against aspirin-induced antral and duodenal damage with enprostil: a double-blind endoscopic study. Gastroenterology 88: 382-286
12. Cohen MM (1987) Role of endogenous prostaglandins in gastric secretion and mucosa defense. Clin Invest Med 10: 226-231

Discussion Following the Report of Prof. Cohen

LANGMAN

Can you justify the statement that damage is not related to cyclooxygenase inhibition, because clinically it looks to me as though it actually fits very well with that hypothesis? And, secondly, I am not aware of any evidence that damage associated with tiaprofenic acid is actually any different from that with indomethacin.

COHEN

The evidence that ulceration is not due to inhibition of cyclo-oxygenase per se is that aspirin can completely block cyclo-oxygenase. However, aspirin administered by mouth leads to gastric mucosal injury. If you give the same amount of aspirin rectally, it produces the same degree of cyclo-oxygenase inhibition in the gastric mucosa and the same blood levels of salycilate and acetylsalicylic acid as by the oral route, and yet causes no gastric mucosa damage whatsoever.

LANGMAN

And with indomethacin and piroxicam and the like?

COHEN

I have not looked at their effects when given by other than the oral route.

LOHANSSEN

Do you really think that the different grades of damage caused by either rectal or oral application of a drug indicate different ways of action? Indomethacin gastric-mucosal concentration will be much lower after rectal versus oral administration. Measurements of prostaglandin biosynthesis in vitro may not represent in vivo conditions due to artificial stimulation and influence from media cofactors, etc. How did you take and treat your biopsies?

COHEN

I do not regard my conclusion as being really all that strong. What I am saying is that you can block cyclooxygenase, and that by itself this does not cause damage. What I am suggesting is that blocking cyclooxygenase is potentially damaging to the mucosa, and there is no doubt in my mind that a mucosa in which the cyclo-oxygenase activity is blocked is a mucosa at risk, and which is susceptible. I agree that you observe lower concentrations in the mucosa for prolonged rectal administration, and that therefore there is less local injury.

JOHANSSEN

You pointed out that ulcerations develop in the prostaglandin-depleted stomach only in the presence of acid. By analogy bile acids may have to be present to produce lesions in the prostaglandin-depleted small intestine, and the presence of colonic bacteria is required for colonic damage by NSAID. In all these situations you need an aggressor in addition to a completely blocked defense mechanism. I believe we agree that cyclo-oxygenase blockers pose a high risk to the mucosa by inhibiting defense mechanisms.

Can Nonantisecretory Doses of Prostaglandins Prevent Mucosal Damage in Nonsteroidal Anti-inflammatory Drugs?

B. SIMON, H. G. DAMANN, and P. MÜLLER

Introduction

Orally effective prostaglandin analogues have been used in the treatment of peptic ulcers for a relatively short time [2]. Through an interaction with the histamine-stimulating adenosine monophosphate formation they inhibit the acid secretion process and speed up the healing of duodenal and gastric ulcers in antisecretory doses. In a direct comparison with H_2-blockers an almost similar effect can be observed.

The prostaglandins, however, are attractive to the gastroenterologist for another reason: in animal experiments it has been shown that they protect the gastric and duodenal mucosal epithelium against a number of chemical and physical oxious agents [28]. This protective effect is inherent to all prostaglandins. It can be found in a concentration which is clearly below that required for acid inhibition. We therefore had great hopes that the human gastric and duodenal mucosal epithelium could be completely protected, for example against nonsteroidal antirheumatic drugs, and in doses which are so low that they have practically no side effects.

Methods

The proof that prostaglandins have a mucosal protective effect is more difficult to achieve in man than in animals. The following methods have been more or less successful:

1. Measuring the transmucosal gastric potential difference
2. Measuring the fecal blood loss
3. Determining the gastric microbleeding rate (Hb content) in the gastric juice
4. The analysis of the gastric epithelial cell desquamation (DNA content) in the gastric juice
5. The endoscopic evaluation of gastric and duodenal mucosa

Measuring the Transmucosal Gastric Potential Difference

Certain mucosal irritants, like aspirin, ethanol, etc., cause a drop in the transmucosal potential difference (PD) of the gastric mucosal. Under certain circumstances this elec-

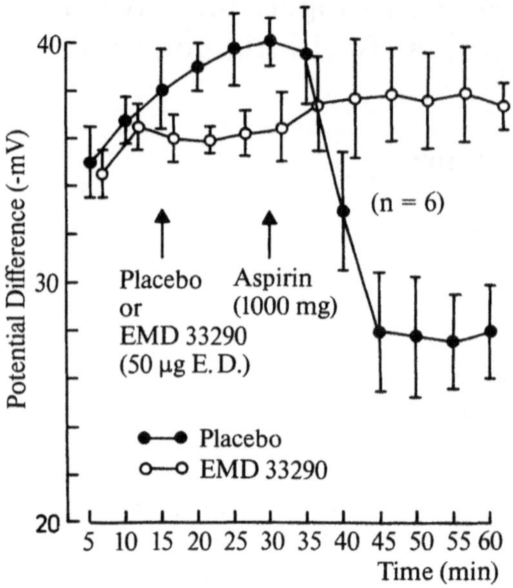

Fig. 1. Behaviour of the transmucosal gastric potential difference of man during administration of 1000 mg aspirin in the presence and absence of the thiaprostaglandin EMD 33290

trophysiological parameter can be seen as an indirect measurement for the integrity of the mucosal barrier. The studies are usually conducted on healthy volunteers following a 12-h fasting period. The potential is measured via electrolytic bridges from the corpus of the stomach or the cubital vein. A moderate PD of − 36 to − 44 mV indicates the correct placement of the probe in the fundus/corpus region.

As shown in Fig. 1, the oral administration of 1000 mg acetylsalicylic acid causes a 35% drop in the potential difference. The PD does not return to the initial values until after 60–90 min. A 15-min pretreatment with 50 µg EMD 33290, a thiaprostaglandin, can prevent the drop in PD caused by the 1000 mg of aspirin throughout the entire period of measurement [10]. A dose of 50 µg EMD 33290 causes no antisecretory activity as supplementary acid secretion studies have shown. This is reference to the fact that prostaglandins exhibit PD-stabilizing characteristics on the human gastric mucosal epithelium [10]. Other authors have confirmed these observations (Table 1) [4, 5, 5a, 6, 11, 13, 24, 26].

Various prostaglandins like misoprostol, mexiprostil, enprostil, rioprostil, 16,16-dimethyl-PGE_2, arbaprostil, FCE 20700, and PGE_2 were used here. The main iritants used were acetylsalicylic acid or taurocholate (TC). In all cases the prostaglandins were able to prevent completely or partially the irritant-induced drop in transmucosal PD and they did so in a dose range which cannot be viewed as nonantisecretory. This effect sets prostaglandins apart from common therapeutic agents used for ulcers. These PD-stabilizing properties are not to be treated as equivalent to the macroscopically or microscopically evident protective effects (see below).

Table 1. PD-stabilizing properties of PG in man

Autor		PG	Irritants	Antisecretory dose	PD stabilization
Carmichael et al.	[5a]	Arbaprostil	ASS	?	+
Müller et al.	[24]	16,16-dm PGE_2	ASS	ja	+
Müller et al.	[24]		TC	ja	+
Cohen	[6]	PGE_2	ASS	ja	+
Fimmel and Blum	[13]	Misoprostol	TC	ja	(+)
Bianchi-Porro et al.	[5]	Mexiprostil	ASS	ja?	+
Bernier et al.	[4]	Enprostil	ASS	ja?	(+)
Demol et al.	[4]	Rioprostil	ASS	ja	+
Müller et al.	[26]	FCE 20700	ASS	ja	+

Measuring the Fecal Blood Loss

After aspirin or other nonsteroidal antirheumatic drugs are administered for several days, an increased excretion of erythrocytes into the lumen of the bowels takes place due to mucosal irritation. This can be calculated by determining the daily loss of radioactively marked erythrocytes in the stool. Table 2 shows the fecal blood loss after administration of various nonsteroidal antirheumatic drugs. While the daily blood excretion after placebo is around 0.7 ml, it increases about ten times with aspirin. Newer nonsteroidal antirheumatic drugs lead to a lower blood excretion than aspirin but to a significantly higher one than placebo. In this connection Ingelfinger [18], for instance, calculated a blood loss of 10 million ml based on an annual consumption of 20–30 billion aspirin tablets taken in the United States. This is equal to twice the transfusion volume for 1 year.

In 1981 Cohen et al. [7] were able to show for the first time that by administering 4 x 1 mg PGE_2 the daily blood loss induced by 2600 mg aspirin could be completely

Table 2. Occult fecal blood loss during administration of nonsteroidal antirheumatic drugs over several days

Substance	Daily dose (mg)	gastrointestinal blood loss (ml/day)
Control	–	0.5
Acemetacin	180	0.7
Piroxicam	20	1.0
Diclofenac	150	1.7
Lonazolac	600	2.0
Indometacin	150	2.9
Asprin	2400	7.0

Table 3. Fecal blood loss

Autor		Irritants	PG	protective Doses (μg)
Ryan et al.	[29]	ASS	Misoprostol	4× 200[a]
Cohen et al.	[9]	ASS	Misoprostol	4× 25[b]
Navert	[27]	ASS	Enprostil	2× 35[a]
Cohen et al.	[9]	ASS	PGE_2	4×1000[a]
Cohen et al.	[9]	ASS	PGE_2	4× 250[b]
Johansson et al.	[20]	Indo	PGE_2	3×1000[a]
Kollberg et al.	[21]	Indo	PGE_2	3× 330[b]
Johansson et al.	[19]	Indo	Arbaprostil	3× 40[a]

[a] Antisecretory, [b] Nonantisecretory

eliminated. The authors attributed this to the so-called mucosal protective properties of PGE_2 since, according to opinions at the time, the natural PGE_2 was not supposed to have an antisecretory effect. A similar reaction to indometacin (3 x 50 mg daily) was also reported for 15-R-15-methyl-PGE_2 [19]. The conclusion that prostaglandins are also mucosally protective in man had to be revised afterwards, however, since the tested prostaglandin doses are capable of inhibiting acid secretion [3a]. The protective effect is based on a reduction of intragastric acidity: acetylsalicylic acid (pH 3.5) is then predominantly present in a dissociated, extremely impermeable form, leading to a considerable reduction of its deleterious effects upon mucosa. It is relevant to say that substances with only antisecretory action, like H_2-blockers, etc., are also able to prevent the aspirin-induced increase in fecal blood loss [33].

Studies with respect to this point have been done using various prostaglandin analogues. In the majority of the studies, doses with an antisecretory effect were used, such as for example 4 x200 μg misoprostol daily, 2 x35 μg enprostil daily, 3 x 40 μg arbaprostil daily. Only in two studies was PGE_2 given in such low doses (4 x 250 μg daily and 4 x 330 μg daily) that no appreciable suppression of the human acid secretion was to be expected (Table 3) [7, 8, 9, 19, 27, 29].

Measuring the Gastric Microbleeding Rate

The increase in the Hb content in gastric fluid after administering irritants serves as a measurement of the mucosal damage. Compared with the measurement of the fecal blood loss, this method has the advantage that it only applies to mucosal damage in the stomach region. However, there are limits set to this method, because only aspirin- and ethanol-induced damages can be recorded. Modern nonsteroidal antirheumatic drugs do not induce any significant increase in the gastric microbleeding rate.

There were some studies in which the efficacy of prostaglandins could be shown using this test model. But in these cases, too, a clear protective effect could only be ensured if antisecretory doses were given. If, for instance, misoprostol is applied in a very weak antisecretory dose (4 x25 μg daily), the aspirin-induced blood loss cannot be

Table 4. Gastric microbleeding following ASS

Autor		PG	Protective doses (μg)
Hunt et al.	[17]	Misoprostol	4× 50[a]
Konturek et al.	[22]	PGE_2	4×500[a]
Hawkey et al.	[16]	Enprostil	2× 35[a]
			No protection
Hunt et al.	[17]	Misoprostol	4× 25[b]
Müller et al.	[25]	Arbaprostil	1× 20[a]

[a] Antisecretory, [b] Nonantisecretory

suppressed. So in this test, too, the protective effect of prostaglandins does not differ from that of the H_2-blockers. In analagously set-up studies doses of 2 x 150 mg ranitidine daily were able to return the increased microbleeding rate back to normal [16] (Table 4) [15, 17, 22, 25].

Endoscopic Evaluation

The above *indirect* methods of proof have the disadvantage that they do not tell us anything about localization, degree, or depth of the mucosal damage following administration of antirheumatic drugs over several days. What is more, they are all relatively complicated methods which are troublesome for the patients and which can only be carried out, for the most part, in special laboratories.

As a result of these drawbacks, over the past few years the *direct* method, i.e., the endoscopic evaluation of the upper gastrointestinal tract following administration over several days of antirheumatic agents has come into the forefront. Test persons or patients are treated over several days with an antirheumatic agent. At fixed times an endoscopic study of the gastric and duodenal mucosa is made. A simple mucosal damage score is tabulated to quantify and qualify the lesions.

Also with this method, nowadays viewed as the method of choice, the facts already described above are found: prostaglandins are only protective against antirheumatic agents and alcohol if they are applied in antisecretory doses (Table 5). Due to their varying strength of antisecretory action enprostil, for instance, prevents aspirin-induced lesions in doses as small as 2 x 35 μg daily, rioprostil at 2 x 300 μg daily, and misoprotol at 4 x 200 μg daily [1, 3, 9a, 12, 14, 23, 27, 30, 32].

With a dose which is still just barely antisecretory (e.g., 2 x 7 μg enprostil daily), the protective action is only partly present, with nonantisecretory doses it is not evident at all.

Table 5. Endoscope studies

Autor		Irritant	PG	Protective dose (μg)
Gilbert et al.	[14]	ASS	Arbaprostil	>20[a]
Silverstein et al.	[30]	ASS	Misoprostol	4×200[a]
Stiel	[32]	ASS	Enprostil	2× 35[a]
				4× 35[a]
Cohen et al.		ASS	Enprostil	2× 70[a]
				2× 7[a]
Navert	[27]	ASS	Enprostil	2× 35[a]
Detweiler et al.	[12]	ASS	Rioprostil	4×300[a]
Lanza	[23]	Tolmetin	Misoprostol	4×200[a]
Aadland et al.		Naproxen	Misoprostol	4×200[a]
Agrawal et al.	[3]	Äthanol	Misoprostol	4×200[a]
Simmons	[3]	NSA	Arbaprostil	3× 40[a]

[a] Antisecretory

Summary

Prostaglandins have various pharmacological effects on gastric mucosal epithelium in man. Besides inhibiting acid secretion (and inhibiting the release of gastrin), they stimulate the mucus and alkali secretion of the surface epithelia, speed up the cell regeneration rate, and promote the gastric mucosal blood flow. In addition we have found in animal experiments that they also have "mucosal protective" properties which concern primarily the deeper layers of the epithelium.

Therefore we have been very interested in pursuing the use of prostaglandins in ulcer treatment. It has been clearly shown that the ulcer-healing effect of these substances is closely linked to the degree of acid inhibition. The supplementary effects (such as alkali and mucus secretion) are of little therapeutic use.

Up to now, no answer has been found to the question of whether prostaglandins can prevent mucosal damage caused by agents other than nonsteroidal antirheumatic agents or other irritants (ethanol). This hypothesis sounds plausible since it has been conjectured that the inhibition of endogenous biosynthesis is at the center of the pathogenetic mechanism of the mucosal-damaging effect of nonsteroidal anti-inflammatory drugs. In this sense the lesions would be an expression of an endogenous shortage of prostaglandin.

In the meantime it has been shown, however, that there are many different causes leading to the formation of these lesions and that there is also a significantly permissive role given to the degree of damage of the hydrochloric acid in the lumen of the stomach.

The findings achieved by various authors using the direct endoscopic method of proof alow us recognize that prostaglandins can only prevent mucosal damage if they are applied in antisecretory doses. Weak antisecretory doses only have a partial, if any, protective action. The endoscopic findings are upheld by the results of the indirect methods of proof (fecal blood loss, etc.).

The PD-stabilizing properties point, however, to an additional effect of prostaglandins on gastric mucosa in man, which is *not* inherent to other ulcer-treating drugs. This effect is already evident in low nonantisecretory doses. The transmucosal PD is an expression of the sum of various ionic flows through the gastric mucosa. It is imaginable that such processes are inhibited by nonsteroidal antirheumatic drugs and restituted by prostaglandins. We cannot, however, infer general protective effects from the PD-stabilizing effects: our own studies with the PGE-analogue FCE 20700 have shown that in nonantisecretory doses it prevents the aspirin-induced drop in PD, but not the indomethacin-induced mucosal damage.

References

1. Aadland E, Fausa O, Vatn M (1986) Misoprostol protection against naproxen-induced gastric damage. In: Advances in Prostaglandins and Gastroenterology. Symposium Sao Paulo, 4.-6. Sept. 1986. Proceeding volume, in press
2. Aenishänslin W, Bärlocher C, Bernoulli R et al. (1985) Misoprostol und Cimetidin bei der Behandlung des Ulkus duodeni. Eine multizentrische Schweizer Doppeltblindstudie. Schweiz med Wschr 115: 1125-1231
3. Agrawal NM, Godiwala T, Arimura A, Dajani EZ (1986) Comparative cytoprotective effects against alcohol insult. Misoprostol versus cimetidine. Digestive Dis Sciences 31(2): 142 S-144
4. Bernier JJ, Florent C, Flourie B, Pfeiffer A (1985) Mesure de la difference de potentiel transepitheliale gastrique. Effect des agents agressifs (aspirine, alcool) and enprostil et des pansements gastriques. Gastroenterol Clin Biol 9 (12): 58-64
5. Bianchi-Porro G, Petrillo M, Lazzaroni M, Fuccella LM, Sassela D (1984) Gastric antisecretory and cytoprotective activity of MDL 646, a new PGE_2 analog, in man. GUT A 580, F. 108

5a Carmichael HA, Nelson ML, Russell RI (1982) Effect of natural prostaglandin E_2 (PGE_2) and derivatives on aspirin-induced fall in gastric mucosal electropotential difference in man GUT 86: A 424

6. Cohen MM (1981) Prevention of aspirin-induced fall in gastric potential difference with prostaglandins. Lancet i: 785
7. Cohen, MM (1981) Prevention of aspirin-induced fecal blood loss with oral prostaglandin E_2: Dose-response studies in man. Prostaglandins 21 (Suppl): 155-160
8. Cohen MM, Clark L, Armstrong L et al (1983) Reduced aspirin-induced fecal blood loss with simultaneous administration of misoprostol. Gastroenterology 84: 1126
9. Cohen MM, Clark L, Armstrong L, d'Souza J (1985) Reduction of aspirin-induced fecal blood loss with low-dose misoprostol tablets in man. Digestive Dis Sciences 30 (7): 605-611

9a Cohen MM (1987) The protective effects of prostaglandins. In: Enprostil: A synthetic prostaglandin for gastrointestinal disorders. Symposium: Sao Paulo. Proceeding Volume, in press

10. Dammann HG, Müller P, Heun J, Simon B (1982) Säurehemmung und Verhinderung des transmukösen Potentialdifferenzabfalls durch das Thiaprostaglandin EMD 33290 beim Menschen. Schweiz med Wschr 112: 829-831
11. Demol Pl, Schmith HD, Weihrauch TR, Kuhlmann J (1986) Prevention of acetylsalicylic acid-induced changes of the gastric potential difference by the new synthetic prostaglandin E_2 analog rioprostil. Arzneimittel-Forschung 36 (II): 1406-1408
12. Detweiler MK, Harrison CA, Rollins DE, Tolman KG, McCormack GH, Simon DM (1984) Effect of rioprostil on aspirin-induced gastrointestinal mucosal changes in normal volunteers. Gastroenterology 86 (5/2): A 1065
13. Fimmel CJ, Blum AL (1983) Acid inhibition, but no protection from bile salt damage by a prostaglandin E_2 analog in man. Gastroenterology 84 (5/2): 1151
14. Gilbert DA, Surawicz CM, Silverstein FE et al (1984) Prevention of acute aspirin-induced gastric mucosal injury by 15 (R)-15 methyl prostaglandin E_2: an endoscopic study. Gastroenterology 86: 339-345

15. Hawkey ChJ (1985) Effect of enprostil on gastric bleeding induced by administration of aspirin to healthy volunteers. In: Protective and therapeutic effects of gastrointestinal prostaglandins. Toronto, Canada, Nov, 12-14
16. Hawkey CJ, Somerville KW, Marshall S (1986) Human gastric mucosal protection by ranitidine. Gastroenterology 90 (5/2): A 1489
17. Hunt JN, Smith JL, Jiang CL, Kessler L (1983) Effect of synthetic prostaglandin E_2 analog on aspirin-induced gastric bleeding and secretion. Digestive Deseases and Sciences 28(10): 897-902
18. Ingelfinger FJ (1974) The side effects of aspirin. New Engl J Med. 290: 1196-1199
19. Johannson, Kollberg B, Nordemar R, Bergström S (1979) Mucosal protection by prostaglandin E_2. Lancet i: 317
20. Johannson C, Kollberg B, Nordemar R, Samuelson K, Bergström S (1980) Protective effect of prostaglandin E_2 in the gastrointestinal tract during indometacin treatment of rheumatic diseases. Gastroenterology 78: 479-483
21. Kollberg B, Nordemar R, Johannson C (1981) Gastrointestinal protection by low dose oral prostaglandin E_2 in rheumatic diseases. Scand J Gastroent. 16: 1005-1008
22. Konturek SJ, Kwiecien N, Obtulowicz W, Polanski M, Kopp B, Olesky J (1983) Comparison of prostaglandin E_2 and ranitidine in prevention of gastric bledding by aspirin in man. GUT 24: 89-93
23. Lanza FL (1986) Misoprostol prevents duodenal mucosal injury induced by tolmetin in humans. Gastroenterology 90 (5/2): 1511
24. Müller P, Fischer N, Kather H, Simon B (1981) Prevention of aspirin-induced drop in gastric potential difference with 16,16-dm-prostaglandin E_2. Lancet i: 333-334
25. Müller P, Kather H, Simon B (1982) Method for testing cytoprotective agents in man. In: Advances in experimental ulcer. Eds S Umehara, H Ito, Tokyo, Japan, 494-498
26. Müller P, Dammann HG, Simon B (1986) Effecte von FCE 20700, einem oral wirksamen Prostaglandin E_2-Analog, auf das menschliche Magenschleimhautepithel. Z. Gastroenterology 24 (10): 612-617
27. Navert H (1985) Protective effect of enprostil during aspirin administration. In: Protective and therapeutic effects of gastrointestinal prostaglandins. Toronto, Canada. Nov. 12-14
28. Robert A (1979) Cytoprotection by prostaglandins. Gastroenterology 77: 761-767
29. Ryan J (1987) Misoprostol reduces aspirin-induced fecal blood loss in osteoarthritic patients. In: Advances in Prostaglandins and Gastroenterology Symposium Sao Paulo, 8. Sept 1986. Proceeding Volume
30. Silverstein FE, Kimmey MB, Saunders DR et al (1985) Misoprostol protects the gastric mucosa from aspirin-induced damage: an endoscopic study. Dig Dis Sciences 30: 642-644
31. Simmons E (1986) Protection of human gastric mucosa by arbaprostil in rheumatics. Gastroenterology 90 (5/2): 1477
32. Stiel D (1985) The protective effect of enprostil, cimetidine, and sucralfate against aspirin-induced damage of the gastric mucosa. In: Protective and therapeutic effects of gastrointestinal prostaglandins. Toronto, Canada. Nov. 12-14
33. Welch RW, Bentsch HL, Harris SC (1978) Reduction of aspirin-induced gastrointestinal bleeding by cimetidine. Gastroenterology 74: 459-463

Clinical Aspects of the Protective Effects of Prostaglandins on Non-Steroidal Anti-Inflammatory Drug-Associated Mucosal Injury

D. Y. GRAHAM

Introduction

Major clinical problems that occur in patients receiving non-steroidal anti-inflammatory drugs (NSAIDs) include dyspepsia, gastric (and possibly duodenal) ulcer, gastrointestinal bleeding, and gastric or duodenal perforation. Another problem is that many physicians feel compelled to treat visible mucosal damage associated with the administration of aspirin or other NSAIDs. The pathogenesis of NSAID-induced mucosal damage is still unclear; important variables include NSAID dosage, dosing interval, route of administration, formulation, and the solubility of the compound in the acid milieu of the stomach.

A large body of information is available from observations derived from studies in which NSAIDs were administered orally to normal healthy volunteers (acute studies) with the effect on the gastric mucosa being evaluated by endoscopy [1-8]. These endoscopic studies have been used to compare various NSAIDs and to investigate whether particular agents could reduce or prevent mucosal damage. It is frequently implied that results from the acute studies can be used to predict the effect of chronic administration of NSAIDs. The acute endoscopic studies have demonstrated that NSAIDs differ in their propensity to damage the gastric mucosa; aspirin is the most damaging drug, while many of the newer agents are difficult to distinguish from placebo [2]. Dose response effects can be demonstrated for most drugs, i.e., the degree of damage increases as the amount of drug administered is increased (the peak damage may vary greatly between agents) (Fig. 1). The degree of mucosal injury produced can be reduced, or in some instances eliminated, by the co-administration of prostaglandins or H_2-receptor antagonists. NSAID-associated mucosal injury is largely acid-dependent; therefore antisecretory doses of H_2-receptor antagonists and prostaglandins usually appear more effective than cytoprotective doses.

Therapy with an NSAID

It could be speculated that chronic therapy with an NSAID, that was rarely associated with acute mucosal damage, should not cause evidence of mucosal damage such as ulcers or gastrointestinal bleeding. Unfortunately, that is not the clinical experience. Endoscopic inspection of the gastric mucosa of arthritic patients reveals mucosal erosions or mucosal hemorrhages in at least half the individuals, with approximately 10%

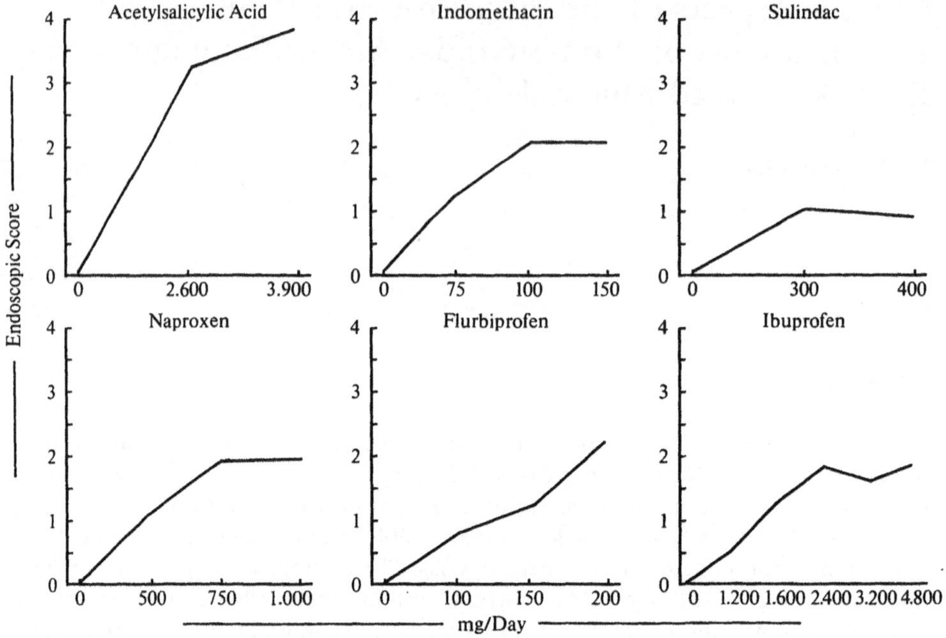

Fig. 1. The dose-response effect relating the severity of gastric mucosal damage to NSAID dosage is shown; adapted from Lanza [1]

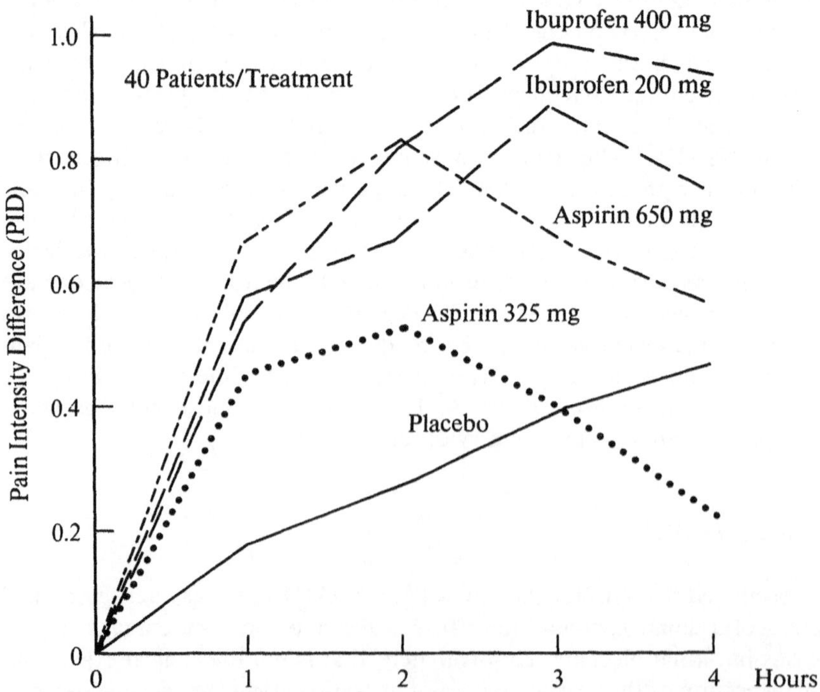

Fig. 3. Time-effect curves from dental impaction pain study comparing ibuprofen, aspirin, and placebo; from Cooper [15]

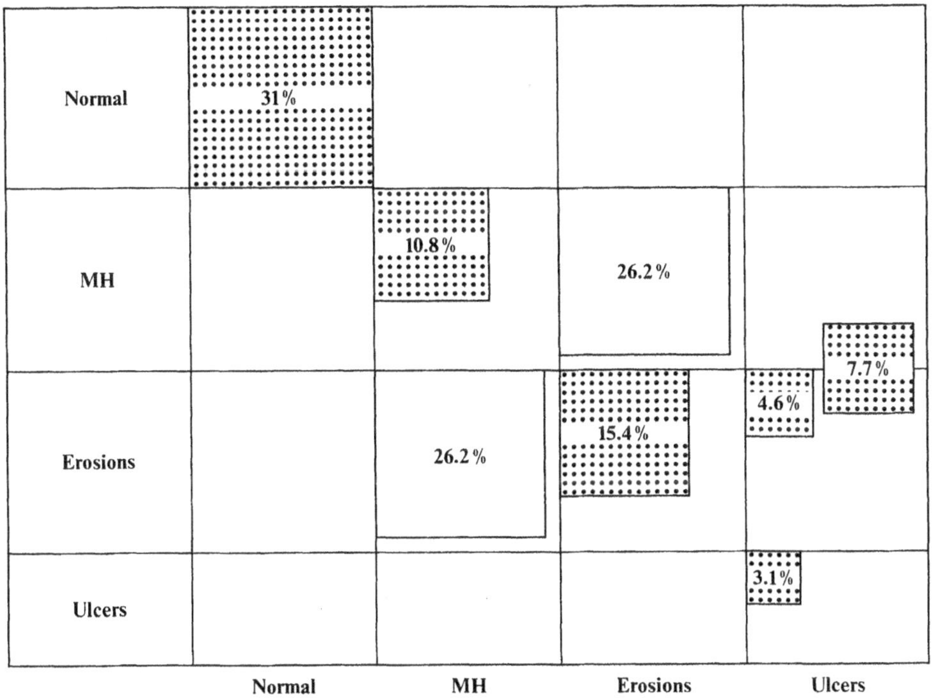

Fig. 2. The proportion of rheumatoid patients with various gastric mucosal lesion. Data derived from 65 patients with rheumatoid or osteoarthritis endoscoped at the VA Medical Center Houston. MH, mucosal hemorrhages

also having a chronic gastric ulcer [9–14, (Fig. 2)]. Thus, the results of acute studies in normal volunteers have little predictive value; there seem to be negligible differences between the prevalence of chronic gastric ulcer in patients receiving aspirin as compared to those receiving one of the new agents. This statement holds even for those drugs that can not be distinguished from placebo in acute studies.

Several facts are worth noting about damage induced by NSAIDs. First, the degree of damage increases with increased dosage (Fig. 1). Similarly, dose response effects are evident for both the analgesic effect of various NSAIDs [15, Fig. 3] and the anti-inflammatory response [16–19]. In general, the dose required to achieve maximum analgesic effect is quite low compared to the dose required to achieve maximum anti-inflammatory effect [20] (the latter may be above the dosages commonly employed in clinical medicine). Finally, the percentage of patients who develop clinically significant side effects, such as gastric ulcers, perforation, or bleeding, is related to drug dose (Fig. 4, 5). As higher levels of drug are needed for anti-inflammatory effect, a method of reducing or preventing the untoward effects associated with NSAID use would be very desirable. One possible approach would be to co-administer small doses of several NSAIDs, thus avoiding a high dose of a single agent. Unfortunately, available evidence suggests that the amount and severity of damage with a combination of agents is at

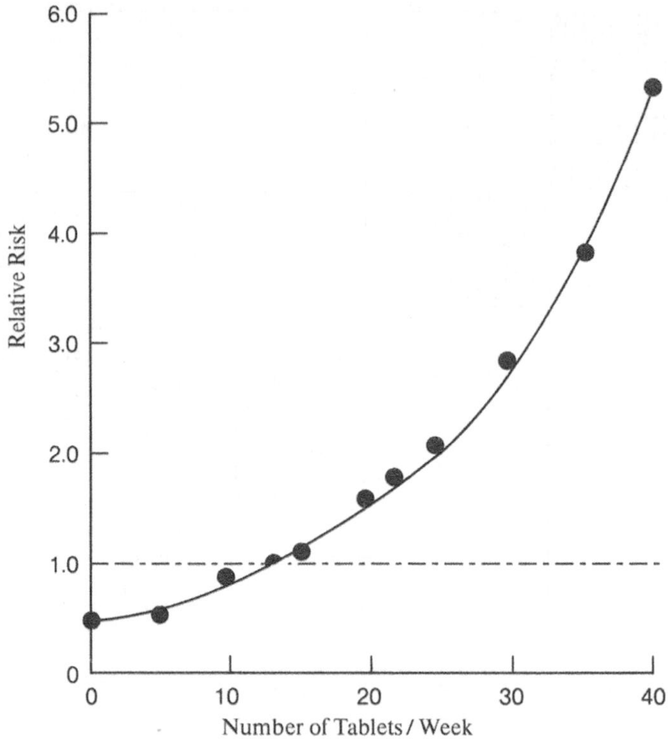

Fig. 4. Risk of developing a chronic gastric ulcer to the amount of aspirin consumed per week. Based on distribution of aspirin use among patients in studies reported by Cameron; from Graham and Smith [8]. The horizontal line shows the relative risk of 1

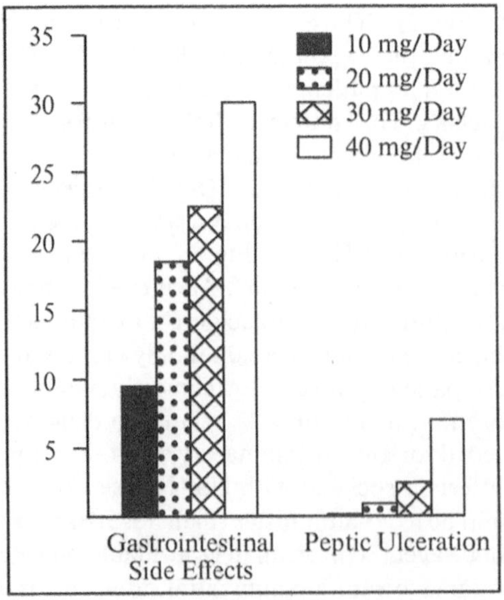

Fig. 5. Frequency of gastrointestinal side effects and peptic ulcer relative to prioxicam dosage in patients with rheumatic disease; from Brogden et al. [16]

least additive [21]. Therefore, the co-administration of several NSAIDs may lead to worse injury than administration of higher doses of a single agent.

Is NSAID-induced gastroduodenal injury a clinically important problem?

Dyspepsia is common and is important in some patients receiving NSAIDs [22]. Although the occurrence of dyspepsia does not predict the presence of gastroduodenal injury, it often precludes use of a particular agent. Dyspepsia usually begins soon after starting therapy with an NSAID; consequently, patients, who take an NSAID chronically, usually have found a product that is both effective and not associated with abdominal discomfort. Some patients can not find an NSAID that does not cause dyspepsia. A drug that would allow such patients to take needed NSAIDs by reducing or eliminating associated dyspepsia would certainly be of value.

The point prevalence of gastric ulcers in arthritic patients receiving NSAIDs is 10–15% [9–14]. Gastric ulcers in these patients are usually silent and become evident only when bleeding or perforation occurs. It is not clear that silent gastric ulcer is a significant clinical problem, or that reduction in the frequency of such lesions would improve the care or the longevity of arthritic patients. It is my personal belief that many newer NSAIDs, although appearing less damaging than aspirin in acute studies, cause more problems than aspirin did in the past. For example, although the consumption of aspirin has steadily fallen in the UK, the frequency of major upper gastrointestinal hemorrhage has increased with much of the increase in bleeding being seen in the older population in whom NSAID use is common [23]. The increase in the frequency of NSAID-associated clinical problems may have several explanations. The newer NSAIDs may be intrinsically more dangerous, doses higher on the dose-response curve may be given, or the dose-response curve for untoward effects may be sharper with newer drugs. It is possible that the actual amount of aspirin taken in the past was less than prescribed. Aspirin is associated with dyspepsia more frequently than are the newer NSAIDs and the presence of aspirin-induced dyspepsia may have reduced the dose actually ingested.

Do arthritic patients frequently die of gastric ulcer, bleeding or perforation?

There has been a slight but steady increase in the proportion of arthritic patients dying because of gastrointestinal problems [24–32]. However, even with the increase in frequency, the magnitude of the problem remains quite small. In the most recent study, gastrointestinal causes accounted for 6% of all deaths in arthritic patients compared to approximately 4% of deaths in the general population [32].

Is it possible to prevent the mucosal damage associated with NSAID use?

Can the lesions that are present be healed? What will be the cost of NSAID-associated mucosal injury measured both in monetary and social units? What will be the cost of prevention both in terms of money and in drug-associated side effects caused by the combination of the NSAID and an agent designed to reduce morbidity and mortality associated with the use of NSAIDs? Can we identify a patient population at special risk for the development of complications related to NSAID use [33-36]?

Conclusion

The ideal agent to prevent NSAID-associated mucosal injury would be one with few side effects of its own, one that would not add to the cost of therapy, and one that could be combined with any NSAIDs. The perfect drug should heal existing mucosal damage and completely prevent new mucosal injury. Are prostaglandins such agents? Cytoprotective doses of prostaglandins have not been shown to yield complete protection against acute mucosal injury associated with NSAID use. It is not clear that an agent able to reduce or eliminate acute changes will be effective in reducing or eliminating the mucosal injury associated with chronic administration of NSAIDs. Preliminary analyses suggest that cytoprotective doses of prostaglandins are not as effective as dosage that mediate significant acid suppression (as monitored on the basis of visible mucosal damage). Reduction in mucosal damage would be a less important achievement than reduction in the frequency of serious side effects of NSAIDs such as hemorrhage or perforation. Unfortunately, it is very difficult to prove reduction in frequency of an already infrequent event. We do not recommend the routine use of any agent with the intent of preventing NSAID-associated gastrointestinal side effects [8]. Ideally, we would prefer to limit treatment to a high-risk population (if such a population could be identified). This approach would at least ensure that the cost of prevention would not be significantly greater than the experience of the problem we are attempting to prevent.

References

1. Lanza FL (1984) Endoscopic studies of gastric and duodenal injury after the use of ibuprofen, aspirin, and other non-steroidal anti-inflammatory agents. Am J Med 77 (suppl 1A): 19-24
2. Graham DY, Smith JL, Holmes GI, Davies RO (1985) Non-steroidal anti-inflammatory effect of sulindac sulfoxide and sulfide on gastric mucosa, Clin Pharmacol Ther 38: 65-70
3. Osnes M, Larsen S, Eidsaunet W, Thom E (1979) Effect of diclofenac and naproxen on gastroduodenal mucosa. Clin Pharmacol Ther 26: 399-405
4. Tronstad RI, Aadland E, Holler T, Olaussen B (1985) Gastroscopic findings after Treatment with enteric-coated and plain naproxen tablets in healthy subjects. Scand J Gastroenterol 20: 239-242.
5. Hradsky M (1981) Endoscopic Evaluation of gastric tolerance to fenclofenac. Upsala J Med Sci 86: 99-103
6. Halvorsen L, Dotevall G, Sevelius H (1973) Comparative effects of aspirin and naproxen on gastric mucosa. Scan J Rheumatol 2: 43-7
7. Lehtola J, Sipponen P (1977) A gastroscopic and histologic doubleblind study of the effects of diclofenac and naproxen on the human gastric mucosa. Scand J Rheumatol 6: 97-102
8. Graham DY, Smith JL (1986) Aspirin and the stomach. Ann Intern Med 104: 390-8
9. Larkai EN, Smith JL, Lidsky MD, Graham DY (1987) Gastroduodenal mucosa and dyspeptic symptoms in arthritic patients during chronic non-steroidal anti-inflammatory drug use. Am J Gastroenterol 82: 1153-1158
10. Silvoso GR, Ivey KJ, Butt JH, Lockard OO, Holt SD, Sisk C et al (1979) Incidence of gastric lesions in patients with rheumatoid disease on chronic aspirin therapy. Ann Intern Med 91: 517-20

11. Bianchi Porro G, Lazzaroni M, Petrillo M (1982) Gastroscopy in elderly patients. Curr Med Res Opin 7 (Suppl 1): 96–103
12. Lockard OO, Ivey KJ, Butt JH, Silvoso GR, Sisk C, Holt S (1980) The prevalence of duodenal lesions in patients with rheumatic diseases on chronic aspirin therapy. Gastrointest Endoscopy 26: 5–7
13. Morris AD, Holt SD, Silvoso GR, Hewitt J, Tatum W, Grandione J, et al (1981) Effect of anti-inflammatory drug administration in patients with rheumatoid arthritis. An endoscopic assessment. Scan J Gastroent 16 (Suppl 67): 131–5
14. Caruso I, Bianchi Porro G (1980) Gastroscopic evaluation of anti-inflammatory agents. Br Med J 280: 75–8
15. Cooper SA (1983) New peripherally-acting oral analgesic agents. Ann Rev Pharmacol Toxicol 23: 617–47
16. Brogden RN, Heel RC, Speight TM, Avery GS (1981) Piroxicam: a review of its pharmacological properties and therapeutic efficacy. Drugs 22: 165–87
17. Luftschein S, Bienenstock H, Varady JC, Stitt FW (1979) Increasing dose of naproxen in rheumatoid arthritis: Use with and without corticosteroids. J Rheumatol 6: 397–404
18. Day RO, Furst DE, Dromgoole SH, Kamm B, Roe R, Paulus HE (1982) Relationship of serum naproxen concentration to efficacy in rheumatoid arthritis. Clin Pharmacol Ther 31: 733–40
19. Berry H, Nichols A (1985) An open study of 1.5 g naproxen daily in osteoarthritis. Curr Med Res Opin 9: 366–70
20. Ekstrand R, Alvan G, L'e Orme M, Lewander R, Palmer L, Sarby B (1980) Double-blind dose-response study of indomethacin in rheumatoid arthritis. Eur J Clin Pharmacol 17: 437–42
21. Baragar FD, Smith TC (1987) Drug interaction studies with sodium meclofenamate (meclomen®). Curr Ther Res 23: S51–9
22. Gibberd FB (1966) Dyspepsia in patients with rheumatoid arthritis. Acta Rheum Scand 12: 112–21
23. Schiller KFR, Truelove SC, Williams DG (1970) Hematemesis and melaena, with special reference to factors influencing the outcome. Br Med J 2: 7–14
24. Uddin J, Kraus AS, Kelly HG (1970) Survivorship and death in rheumatoid arthritis. Arth Rheum 13: 125–30
25. Mutru O, Koota K, Isomaki H (1976) Causes of death in autopsied RA patients. Scand J Rheumatology 5: 239–40
26. Monson RR, Hall AP (1979) Mortality among arthritics. J Chron Dis 29: 459–67
27. Rasker JJ, Cosh JA (1981) Cause and age at death in a prospective study of 100 patients with rheumatoid arthritis. Ann Rheum Dis 40: 115–20
28. Morris AD, Holt SD, Silvoso GR, Hewitt J, Tatum W, Grandione J, Butt JH, Ivey KJ (1981) Effect of anti-inflammatory drug administration in patients with rheumatoid arthritis. An endoscopic assessment. Scand J Gastroenterol 16: 131–5
29. Abruzzo JL (1982) Rheumatoid arthritis and mortality. Arth Rheum 25: 1020–3
30. VanDenbrouche JP, Hazevoet HM, Cats A (1984) Survival and cause of death in gherumtroid arthritis: a 25-year prospective follow-up. J Rheumatol 11: 158–61
31. Mutru O, Laakso M, Isomaki H, Koota K (1985) Ten-year mortality and causes of death in patients with rheumatoid arthritis. Br Med J 290: 1811–13
32. Mitchell DM, Spritz PW, Young DY, Bloch DA, McShane DJ, Fries JF (1986) Survival, prognosis and causes of death in rheumatoid arthritis. Arth Rheum 29: 706–14
33. Collier DSTJ, Pain JA (1985) Non-steroidal anti-inflammatory drugs and peptic ulcer perforation. Gut 26: 359–63
34. Alexander AM, Veitch GBA, Wood JB (1985) Anti-rheumatic and analgesic drug usage and acute gastrointestinal bleeding in elderly patients. J Clin Hosp Pharm 10: 89–93
35. Clinch D, Banergee AK, Ostick G, Levy DW (1983) Non-steroidal anti-inflammatory drugs and gastrointestinal adverse effects. J R Coll Physicians (London) 17: 228–30
36. Llewelyn JG, Pritchard MH (1983) Acute gastric haemorrhage and its relationship to the use of anti-inflammatory analgesics (NSAIDs). Ann Rheum Dis 42: 228–9

Discussion Following the Report of Prof. Graham

LANGMAN

If I look at the United Kingdom, there is no doubt that a group of patients for whom a prophylactic prevention of NSAID-induced adverse reactions seems more important than for other groups of the population. And I am fortified in my belief that the rate of adverse reactions in the elderly is probably unacceptable. I think in younger patients the rate of side effects is so low that one could never show conclusively the benefit of prevention. In the elderly this could more likely be done. In this group 2000–3000 admissions a year with serious bleeding and perforations is a relevant problem. I do not think it really matters whether they have an ulcer history or not.

SIMON

You have described an adaptation of the gastric mucosa to the damaging effect of aspirin when given over some weeks. Did you see the same adaptive mechanisms with newer nonsteroidal anti-inflammatory drugs?

GRAHAM

We have shown in a prospective study that mucosal adaptation to ASA does occur, but it is dose-dependent. The gastric mucosa will not adapt to very high doses of aspirin. With other NSAID the occurrence of lesions may be basically different. While during short-term treatment no lesions may be observed, however they do appear under long-term treatment. I do not know how to explain why gastric mucosal lesions occur almost exclusively under long-term treatment with NSAID. Prostaglandin inhibition and the other changes we have talked about may offer the answer to this phenomenon.

RACHMILEWITZ

Would you recommend a concomitant administration of a protecting agent during NSAID treatment?

GRAHAM

I would not take a drug to prevent something that probably is not going to occur. I think the nonsteroidal anti-inflammatory drugs can be made safer by formulation changes alone. I would not take anything unless I had had an NSAID side effect. And those who have had side effects under NSAID treatment may represent a subgroup which concomitantly needs protective drugs.

BIANCHI PORRO

I perfectly agree with you. According to our experience there is in fact one subgroup of patients in whom we always expect troublesome side effects, namely those with a history of duodenal or gastric ulcer (especially duodenal ulcer). When we perform endoscopy and find a scar, and the patient has to take anti-inflammatory drugs, we always fear major clinical problems due to a recurrence of the ulcer. I think in this subgroup it would be worthwhile to prescribe a "protective" drug (of any kind).

GRAHAM

Let me add one thing about aspirin I have not mentioned. I think that aspirin is much safer than the new NSAID. If you consider the United Kingdom data, it is evident, that the frequency of aspirin used has gone down remarkably. Yet the frequency of bleeding has increased. I thing aspirin is probably intrinsically safer, partially because you cannot increase the dose too much without developing marked symptoms, which in turn prevents patients from taking very high doses. But this is not true for the other NSAID. Also the combination of low doses of aspirin and another NSAID is not necessarily safe. On the contrary, you can even expect a higher frequency of untoward events.

WALAN

Dr. Langman, did you find an increased incidence of peptic ulcer history in patients who bled or perforated under NSAID treatment compared to those NSAID users who had no bleeding history?

LANGMAN

I cannot answer the question properly. But there is a fair proportion of NSAID users with no gastrointestinal history at all who turn up with lesions out of the blue.

Prostaglandins and Leukotrienes in Gastrointestinal Diseases – Present Clinical Role

Gastrointestinal Microbleeding and Ulcerogenic Drugs: Prevention by Co-Administration of Prostaglandins

C. JOHANSSON

Introduction

It is known empirically and from a larger number of clinical studies that treatments with steroids or non-steroidal anti-inflammatory drugs (NSAIDs) are associated with development of bleeding erosions and peptic ulcerations in the upper gastrointestinal tract [1, 2, 3]. More recently it was demonstrated that such treatments are ulcerogenic also to the human colonic mucosa [4, 5]. This is a brief summary of some clinical and pathophysiological aspects on drug-induced mucosal lesions and their prevention particularly by co-administration of prostaglandins.

Clinical Studies of Drug-Induced Damage

Damage of the human gastric mucosa following intake of acetylsalicylic acid was recognized in 1935 [6]. Since then, many clinical studies have confirmed the ulcerogenic effects of steroids and NSAIDs. Different approaches have been used, such as systemic registration of side effects during drug therapy [7], endoscopic examination with grading of lesions [8], measurements of fecal blood loss [9, 10], and determination of hemoglobin [11] or DNA [12] in gastric washings.

In short term studies with aspirin or indomethacin almost all healthy subjects have signs of mucosal damage [2, 3, 8, 9–11].

Long-term treatment with NSAIDs or steroids is associated with a high prevalence of gastric ulcers and erosions [13, 14], 50–86% of the patients having endoscopically verified lesions. Others have failed to find a connection between steroid treatment and gastric ulcerations [15], but after correction for variable treatment times these data demonstrated that long-term steroid treatment did, indeed, increase the risk to have a peptic ulcer [16].

Studies, like those cited, have met with criticism due to their retrospective design, small patient groups, lack of adequate controls, and failure to separate prevalence from incidence. In the single large prospective and controlled American aspirin myocardial infarction study a more than fivefold incidence of peptic ulcer was found in patients on active treatment [17].

The study does not provide a safe estimate of the incidence of ulcerations during long-term aspirin treatment, since in this polulation the incidence of ulcerations in placebo treatment patients was only 1/3 of that usually reported for western populations.

Thus, even if criticism can be raised against single resports, the summarized information from a large number of short- and long-term clinical studies is convincing. It is safe to conclude that NSAIDs and steroids are ulcerogenic to the gastroduodenal mucosa. The exact incidence of drug-induced lesions in patients on long-term treatment remains to be determined.

Clinical Relevance of Drug-Induced Lesions

The impact of drug-induced lesions for clinical medicine, as questioned by Ingelfinger, may partially be a matter of position [16]. Prescription of a drug that increases peptic ulcer incidence tenfold means that a rheumatologist will encounter 18 peptic ulcers per 1000 patients annually of which 6 are asymptomatic. Understandably, he will tend to overlook the problem. In contrast, the gastroenterologist, who finds that up to 30% of severe bleedings from the GI tract were preceded by aspirin intake [18], is probably more apt to emphasize the morbidity following antiphlogistic drugs. For patients on continuous treatment with NSAIDs even a moderate daily increase of fecal blood loss may contribute to anemia. As pointed out [4], the very old seem to be more sensitive to ulcerogenecity by NSAIDs.

Physiological Aspects on Drug-Induced Mucosal Lesions

It is assumed that NSAIDs and steroids are ulcerogenic because they inhibit the endogenous prostaglandin formation, thereby reducing the mucosal resistance to normally present and potentially harmful agents.

The human gastroduodenal mucosa has a large capacity to metabolize arachidonic acid. The formation of prostaglandins *in vivo* can be followed in luminal contents, that can be atraumatically sampled [19]. Indomethacin reduced luminal concentrations of PGE_2 in the basal state [2] and less so after challenge [20]. Arachidonic acid metabolism in human mucosal biopsies is suppressed [2, 3]. Direct support for the hypothesis that NSAIDs are ulcerogenic because they inhibit the endogenous prostaglandin formation and not because of other unspecific properties is provided by studies demonstrating that NSAID-induced gastroduodenal lesions or bleeding in experimental animals [21] and in man [9, 10] can be prevented by concomitant supplementation with a prostaglandin devoid of acid antisecretory action.

Blocking of the mucosal prostaglandin formation with NSAIDs is followed by suppression of several recognized mucosal defense factors. The drugs inhibit basal and stimulated bicarbonate transport in various species including man [19, 22] and reduce the thickness of the protective pH-mucus barrier that overlays the mucosal cells [23]. Indomethacin-treated experimental animals have reduced production and release of mucus glucoproteins [24] and atrophic changes of gastroduodenal epithelia (Uribe et al 1986 personal communication). In addition, indomethacin reduces cytoprotection by certain endogenous compounds, which partially act by increasing endogenous prostaglandin levels.

Animal studies suggest that reduction of mucosal resistance through suppression of defense factors can not alone account for the ulcerogenic actions of cyclooxygenase-blockers. NSAIDs produce bleeding gastric erosions in the rat only when gastric acid is present [25]. In analogy, NSAIDs are not ulcerogenic in the small intestine if the bile is diverted [26] and is not harmful to the colonic mucosa of germ-free animals [27].

Role of Endogenous Prostaglandins in Mucosal Defense

The ulcerogenic actions of cyclooxygenase-blockers is indirect evidence that endogenous formation of certain prostaglandins may be the key event in the defense of the gastroduodenal mucosa. Exogenous prostaglandins, in particularly E- and I-series, stimulate bicarbonate secretion in experimental animals and in man [20, 22] and increase the thickness of the gastric pH-mucus barrier [23] and luminal mucus content [28]. Natural PGE and stable analogs have trophic actions on gastrointestinal epithelia in the rat [29] and in man [30] by reducing cell losses from the mucosal surface with secondary slowing of cell migration and reduced new cell production [31]. Prostaglandins, including those without acid antisecretory action, are cytoprotecitve [32], that is, they prevent mucosal damage in lesion models resistant to gastric acid inhibition.

Challenge of the mucosal defense is associated with increased endogenous prostaglandin formation. Brief exposures of the duodenal mucosa to acid in experimental animals [33] and in man [20] result in dose-related stimulation of the bicarbonate secretion with a parallel increase of luminal PGE_2, whereas indomethacin produces the reverse effects.

Prevention of Drug-Induced Gastrointestinal Lesions

Since blockers of prostaglandin biosynthesis are ulcerogenic in the gastroduodenal mucosa only in the presence of acid, such damage is expectedly prevented both by stimulators of defense mechanisms and by inhibitors of gastric acid. In contrast, several drastic agents like absolute ethanol, hyprosmotic solutions of hydrochloric acid, and sodium hydroxide, will induce gross mucosal damage irrespective of gastric pH and secretory state. Such gross damage may be prevented by cytoprotective agents like prostaglandins [32]. The nature of cytoprotection is yet not known; cytoprotection by prostaglandins is established within moments and has been demonstrated against damage of several organs outside the GI tract and with isolated cells [34]. A suggested association between cytoprotection and the mentioned mucosal defense factors is therefore less likely. The importance of cytoprotection for gastroduodenal mucosal defense in man is difficult to evaluate. The only valid model is acute challenge of the human gastric mucosa with 40–50% ethanol [35, 36]. One approach has been to use natural PGE_2 that has little acid antisecretory effect. It has been repeatedly demonstrated that drug-induced mucosal erosions of gastrointestinal bleeding are prevented by co-administration of small doses of PGE_2 in healthy subjects [3, 10, 35] and in patients with rheumatic disease [9]. In addition, natural PGE_2 seems to accelerate healing of ulcerations [34].

Stable analogs of PGE share the defense-stimulation properties, are cytoprotective and, in addition, have acid antisecretory actions. Such compounds should be even more effective in preventing gastroduodenal lesions and gastrointestinal blood loss following prostaglandin depletion.

Several other endogenous compounds [37, 38] and drugs [36, 39, 40, 41] have prostaglandin – like cytoprotective properties in animal and human experimental models. Their effects are at least partially exerted by stimulation of prostaglandin biosynthesis and their long-term efficacy in the prostaglandin-depleted stomach remains to be examined.

References

1. Simon LE, Mills JA (1980) Nonsteroidal antiinflammatory drugs I. New Engl J Med 302: 1179–1185
2. Cohen MM, MacDonald WC (1982) Mechanism of aspirin injury to human gastric mucosa 9: 241–255
3. Konturek SJ, Kwiecen N, Obtulowicz, Kiec Dewbinska A, Polanski M, Kopp B, Sito E, Oleksy J (1982) Effect of Carprofen and Indomethacin on Gastric Function, Mucosal Integrity and Generation of Prostaglandins in Man. Hepatogastroenterology 29: 267–270
4. Langman MJS, Morgan L, Worall A (1985) Use of anti-inflammatory drugs by patients admitted with small or large bowel preforations and haemorrhage. Br Med J 290: 347–349
5. Uribe A, Johansson C, Slezak P, Rubio C (1986) Ulceration of the colon associated with naproxen and acetyl salicylic acid treatment; an overlooked complication 32: 242–244
6. Wyllie AM (1935) Fatal case of aspirin poisoning with post mortem findings 2: 768–769
7. Paulus HE (1985) Postmarketing surveillance of nonsteroidal antiinflammatory drugs Arthritis Rheumatism 28: 1168–1169
8. Lanza FL, Royer Gl, Nelson RS (1980) Endoscopic evaluation of the effects of aspirin, buffered aspirin and enteric-coated aspirin on gastic and duodenal mucosa. New Engl J Med 303: 136–138
9. Johansson C, Kollberg B, Nordemar R, Samuelsson K, Bergström S (1980) Reduction of gastrointestinal bleeding by oral prostaglandin E_2 during indomethacain treatment of rheumatic patients. Gastroenterology 78: 479–783
10. Cohen MM, Cheung G, Lyster DM (1980) Prevention of aspirin-induced faecal blood loss by prostaglandin E_2. Gut 21: 602–606
11. Hunt JN, Franz DR (1981) Effect of prostaglandin E_2 on gastric mucosal bleeding caused by aspirin. Dig Dis Sci 26: 301–306
12. Garner A (1977) Influence of Salicylates on the Rate of Accumulation of deoxyribonuchic acid in gastric washings from the guinea pig. Toxical and Pharmacol 42: 119–128
13. Silvoso GR, Ivery KJ, Butt JH, Lockard OO, Holt SD, Sisk C, Baskin WN, Mackercher PA, Hewett J (1979) Incidence of gastric lesions in patients with rheumatic disease on chronic aspirin therapy. Ann Int Med 91: 517–520
14. Tympner F (1981) Gastroscopic findings after therapy with non-steroidal antirheumatic drugs. Z Rheumatol 40: 179–181
15. Conn HO, Blitzer BL (1976) Nonassociation of adrenocorticosteroid therapy and peptic ulcer. New Engl J Med 294: 473–479
16. Kurata JH, Elashoff JD, Grossman M (1982) Inadequacy of the literature on the relationship between drugs, ulcers, and gastrointestinal bleeding. Gastroenterology 82: 372–382
17. Aspirin Myocardial Infarction Study Group (1980) a randomized controlled trial of aspirin in persons recovered from myocardial infarction. J Am Med Assoc 243: 661–669
18. Levy M (1974) Aspirin use in patients with major upper gastrointestinal bleeding and peptic-ulcer disease. New Engl J Med 290: 1158–1162
19. Aly A, Green K, Johansson C (1984) Prostaglandin E_2 in basal gastric secretion and during stimulation of muscarinic receptors in man; measurements with gas chromatography – mass-spectrometry. Acta Physiol 122: 583–584
20. Aly A, Selling JA, Hogan DL, Isenberg J, Koss MA, Johansson C (1985) Gastric and duodenal prostaglandin E_2 in humans. Gastroenterology 88: 1305

21. Whittle BJR (1976) Relationship between the prevention of rat gastric erosions and the inhibition of acid secretion of prostaglandins. Eur J Pharmac 40: 233–239
22. Flemström G (1981) Gastric secretion of bicarbonate. In: Physiology of the Gastrointestinal tract. (Ed Johnsson RL, Christensson J, Grossman MI, Jacobsson ED, Schultz SG). Raven Press, N.Y. 603–616
23. Ros IN, Bahari HMM, Turnberg LA (1981) The pH gradient across mucus adherent to rat fundic mucus in vivo and the effects of potential damaging agents. Gastroenterology 81: 713–718
24. Parke DV, Lindup WE, Shillingford JS (1975) The effects of ulcerugenic and ulcerhealing drugs on gastric mucus. Gut 16: 316
25. Brodie DA, Chase BJ (1967) Role of gastric acid in aspirin-induced gastric irritation in the rat. Gastroenterology 53: 604–610
26. Brodie DA, Cook PG, Bauer BJ, Dayle GE (1970) Indimethacin-induced interstinal lesions in the rat. Toxicol Appl Pharmacol 17: 615–624
27. Robert A (1977) Resistance of germfree rats to indomethacain-induced intestinal lesion in Prostaglandins 14: 333–341
28. Domschke W, Domschke S, Hornig D, Demling L (1978) Prostaglanding-stimulated gastric mucus secretion in man. Acta Hepato Gastroenterol 25: 292–294
29. Johansson C, Aly A, Kollberg B, Rubio C, Erikoinen T, Helander HF (1982) Oral E_2 prostaglandins stimulato growth of the rat stomach, small intestine and colon. Advances in Prostaglandin, Thromboxane and Leukotriene Research 12: 403–407
30. Tytgat GN, Henzen Logmans SC, van Minnen AJ (1984) Human gastric mucosal changes after oral 15(R)15 methyl prostaglandin E_2 adminatration. Gastroenterology 82: 1200
31. Uribe A, Rubio C, Johansson C (1986) Action of E_2 prostaglandins on cell kinetics in rat gastric and intestinal epithelia. Sc J Gastroenterol 21: 246–252
32. Robert A, Nezamis JE, Lancaster C, Hachar AJ (1979) Cytoprotection by prostaglandins in rats. 77: 433–443
33. Isenberg JI, Smedfors B, Johansson C (1985) The effects of graded doses of intraluminal H^+ prostaglandins E_2 and inhibition of prostaglandin synthesis on proximal duodenal bicarbonate secretion in the unanesthetized rat. Gastroenterology 88: 303–307
34. Johansson C, Bergström S (1982) Prostaglandins and protection of the gastroduodenal mucosa. Scand J Gastroenterol suppl 77: 21–46
35. Ruppin H, Person B, Robert A, Domschke W (1981) Gastric cytoprotection in man by prostaglandin E_2. Scand J Gastroenterol 16: 647–652
36. Hollander D, Tarnawski A, Gergety H, (1984) Sucralfate protection of the gastric mucosa against ethanol induced injury. Scand J Gastroenterol 19: 97–102
37. Szabo S, Trier JS, Frankel PW (1981) Sulfhydryl components may mediate gastric cytoprotection. Science 214: 200–203
38. Konturek SJ, Radecki T, Brzozowski T, Piasticki I, Dembinski A, Dembiaska-Kie A, Zmuda A, Gryglewski R, Gregory H (1981) Role of mucosal prostaglandins and DNA synthesis in gastric cytoprotection by luminal epidermal growth factor. Gut 22: 927–932
39. Derelnako MJ, Long JF (1981) Carbenoxolone Sodium protects rat gastric mucosa against ethanol induced necrosis. Proc Exp Biol Sci 166: 394–397
40. Malandrino S, Fumagilli G, Melillo G, Caselli G, Borsa M, Tonon EC (1986) Int Conf on Prostaglandins Abstract Florence p 210
41. Kollberg B, Isenberg JI, Johansson C (1984) Cytoprotective effect of oral omeprazole in the rat gastric mucose. Medianisms of mucosal protection Allen A et el. (eds). Raven Press, New York 351–356

Discussion Following the Report of Prof. Johansson

DOMSCHKE

How shall we proceed in the clinical setting until the problem has been definitely resolved? Shall a patient who is to be put on a long-term treatment with nonsteroidal anti-inflammatory drugs be advised to take simultaneously H_2 blockers, or shall he take concomitantly a prostaglandin preparation? What would you recommend?

JOHANSSON

I am not prepared to answer this question. There are too few clinical studies to support coadministration with H_2-receptor blockers or with prostaglandins. Of course, if you deplete the stomach of prostaglandins, it seems more logical to give a prostaglandin as supplementary therapy than any other compound. Yet, this has to be found out in clinical trials.

DOMSCHKE

So at present it seems to be an open question as to which prophylactic means should be preferred in NSAID therapy, either concomitant H_2 blocker or prostaglandin administration. Is this correct?

JOHANSSON

We do not have sufficent clinical data. There is no study in rheumatoid arthritis patients in which long-term treatment with NSAID has been combined with either an H_2 receptor-blocking agent or a prostaglandin. We have coadministered PGE_2 for a period of 6 weeks in an open study of a limited number of RA patients. Apparently, 2.5 mg PGE_2 daily does not counteract the beneficial effect of the nonsteroidal anti-inflammatory drug on the joint symptoms.

COHEN

I have a comment on the question that you have just asked, whether an H_2 blocker would be an appropriate drug to use for the prevention of injury in a patient taking non-steroidals. I think we should remember that there is at least theoretical evidence that an H_2 blocker might, in fact, be harmful here; while, on the one hand, it reduces the amount of acid present in the lumen, on the other, it turns off active secretion. There is also at least experimental evidence that a mucosa, where secretion is inhibited, is a mucosa which is more susceptible to damage by non-steroidal anti-inflammatory drugs.

JOHANSSON

This is an acute experiment, and it still has to be proven whether also correct in the long run. Achlorhydria is common in patients with rheumatoid arthritis, which may account for the fairly low prevalence of gastric lesions. For this reason such patients may have less, not more, need of protection against lesions during NSAID treatment.

BIANCHI PORRO

Also concerning this specific point, it could be interesting to know the results of a double-blind trial that we have just completed. We treated more than 250 patients with osteoarthritis and rheumatoid arthritis. They were endoscoped at the beginning, showing a normal gastroduodenal state, and then were randomized to ranitidine or to placebo and treated with anti-inflammatory drugs for 4 weeks, after which time endoscopy was repeated. In summary, we were not able to show any difference between the group "protected" with ranitidine and the group treated with placebo. The percentage of lesions of different degrees of severity was very similar; it was even a little higher in the ranitidine group.

JOHANSSON

This is the sort of studies we need in order to evaluate a possible beneficial effect of coadministered protective drugs.

RACHMILEWITZ

Just to complete the issue. Yesterday Professor Simon showed data, which we have recently collected in patients treated for 1 week either with indomethacin (150 mg/day) and concomitantly with cimetidine (400 mg, 800 mg) or placebo. We managed to show in an endoscopic study that cimetidine, but only the 800 mg dose, very significantly decreased the number of patients affected, and that in those affected, the severity of the damage was reduced. We also did a similar study with randitidine showing no protective effect.

DOMSCHKE

This is quite an interesting aspect, as it shows in this specific situation a superiority of cimetidine over ranitidine.

JOHANSSON

Or just different proportions of achlorhydric patients, in the two treated groups.

GRAHAM

I have a question for Dr. Rachmilewitz. Not that you have done that study, but what have you learned?

RACHMILEWITZ

I believe this is related to the quesion I asked you yesterday. I think that if I had to take a nonsteroidal anti-inflammatory drug for an acute reason today, I would take it together with cimetidine 800 mg/day.

DOMSCHKE

Thank you for this very definite answer.

SZABO

You presented a nice review, and you seem to ascribe a general role to bicarbonate secretion, but Dr. Flemström was more specific yesterday. He made the point that bicarbonate and mucus are the first defense against acid and pepsin but not against ethanol and lesion-inducing drugs. I am surprised that you did not mention your own nice model and study, which you published recently in a letter to the *Lancet*, showing that local application of prostaglandins to leg ulcers accelerated the healing. Firstly, this was a human model, and, secondly, you could exclude bicarbonate and mucus and nevertheless had an accelerated healing – probably due to epithelialization, granular-tissue proliferation, or increased blood flow. What is the bottom line there? What do you think is the mechanism of action, and did you continue your studies?

JOHANSSON

The reason for using PGE_2 as a local treatment of skin ulcers was to examine whether ulcer-healing properties of the compound were a general phenomenon. If locally applied PGE_2 accelerates healing of a long-standing leg ulcer, it can hardly be attributed to its acid (HCl) antisecretory effects. This was an open study, including 14 patients with chronic leg ulcers resistant to all other medical treatment for at least 2.5 years. The results are promising and a controlled study is now planned. Moreover, it is a clinical situation, in which one knows that the given compound reaches the ulceration.

SZABO

Have you included new patients into the study?

JOHANSSON

Only 14 so far. These studies last very long, for healing in skin ulcers is much slower than in peptic ulcers. One therefore needs a lot of patience.

REES

May I just come back to your slide on the American myocardial infarction study? It is a small point, but I think we have to be very careful when interpreting these findings. I have been in correspondence with an author of this study, and it is a shame that, while this was potentially a superb study to look prospectively at the effects of aspirin on the healthy stomach, the study was designed by cardiologists and not by gastroenterologists, and the incidence of peptic ulcer disease was evaluated using barium meal and not endoscopy. This may well account for the very low incidence of PU in the groups. Secondly, they examined different numbers of placebo-treated and aspirin-treated patients, i.e., they studied symptomatic subjects and not equal numbers of each group. So I think we have to be very careful in the interpretion because of the methods used and the way in which they analyzed the patient groups. If you look at it in further detail, there are also some curious findings. For example, the incidence of hematemesis and melena was not different in the two groups, while acute rectal bleeding was significantly higher in the aspirin group.

JOHANSSON

You are perfectly correct. It was a study just of ulcer symptoms during aspirin treatment. However, it is the only prospective study available. It seems improbable that the very low incidence of peptic ulcers in treated patients (compared to the incidence in most Western countries) could be attributed entirely to methodology.

GRAHAM

One other point about the same study, the one I showed yesterday, is that the relative risk for a diagnosable ulcer, relates to dosage intake. The cardiovascular studies by and large used relatively low doses. The fact is that there is a dose-response curve responsible for the FDA recommending even a lower dose for the prevention of cardiovascular events. So I think it also explains the low ulcer frequency.

LANGMAN

In examining aspirin studies, you come back to what the risk is. And if this is only a doubling or a tripling, then, as we said yesterday, you must have an enormous study to show something is there. This is why nonsteroidal anti-inflammatories are shown to be free of gastric side effects when they are released.

DOMSCHKE

Just an extension of this topic: What do you think of starting with low doses of aspirin, to take advantage of this potential adaptation phenomenon which you have alluded to during your presentation? Moreover, with regard to clinical practice, I should like to ask: What do you think about these microencapsulated formulations of acetylsalicylic acid? Are they less harmful?

JOHANSSON

As to your first question, I think this has to be clinically investigated before we can answer to it. As to the second, I am not so sure. Intestinal lesions have been reported following treatment with nonsteroidal anti-inflammatory drugs. If you take a slow-release drug and happen to swallow it just before an interdigestive migrating complex, you will propulse the drug to a certain level in the intestine, where it will stay for another 90–150 min., probably giving rise to a very high local concentration of the ulcerogenic drug. This is likewise the case with slow-release potassium tablets. Personally, I would rather take soluble aspirin than any slow-release form.

Exogenous Prostaglandins and Their Analogues in Gastric Ulcer Therapy

D. RACHMILEWITZ

Introduction

Prostanoids inhibit gastric acid secretion and exert cytoprotective properties. In patients with active duodenal and gastric ulcers [1, 2] decreased endogenous prostanoid synthesis was reported. Synthetic prostanoids are effective in the treatment of duodenal ulcer though healing rates are somewhat lower than those achieved with H_2-blockers [3]. In patients with gastric ulcer, hyperacidity is probably less important than in patients with duodenal ulcer, and therefore synthetic prostanoids may be of special value in the induction of healing.

The present report summarizes the results of published [4–6] clinical trials in which the efficacy of synthetic prostanoid analogues, misoprostol and enprostil, in the healing of gastric ulcer was compared to that of placebo and H_2-blockers.

Misoprostol, a synthetic PGE_1 analogue, inhibits the secretion of gastric acid and pepsin in man [7] and increases duodenal bicarbonate and mucus secretion [7–8]. It does not decrease gastric blood flow [9] nor modify the gastrin response to a standard test meal [10]. Misoprostol protects against the damaging effects of bile [11], alcohol [12], and aspirin [13, 14]. Enprostil is a synthetic analogue of PGE_2. It also inhibits gastric acid secretion, stimulates mucus secretion, but is claimed to inhibit antral gastrin release.

Comparison of Misoprostol and Cimetidine

Patients had at least one benign gastric ulcer with a diameter of 0.5–2.5 cm which was proven endoscopically. The study was a multicenter double-blind, parallel-group comparison of two doses of misoprostol (50 μg and 200 μg) with 300 mg of cimetidine. Patients were treated four times daily and the duration of treatment was 4 weeks when endoscopic assessment was repeated. Healing rates were analyzed for three cohorts of patients:

1. the intent-to-treat group, in which all eligible patients who received at least one dose of study medication were included and all withdrawals and losses to follow-up were regarded as failures;
2. similar to the first cohort but excluding petients lost to follow-up and
3. similar to cohort 2, but also excluding patients withdrawn for reasons unrelated to treatment.

The healing rate was analyzed using log linear models to examine treatment differences. Global pain was graded as none, mild, moderate, or severe at each visit. The two-paired comparisons were performed separately at 2 and at 4 weeks using the Mann-Whitney test.

Study Population

A total of 628 patients received treatment, 14 of them did not meet the inclusion criteria and were therefore ineligible. As a result, the intent-to-treat cohort consisted of 178 patients in the misoprostol 50 μg group and 218 in each of the other two treatment groups. Five patients in each group were lost to follow-up. Seven patients in the misoprostol 50 μg group and five in each of the other two groups were withdrawn for reasons unrelated to treatment. Thus cohort 3 comprised 166 patients in the misoprostol 50 μg group and 208 patients in each of the other two groups.

Demographic Details. There were no marked differences in age or occupation between the three groups, but there were more men than women in each group. The proportion of men in the misoprostol 50 μg, 200 μg, and cimetidine groups was 67%, 63%, and 59%, respectively. The distribution of cigarette smokers to nonsmokers and of alcohol consumption was also similar in the three treatment groups.

Healing Rates

The difference in healing rates was similar in all three cohorts: misoprostol 200 μg was significantly better than 50 μg but not different from cimetidine (Table 1). Tobacco, alcohol usage, and gender had no statistically significant effect on treatment comparison (Table 2). At 4 weeks, however, the differences in the healing rates in smokers were quite marked, at 32% for misoprostol 50 μg, 46% for misoprostol 200 μg, and 58% for cimetidine.

In all three treatment groups, the incidence and severity of pain before therapy was similar, and there was a reduction in pain over time. At 2 weeks, cimetidine relieved

Table 1. Healing effect of 4-weekly therapy with misoprostol and cimetidine on gastric ulcer healing

Treatment group	Cohort 1		Cohort 2		Cohort 3	
	(*n*)	(%)	(*n*)	(%)	(*n*)	(%)
Misoprostol (50 μg)	70/178	39.3	70/173	40.5	70/166	42.2
Misoprostol (200 μg)	112/218	51.4	112/213	52.6	112/208	53.9
Cimetidine (300 mg)	126/218	57.8	126/213	59.2	126/208	60.6
Statistical significance						
Misoprostol (200 μg) vs. 50 μg (one-sided)	$P = 0.008$		$P = 0.008$		$P = 0.013$	
Misoprostol vs. cimetidine (two-sided)	$P = 0.16$		$P = 0.15$		$P = 0.13$	

Table 2. Effects of tobacco, alcohol consumption, and gender on gastric ulcer healing

	Healing rate			
	Misoprostol (50 μg) (%)	Misoprostol (200 μg) (%)	Cimetidine (300 μg) (%)	Overall (%)
Tobacco	32	46	58	46
No tobacco	54	60	57	57
Alcohol	37	58	61	53
No alcohol	40	49	57	49
Men	41	48	60	50
Women	36	57	55	51

pain significantly better than misoprostol 200 μg ($P = 0.047$), but at 4 weeks there was no significant difference. Misoprostol 200 μg relieved pain significantly better at 4 weeks than did the 50 μg dose ($P = 0.019$). However, pain is not always present when there is an active ulcer, and sometimes it is present when there is no ulcer [15, 16].

Side Effects

The number of patients reporting increased frequency of bowel function at 2 and 4 weeks was not significantly different between the treatment groups. The bowel habits of the majority of patients did not change. The only potentially important change in the biochemical variables was an increase in mean serum creatinine in the cimetidine group from 83.5 μmol/liter to 90.0 μmol/liter and 88.8 μmol/liter at 2 and 4 weeks, respectively. The increase was statistically significant in the misoprostol groups.

Comparison of Misoprostol and placebo

This was a multicenter randomized double-blind study in which two doses of misoprostol 25 μg q.i.d and 100 μg q.i.d were compared at 2, 4, and 8 weeks. Healing rates were analyzed according to the three cohorts previously described. A total of 304 patients entered the trial, five of whom were not eligible for analysis. The proportion

Table 3. Healing effect of 8-weekly therapy with misoprostol and placebo on gastric ulcer healing

Treatment group	Cohort 1		Cohort 2		Cohort 3	
	(*n*)	(%)	(*n*)	(%)	(*n*)	(%)
Misoprostol 25 μg	52/104	50.0	52/95	54,7	59/94	54.3
Misoprostol 100 μg	57/92*	62.0	57/85	67.1	54/79	68.4
Placebo	46/103	44.7	46/86	53.5	44/80	55.0

* $P < 0.042$ between treatment groups

of subjects healed at 2 and 4 weeks was greater in the misoprostol 100 μg q. i. d group, though it reached statistical significance only at 8 weeks and only in the intent-to-treat group, i.e., cohort 1 (Table 3). There was no difference among the three treatment groups in the decrease of ulcer pain. Mild self-limiting diarrhea was noted in 9.8% of patients treated with the high misoprostol dose, in 7.7% of patients treated with the low dose and in 1.9% of placebo – treated patients.

Efficacy of Enprostil

A total of 128 gastric ulcer patients were randomly assigned to receive treatment with either enprostil 70 μg b. i. d., enprostil 35 μg b. i. d., or with placebo. Patients were endoscoped following 2, 4, and 6 weeks of treatment. Ulcer healing rates are detailed in Table 4: there were no statistically significant differences in healing rates among the three groups at 2 and 4 weeks. At 6 weeks, the healing rate with enprostil 35 μg b. i. d was significantly better than with placebo ($P < 0.008$). The most common side effect was diarrhea which was mild and transient. In a second study 50 patients with gastric ulcer were randomly allocated to receive treatment with enprostil 70 μg b. i. d or with ranitidine. Endoscopy was repeated monthly for 3 months or until healing. Healing rates were similar in the two treatment groups.

In a third study, 100 patients with active gastric ulcer were randomized to receive enprostil 35 μg b. i. d. or ranitidine 150 mg b. i. d.. Endoscopy was performed biweekly for 2 months or until healing. Healing rates in the enprostil group were 22%, 58%, 80%, and 86% at 2, 4, 6, and 8 weeks. In the ranitidine-treated patients the corresponding healing rates were 22%, 66%, 84%, and 89% (Table 4). The differences were not statistically significant.

In conclusion, the synthetic prostanoids misoprostol and enprostil appear to be safe and effective in the treatment of gastric ulcer. However, their effects do not seem to be different from those of H_2-blockers.

Table 4. Effect of enprostil and ranitidine on gastric ulcer healing

		Healed ulcer at week				
Treatment group	*(n)*	2	4	6	8	12
	(%)	(%)	(%)	(%)	(%)	(%)
Enprostil 70 μg b.i.d.	36	17	50	71		
Enprostil 35 μg b.i.d.	35	17	53	82		
Placebo	32	16	35	52		
Enprostil 70 μg b.i.d.	25		64		92	92
Ranitidine 150 mg b.i.d.	25		52		88	100
Enprostil 35 μg b.i.d.	50	22	58	80	86	
Ranitidine 150 mg b.i.d.	50	22	66	84	89	

References

1. Rachmilewitz D, Ligumsky M, Fich A, Goldin E, Eliakim A, Karmeli F (1986) Role of endogenous gastric prostanoids in the pathogenesis and therapy of duodenal ulcer. Gastroenterology; 90: 963-9
2. Wright JP, Young GO, Klaff CJ, Weers LA, Price SK, Marks IN (1982) Gastric mucosal prostaglandin E levels in patients with gastric ulcer disease and carcinoma. Gastroenterology; 82: 263-7
3. Nicholson PA (1985) A multicentre international controlled comparison of two dosage regimens of misoprostol and cimetidine in the treatment of duodenal ulcer in outpatients. Dig Dis Sci; 30: 171S-177S
4. Agrawal NM, Saffouri B, Kruss DM, Callison DA, Dajani EZ (1985) Healing of benign gastric ulcer: a placebo-controlled comparison of two dosage regimens of misoprostol – a synthetic analogue of prostaglandin E_1. Dig Dis Sci 30: 164S-170S
5. Rachmilewitz D, Chapman JW, Nicholson PA (1986) A multicentre international controlled comparison of two dosage regimens of misoprostol with cimetidine in treatment of gastric ulcer in outpatients. Dig Dis Sci 31: 75S-80S
6. Proceedings of Symposium "Protective and therapeutic effects of gastrointestinal prostaglandins. Enprostil: a new therapeutic modality", Toronto, Canada (Nov 1985)
7. Wilson DE, Quadros E, Rajapaksa T, Adams A, Noar M (1986) Effects of misoprostol on gastric acid and mucus secretion in man. Dig Dis Sci; 31: 1269-1299
8. Isenberg JI, Hogan DL, Selling JA, Koss MA (1986) Duodenal bicarbonate secretion in humans: role of prostaglandins. Dig Dis Sci; 31: 130S (Abstract)
9. Leung FW, Miller JC, Guth PH (1986) Dissociated effects of misoprostol on gastric acid secretion and mucosal blood flow. Dig Dis Sci; 31: 86S-90S
10. McGuigan JE, Chang Y, Dajani EZ (1986) Effect of misoprostol, an antiulcer prostaglandin on serum gastrin in patients with diodenal ulcer. Dig Dis Sci; 31: 120S-125S
11. Fimme CJ, Blum AI (1983) Acid inhibition but no protection from bile salt damage by a prostaglandin E_1 analog in man. Gastroenterology; 84: 1151 (Abstract)
12. Agrawal NM, Godiwala T, Arimura A, Dajani EZ (1986) Comparative cytoprotective effects against alcohol insult: Misoprostol versus cimetidine. Dig Dis Sci; 31: 142S (Abstract)
13. Cohen MM, Clark L, Armstrong L, D'Souza J (1985) Reduction of aspirin-induced fecal blood loss with low dose of misoprostol tablets in man. Dig Dis Sci 30: 605-611
14. Hunt JN, Smith JL, Jiang CL, Kessler L (1984) Effect of synthetic prostaglandin E_1 analogue on aspirin-induced gastric bleeding and secretion. Dig Dis Sci; 28: 897-902
15. Misiewicz JJ (1978) Peptic ulceration and its correlation with symptoms. Clin Gastroenterology; 7: 571-582
16. Frost F, Ratibek I, Rune SJ, Birger-Jensen K, Godmand-Hoyer E, Krag E, Rask-Madsen J, Wulff HR, Garbol J, Gotlieb-Jensen K, Hojlung M, Nissen VR (1977) Cimetidine in patients with gastric ulcer: a multicentre controlled trial. Br Med J 2: 795-797

Exogenous Prostaglandins and their Analogues in Duodenal Ulcer Therapy

S. J. SONTAG

Introduction

The role of prostaglandins (PGs) in the gastrointestinal tract, especially concerning regulation of gastric secretion and protection of the mucosa, has recently captured the interest of the scientific community [1, 2].

After PGs of the E series were found to be potent inhibitors of basal and stimulated gastric acid in man [3, 4], investigation of their effects on ulcer disease followed. These naturally occurring PGs, however, were short lived and were rapidly inactivated by enzymes in human tissues [5]. Therapeutically useful compounds would have to be longer acting and able to resist rapid destruction. To solve this problem, various PG analogs were developed that were resistant to normal enzymatic metabolism, making them active in oral form and more potent than their naturally occurring counterparts. These synthetic analogs of PGE_1 and PGE_2, when administered orally in microgram amounts, inhibited histamine-, pentagastrin-, and food-stimulated gastric acid for up to five hours [6, 7].

The antisecretory properties of PGs, the ability of PGs to protect the gastric mucosa aganist a variety of noxious agents [8–12], and the evidence suggesting that ulcer is a PG deficiency state [13–15] theoretically provide a rationale for the therapeutic use of exogenous PGs in ulcer disease.

In an effort to determine whether administration of PG analogues would heal gastroduodenal ulcers, a number of pharmaceutical companies have begun clinical ulcer healing trials with newly developed synthetic PGs of the E series (Fig. 1).

To date, only four PG analogues have been subjected to double-blind controlled duodenal ulcer trials large enough to provide meaningful efficacy data: arbaprostil, enprostil, misoprostol, and rioprostil. Entrance and exclusion criteria were essentially similar for all studies. The characteristics of the study designs are shown in Table 1.

Overall Healing Rates

Figures 2–5 show the 4 week duodenal ulcer healing rates for the PG analogs enprostil, misoprostol, arbaprostil, and rioprostil and the comparative drugs, placebo, cimetidine, and ranitidine.

Table 1. Characteristics of double-blind controlled prostaglandin trials in duodenal and gastric ulcers. DU duodenal ulcer; MISO misoprostol; ARBA arbaprostil; ENP enprostil; CIM cimetidine; RAN ranitidine; PLA placebo; * statistically better than placebo; ** statistically better than 50 mcg misoprostol; + statistically better than enprostil.

Ref.	Ulcer type	PG analogue	Comparator.	Dose	Timing	Percent healed weeks 2	4	6	8	12	Antacids allowed	Countries	No. of evaluable patients	No. of invest
[16]	DU	MISO	PLA	50 mcg M	QID		45				yes	USA, Can., Arg., Kuwait	272	23
				200 mcg M			80*							
				P			54							
[17]	DU	MISO	PLA	100 mcg M	QID		65*				no	USA, Brazil Arg, Venez	227	15
				P			47							
[18]	DU	MISO	PLA	200 mcg M	BID		53				yes	USA, Canada	280	29
				400 mcg M			65*							
				P			42							
[19]	DU	MISO	PLA	200 mcg M	QID		61*			83*	yes	Hong Kong	229	1
				300 mcg M			71*			88*				
				P			36			59				
[20]	DU	MISO	CIM	50 mcg M	QID		43				no	Austrl., GB, Belg., Can., Fin, NL, Isr. Gre., Kor., Nor., S, Afr, Swe., W. Ger.	640	22
				200 mcg M			62*							
				300 mg C			72**							
[21]	DU	MISO	NONE	200 mcg M	QID		65		87		yes	GB, Ire.	416	16
				400 mcg M	BID		69		88					
[22]	DU	ARBA	PLA	150 mcg A	QID		67*				yes	Belg., Pol., Hol., Fra.	173	4
				P			39							

Table 1. (Continued)

Ref.	Ulcer type	PG analogue	Comparator.	Dose	Timing	Percent healed weeks 2	4	6	8	12	Antacids allowed	Countries	No. of evaluable patients	No. of invest
				35 mcg E		20	65*					Can., N. Zea.,		
[23]	DU	ENP	PLA	70 mcg E	BID	37*	78*				yes	GB, Nor.	114	5
				P		14	39							
				35 mcg E		38	70*							
[24]	DU	ENP	PLA	P	BID	23	48				yes	USA	87 5	
				35 mcg E		40	75	84				Belg., Fra.		
[25]	DU	ENP	CIM	400 mg C	BID	42	77	87			yes	Swe., GB.	348	24
	DU	RIO	RAN	35 mcg E		51	74	85						
[26]				150 mcg R	BID	65^{+}	89^{+}	88^{+}			yes	Denmark	163	2
	DU	RIO	RAN	600 mcg Rio	HS	54	84							
[27]				300 mg R		54	90				no	W. Ger.	208	4

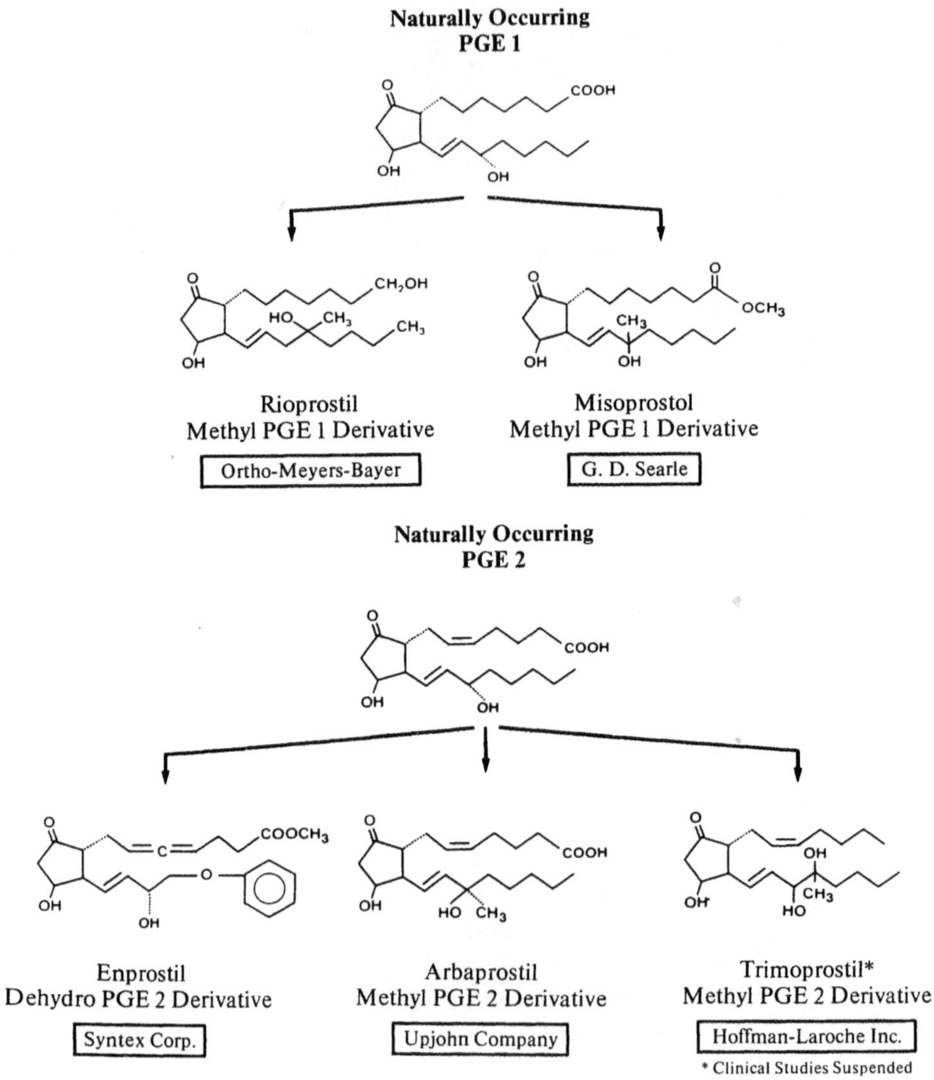

Fig. 1. Newly developed synthetic PGs of the E series

Enprostil

More than 700 patients from 10 countries have been enrolled in 4 controlled duodenal ulcer trials of enprostil. Enprostil 35 mcg twice daily resulted in healing rates at 4 weeks of between 65% and 75% [23–26]. Although 70 mcg twice daily of enprostil had a healing rate at 4 weeks of almost 80% [23], the high incidence of diarrhea (51%) prevents its therapeutic usefulness. In 2 non-placebo controlled trials the 4 week healing rates of 35 mcg enprostil bid were similar to 400 mg cimetidine bid in one [25], but statistically inferior to 150 mg ranitidine bid in the other [26].

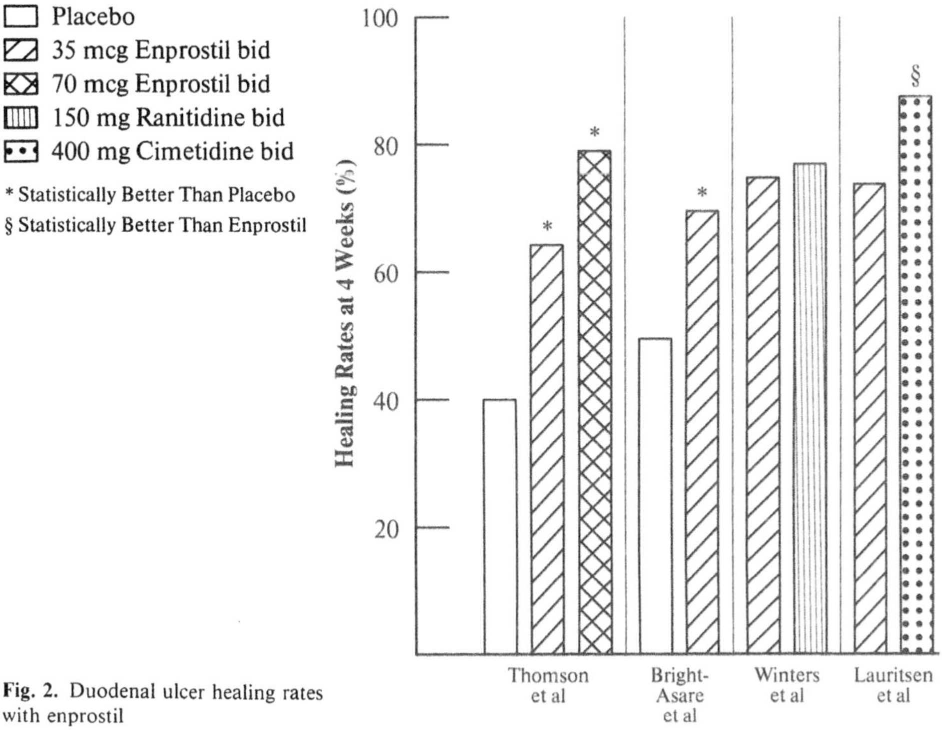

Fig. 2. Duodenal ulcer healing rates with enprostil

Misoprostol

More than 2,000 patients from 20 countries have been enrolled in 6 controlled duodenal ulcer trials. Four times daily of 50 mcg misoprostil, a dosage considered to be non-antisecretory, was no better than placebo in healing duodenal ulcers [16, 20]. Healing rates expressed in terms of percent difference greater than placebo show a definite dose response curve with virtually all qid doses above 50 mcg and the bid dose of 400 mcg being effective in healing ulcers (Fig. 4).

Arbaprostil

One hundred seventy-three patients from 4 countries were enrolled in one duodenal ulcer trial [22]. Although superiority of arbaprostil over placebo was demonstrated, the trial was marred by inconsistent healing rates among investigators. Indeed, one center entered only patients with refractory ulcers, resulting in considerably lower healing rates.

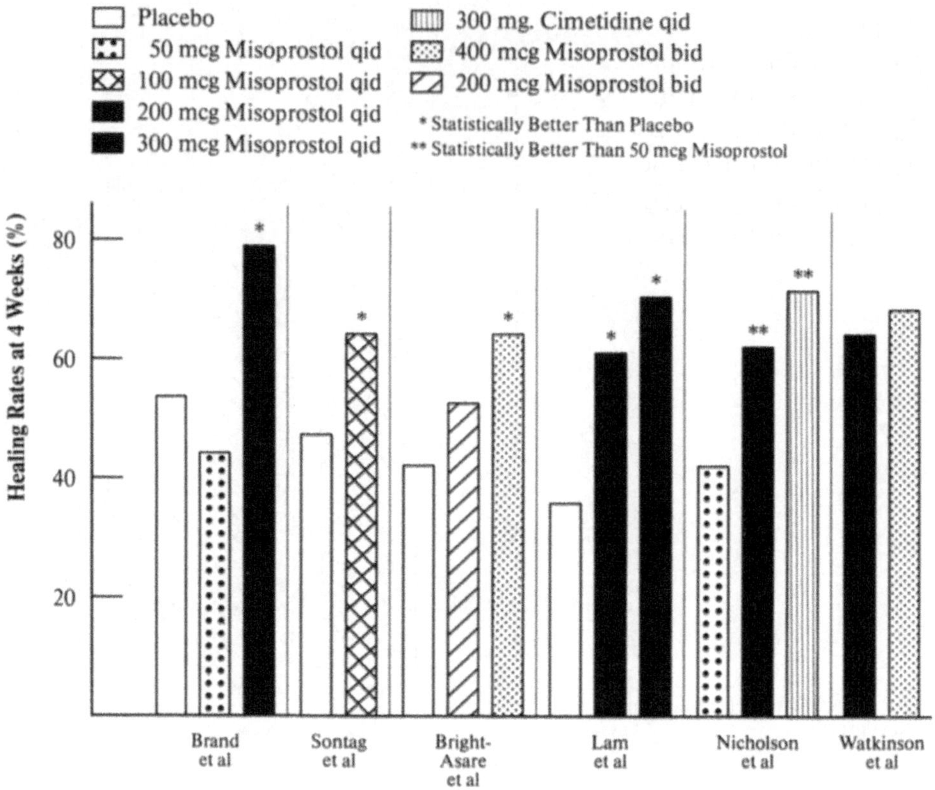

Fig. 3. Duodenal ulcer healing rates with misoprostol

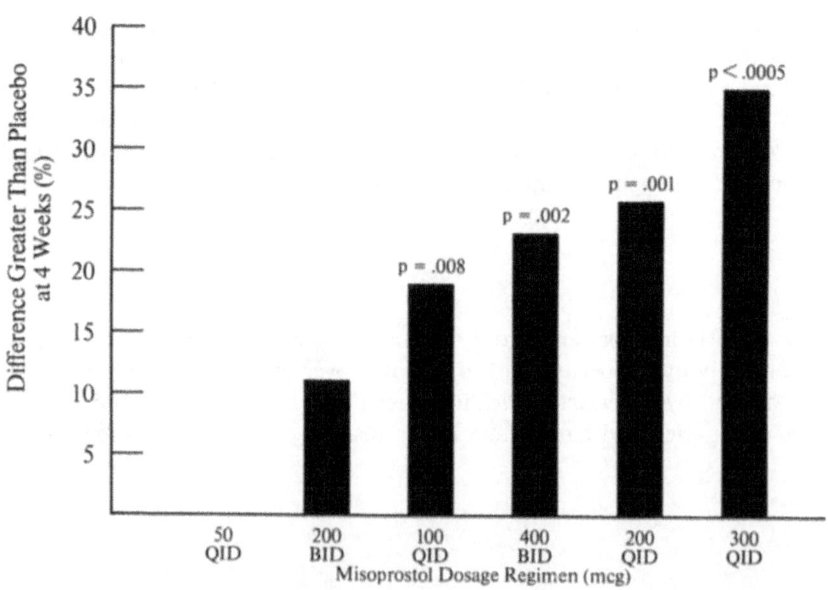

Fig. 4. Misoprostol healing as expressed as percent healed greater than placebo

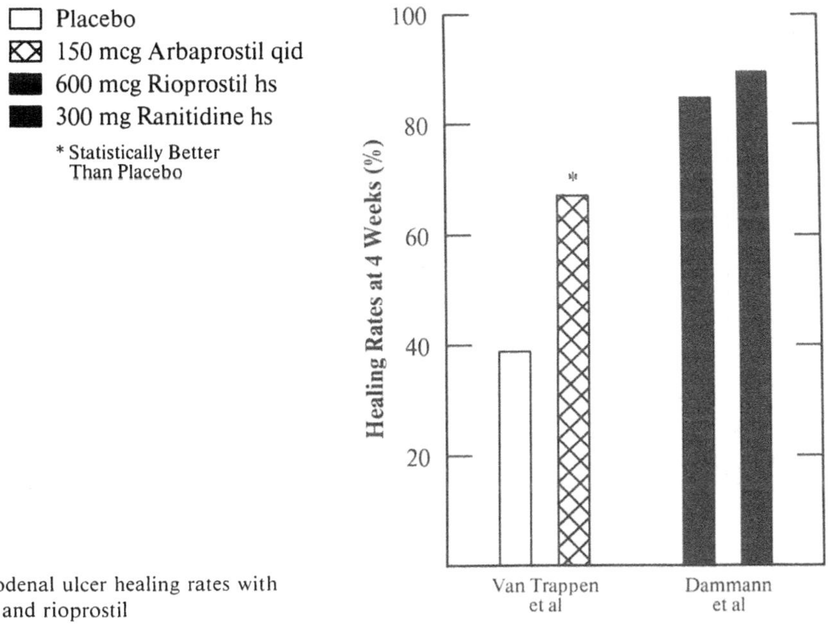

Fig. 5. Duodenal ulcer healing rates with arbaprostil and rioprostil

Rioprostil

Two hundred and eight patients were enrolled in a controlled clinical trial of night-time therapy only [27]. Ranitidine 300 mg hs was compared to rioprostil 600 mcg hs (Fig. 5). Healing rates at 4 weeks were similar in both groups (90% vs 84%) suggesting that one dose at night of a PG analog may be effective in healing duodenal ulcers.

From these studies, PGs are indeed effective in healing duodenal ulcers. The mechanism by which healing occurs, however, is still not certain. For instance, for misoprostol, the non-antisecretory doses that in other studies protected against aspirin injury were not effective in healing duodenal ulcers. For duodenal ulcers, at least, it appears that antisecretory doses of PGs are needed to speed healing. Although it is possible that mucosal protection occurs only with some acid reduction, mucosal protection as the mechanism of ulcer healing in these studies remains theoretical. For enprostil, both doses (35 mcg and 70 mcg) that were effective in healing ulcers [23–26] also significantly inhibited gastric acid secretion; non-antisecretory doses were not studied. Once again, mucosal protection alone as an ulcer healing mechanism was not demonstrated with enprostil. For rioprostil, ulcers healed with a single antisecretory dose at night; daytime gastric acid was not significantly suppressed.

Effect of Smoking on Healing Rates

Cigarette smoking is a major risk factor for the development [28] and recurrence [29, 30] of peptic ulcer. The effect of smoking on ulcer healing in studies large enough to provide adequate data is shown in Figures 6–8.

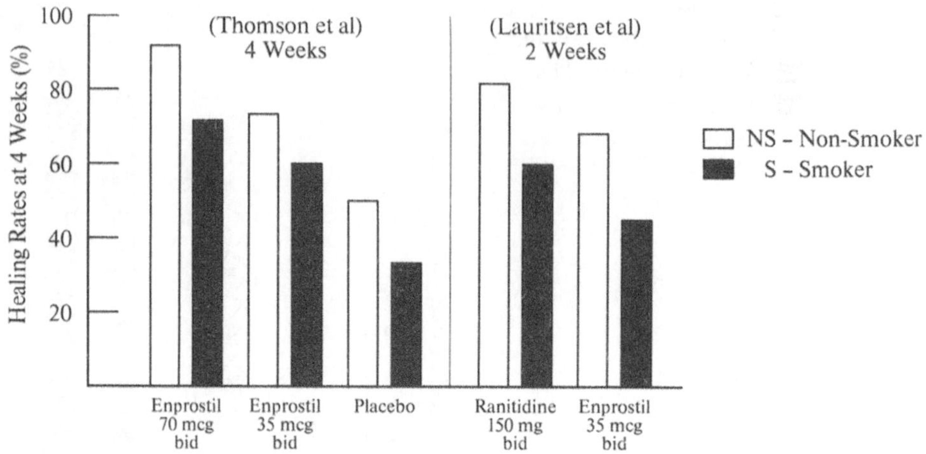

Fig. 6. Effect of smoking on ulcer healing: Enprostil trials

In the enprostil studies (Fig. 6), smokers consistently had lower healing rates than non-smokers. Neither enprostil nor ranitidine appeared to protect smokers.

Misoprostol, on the other hand, at high doses appeared to provide some protection for smokers (Fig. 7), with similar healing rates for smokers and non-smokers only at the 200 mcg qid dose. It is interesting to note that smokers required 200 mcg misoprostol qid to accomplish what misoprostol did in non-smokers at 100 mcg qid. A second study [19] also showed that smokers and non-smokers had similar healing rates when misoprostol was taken at a dose of 200 mcg or 300 mcg qid.

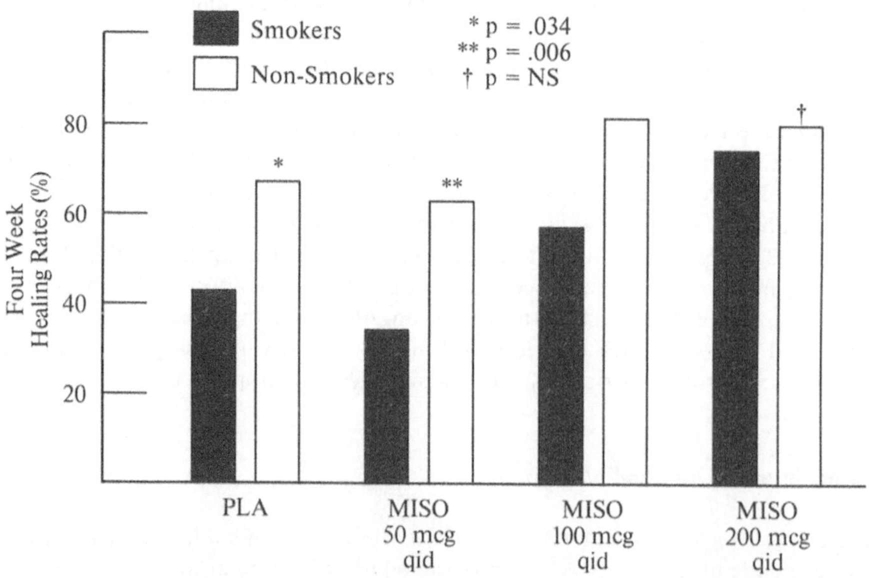

Fig. 7. Effect of smoking on ulcer healing

Table 2. Effect of PGs on pain relief and antacid consumption

Study		Pain relief	Antacid consumption	Ref.
E-35, *E*-70	*P* (b.i.d.)	*E*-35 Superior to *P* at 2 & 4 wks at night	No differences (*E*-70 b.i.d Trend)	[23]
E-35	*P* (b.i.d.)	No differences	No differences	[24]
E-35, *C*-400	(b.i.d.)	*C* Superior to *E* only at night	Data not analyzable	[25]
E-35, *R*-150	(b.i.d.)	*R* Superior to *E* only at weeks 5 & 6	–	[26]
RIO-600, *RAN*300 (hs)		No differences	–	
M-50, *M*-200	*P* (q.i.d.)	No differences	Signif for *M*-200 only during third week	[16]
M-100	*P* (q.i.d.)	No differences	–	[17]
M-200, *M*-300	*P* (q.i.d.)*	*M* Superior to *P* at 4 weeks and beyond	*M* Superior to *P* at 4 weeks and beyond	[19]
M-50, *M*-200, *C*-300	(q.i.d.)*	*C* Superior to *M* at 2 and 4 weeks	–	[20]
M-200, *M*-400	*P* (b.i.d.)	No differences	No differences	[18]

Effect of PGs on Ulcer Symptoms

The effect on ulcer symptoms of PGs, H_2 blockers, and placebo is shown in Table 2. Misoprostol [19] 200 mcg or 300 mcg, qid was superior to placebo in relieving pain at 4 weeks and beyond (Fig. 8). In another study [20], cimetidine 300 mg qid was superior

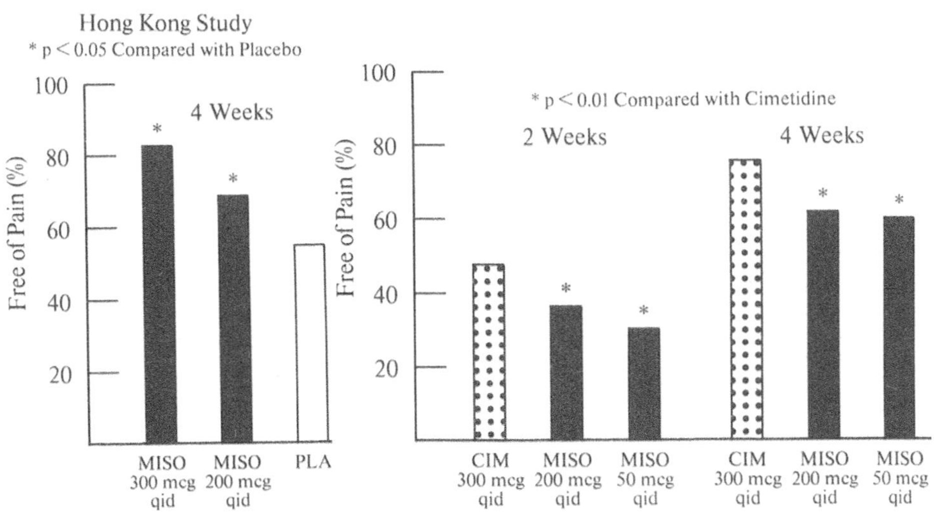

Fig. 8. Effect of cimetidine and misoprostol on ulcer pain

to misoprostol 200 mcg qid in relieving pain. In the remaining 8 studies, no important differences were apparent between the PG analog and either placebo or H_2 blocker.

Summary

Evidence available to date indicates that synthetic analogues of PGs heal duodenal ulcers only in doses that suppress gastric acid. There has not yet been demonstrated any consistent benefit to this class of drugs compared to already available conventional agents in the treatment of duodenal ulcer disease. It is possible, however, that non-antisecretory doses of PGs, by maintaining mucosal integrity and preventing ulcer recurrence, may eventually have a role in the treatment of ulcer desease.

Acknowledgments: The author wishes to acknowledge the assistance of Jean Seidel and the Loyola Medical Photography Department for their assistance in preparing this manuscript.

References

1. Miller TA (1983) Protective effects of prostaglandins against gastric mucosal damage: current knowledge and proposed mechanisms. Am J Physiol 245: 601–23
2. Hawkey CJ, Rampton DS (1985) Prostaglandins and the gastrointestinal mucosa: Are they important in its function, disease, or treatment? Gastroenterology 89: 1162–88
3. Robert A, Nezamis JE, Phillips JP (1967) Inhibition of gastric secretion by prostaglandins. Am J Dig Dis 12: 1073–6
4. Wilson DE, Phillips C, Levine RA (1971) Inhibition of gastric secretion in man by prostaglandin A_1. Gastroenterology 61: 201–6
5. Nelson NA, Kelly RC, Johnson RA (1982) Prostaglandins and the arachidonic acid cascade. Chemical & Engineering News 60: 30
6. Wilson DE, Winnan G, Quertermus J, et al (1965) Effects of an orally administered prostaglandin analog (16,16-dimethyl prostaglandin E_2) on human gastric secretion. Gastroenterology 69: 607–11
7. Konturek SJ, Kwiecien N, Swierczek J, et al (1976) Comparison of methylated prostaglandin E_2 analog given orally in the inhibition of gastric responses to pentagastrin and peptone meal in man. Gastroenterology 70: 683–7
8. Robert A, Nezamis JE, Lancaster C, et al (1979) Cytoprotection by prostaglandins in rats: Prevention of gastric necrosis produced by alcohol, HCl, NaOH, hypertonic NaCl, and thermal injury. Gastroenterology 77: 433–43
9. Jacobson ED, Chaudhury TK, Thompson WJ (1976) Mechanism of gastric mucosal cytoprotection by prostaglandins. Gastroenterology 70: A897
10. Robert A (1979) Cytoprotection by prostaglandins. Gastroenterology 77: 761–7
11. Ito S, Lacy ER (1985) Morphology of rat gastric mucosal damage, defense, and restitution in the presence of luminal ethanol. Gastroenterology 88: 250–60
12. Chaudhury TK, Jacobson ED (1978) Prostaglandin cytoprotection of gastric mucosa. Gastroenterology 74: 58–63
13. Dajani EZ, Callison DA, Bertermann RE (1978) Effects of E prostaglandins on canine gastric potential difference. Dig Dis Sci 436–42
14. Smith CL, Hillier K (1985) Duodenal mucosa synthesis of prostaglandins in duodenal ulcer disease. Gut 26: 237–40
15. Ahlquist DA, Dozois RR, Zinsmeister AR, Malagelada JR (1983) Duodenal prostaglandin synthesis and acid load in health and in duodenal ulcer disease. Gastroenterology 85: 522–9
16. Brand DL, Roufail WM, Thomson ABR, Tapper EJ (1985) Misoprostol, a synthetic PGE_1 analogue, in the treatment of duodenal ulcers: a multicentre double-blind study. Dig Dis Sci 30 (Suppl): 147–58

17. Sontag SJ, Mazure PA, Pontes JF, Beker SG, Dajani EZ (1985) Misoprostol in the treatment of duodenal ulcer. A multicentre double-blind, placebo-controlled study. Dig Dis Sci 30 (Suppl): 159–63
18. Bright-Asare P, Sontag SJ, Gould RJ, Brand DL, Roufail WM (1986) Efficacy of misoprostol (twice daily dosage) in acute healing of duodenal ulcer. A multicentre double-blind controlled trial. Dig Dis Sci 31 (Suppl): 63–7
19. Lam SK, Lau WY, Choi TK, et al (1986) Prostaglandin E_1 (misoprostol) overcomes the adverse effect of chronic cigarette smoking on duodenal ulcer healing. Dig Dis Sci 31 (Suppl): 68–74
20. Nicholson PA (1985) A multicentre international controlled comparison of two dosage regimes of misoprostol and cimetidine in the treatment of duodenal ulcer in outpatients. Dig Dis Sci 30 (Suppl): 171–7
21. Watkinson G, Shroff NE, Akbar FA (June 3–6, 1986) Misoprostol in peptic ulcer disease. International conference on prostaglandins and related compounds. Florence (Italy)
22. Vantrappen G, Janssens J, Popiela T, et al (1982) Effect of 15(R)-15-methyl prostaglandin E_2 (arbaprostil) on the healing of duodenal ulcer: A double-blind multicenter study. Gastroenterology 83: 357–63
23. Thomson ABR, Navert H, Halvorsen L, et al (1986) Treatment of duodenal ulcer with enprostil, a prostaglandin E_2 analog. Am J Med 81 (Suppl): 59–63
24. Bright-Asare P, Krejs GJ, Santangelo WC, et al (1986) Treatment of duodenal ulcer with enprostil, a prostaglandin E_2 analog. Am J Med 1986; 81 (Suppl): 64–8
25. Winters L, Willcox R, Ligny G, et al (1986) Comparison of enprostil and cimetidine in active duodenal ulcer disease: Summary of pooled European studies. Am J Med 81 (Suppl): 69–74
26. Lauritsen K, Laurits SL, Havelund T, et al (1986) Enprostil and ranitidine in duodenal ulcer healing: double-blind comparative trial. Brit Med J 292: 864–6
27. Dammann HG, Walter TA, Müller P, Simon B (1986) Night-time rioprostil versus ranitidine in duodenal ulcer healing. Lancet 2: 335–6 [LETTER]
28. Friedman GD, Seiglaub AB, Seltzer CC (1974) Cigarettes, alcohol, coffee, and peptic ulcer. N Engl J of Med 290: 469–73
29. Sonnenberg A, Müller-Lissner SA, Vogel E, et al (1981) Predictors of duodenal ulcer healing and relapse. Gastroenterology 1061–7
30. Sontag SJ, Graham DY, Belsito A, et al (1984) Cimetidine, cigarette smoking, and recurrence of duodenal ulcer. N Engl J of Med; 311: 689–93

Discussion Following the Reports of Prof. Rachmilewitz and Dr. Sontag

LANGMAN

Firstly, the evidence of prostaglandin deficiency in gastric ulcer is by no means complete; Chris Hawkey in our laboratory, for example, shows mainly a difference between having gastritis and not having gastritis, not related to ulcer. Secondly, I would like to attribute the findings in Jerusalem to intervention by Jehovah, as you do, but I think I must really attribute them to the failure of intervention by a statistician. What you need, is to quote confidence intervals; I think this is true for all the studies, and you can then get a better appreciation of different means between studies. The third point I would like to make is in relation to enprostil. We have looked at relapse rates after stopping treatment, and these do not look very different from the relapse curves for ranitidine. It looks as though they are fundamentally the same (Hawkey CJ (1986) Synthesis of prostaglandin E_2, thromboxane B_2 and prostaglandin catabolism in gastritis and gastric ulcer. Gut 27: 1484–1492).

RACHMILEWITZ

Just two comments. I definitely agree with you that the data about prostaglandin production in gastric ulcer are not complete. As to your second point: I thought that as a Briton you would have a sense of humor. No further comments.

WEIHRAUCH

I think, since the data on misoprostol and enprostil have been extensively reviewed, and the rioprostil nocte study has been mentioned, it would be appropriate and maybe of interest if Dr. Demol would give a short comment on the efficacy of rioprostil in placebo-controlled studies and in studies contrasting cimetidine and ranitidine, for this clinical program is also finished.

DEMOL

Two slides, please. Here are some of the results that we obtained in gastric ulcer. This is a multicenter European study comparing rioprostil (300 µg twice a day) with ranitidine (150 mg twice a day). Endoscopy was done at 4 and 8 weeks; in the first slide are the patients with healed ulcer. As you can see, there was no difference between the two treatments: 50% of patients were healed after 4 weeks and about 80% in both groups after 8 weeks. Here we have done analyses with confidence intervals, and there were no significant differences. The second slide shows the percentages of patients with pain. As you can once again see, in gastric ulcer there was no difference between rioprostil and ranitidine in relieving pain.

RASK-MADSEN

I should like to comment on Dr. Sontag's contribution since we have just finished our trial on ulcer recurrence during maintenance treatment with enprostil, 35 µg daily, versus ranitidine, 150 mg daily, for up to 12 months in 142 patients who had healed on either drug. There was a highly significant difference in recurrence rates at 3, 6, and

12 months, as judged by endoscopy (intent-to-treat cohorts), favoring ranitidine treatment also in the long term, since the recurrence rates observed in the enprostil group were not different from those observed during folow-up off treatment. I would also like to comment on the high healing rates observed in the Danish study. First of all, we have observed similar healing rates in duodenal ulcer patients following treatment with H_2 blockers in all trials based on patients from the Island of Funen, which has a population of some 400000.

SONTAG

Were all the patients referred from the X-ray department?

RASK-MADSEN

No, they were not referred from the X-ray department but directly from general practitioners who had no access tox-ray and did not have a specialist to refer to for endoscopy.

SONTAG

Were these patients the ones with the more difficult ulcers or did they more accurately represent the general population?

RASK-MADSEN

As you suggest, the study reflected what is daily life among patients.

DOMSCHKE

This is in direct association with the differences in the placebo healing rates found in Israel and the United States. Do you think this is a real difference, or could this rather be due to the endoscopic activity which might be different in Israel and in the US? To all evidence North Americans seem a bit more reluctant to perform endoscopies and do them a bit later than is the case in most European countries. So it might be that a negative selection of peptic ulcers is under therapy in the American studies as compared to the Israeli. Would you be kind enough as to speculate on this point?

RACHMILEWITZ

I really do not know the answer. In duodenal ulcers we have recruited about 400 patients for various trials in the past 2 or 3 years. We had a healing rate with placebo which reached about 66%; with cimetidine we had 93%. Worldwide the mean healing rate with H_2 blocker therapy is around 75%. I really do not have an explanation for the fact that in Israel healing rates are higher, and I therefore used a joke in presenting the data.

LANGMAN

I do agree fully with your point of view, because the situation in your country is quite comparable to that in Central Europe. I should like to ask Dr. Sontag: How are the endoscopic activities practiced in your Veterans' Administration Hospital in Hines?

SONTAG

At Hines we offer endoscopy to almost everyone with abdominal pain, and the X-ray department has much less work to do now. We usually perform endoscopy on the same day as they present to us, because patients may have travelled for 20 miles to get to Hines. If they come that far, they should have a definite answer. The placebo healing rate may be lower in Chicago than in Jerusalem or Europe because many patients in clinical trials in the United States are from lower socioeconomic groups; they may have more resistant ulcers.

RACHMILEWITZ

In America, as you know, at least from the physicians' own economic point of view, patients are endoscoped with great enthusiasm – though not in the VA system.

SONTAG

However, they do not often refer their private patients for the studies.

RACHMILEWITZ

That is correct.

REES

A question to both speakers. In the past, for the sake of cleanliness of the study, patients on nonsteroidal anti-inflammatory drugs have often been excluded from various placebo-controlled studies of H_2 antagonists. Do you have any data to suggest that patients with gastric ulcer or duodenal ulcer who are taking nonsteroidal anti-inflammatory drugs behave any differently in response to prostaglandin analogues? Clearly, as we have already heard, this may be an important group of patients in the future for clinicians to treat. Theoretically, I suppose this is an area in which prostaglandin analogues may play an important role.

RACHMILEWITZ

This is a different matter; you are right. They do not allow in all studies recruitment of patients who are to receive a nonsteroidal anti-inflammatory drug while on the study. And, to the best of my knowledge, there are no data available on healing rates achieved in this group of patients.

SONTAG

We exclude from most studies the people who really need the drug, such as those who have multisystem disease or who are taking NSAIDs. Therefore, the results of many studies are not representative for the general population.

DOMSCHKE

This discussion brings me to the central point, namely what are the indications for prostaglandin therapy at the present? As I see the situation, H_2 blockers remain the gold standard in peptic ulcer therapy, but there may be subpopulations of our peptic ulcer patients who might benefit from prostaglandin therapy. Among these may be patients taking long-term nonsteroidal anti-inflammatory drugs. A second group may include patients who are heavy smokers. And a third group of patients may be those with H_2 blocker refractory peptic ulceration. I should like to ask whether you share this view? Do you see additional subgroups of peptic ulcer patients who might be particulary susceptible to prostaglandin therapy? Let us concentrate the discussion on the question of indications for prostaglandin therapy. Would you be kind enough as to help me in answering this question, both of you, Dr. Sontag as well as Dr. Rachmilewitz?

SONTAG

I will be kind, but I can not help you answer the question. The specific indications for prostaglandin therapy in ulcer therapies are strictly theoretical. To my knowledge, there has been no study that has properly addressed this question. Patients who might benefit from prostaglandin therapy include smokers and patients who have refractory ulcers after 8 weeks of H_2 blocker therapy. The problem I see with prostaglandins is that they came after H_2 blockers. Had they come 15 years ago, then H_2 blockers may be having the same difficulty gaining acceptance. If one compares the healing rates in most studies, one sees that the results of H_2 blockers and those of prostaglandins are similar. There are no data to suggest that PGs are superior to available therapy, and there are, as far as I know, no properly planned studies to answer this question. There are studies appearing now, but I am not sure that they are designed to answer this question.

RACHMILEWITZ

I think you have outlined the problem very well. And really, unless one is a shareholder of Syntex or Searle, I think there is no real, objective justification to use any of the synthetic prostanoids available as a first-line choice at present. All the other possibilities have an "if" before them. Moreover, do not forget that with H_2 blockers we have great experience. They have been given to millions of people, and billions of tablets have been consumed, and I think we should be very happy with that. I think that objectively there is no justification to prescribe anything else as a first drug choice, except for one of the H_2 blockers.

GRAHAM

We have only anecdotal experience with nonsteroidal drug-associated ulcer patients. We are endoscoping symptomatic patients and do treat a few. It is my impression that they do heal quite well, despite the fact that a nonsteroidal anti-inflammatory drug is continued. Some of the patients we give no therapy, and their ulcers also heal, but more slowly. But the impression that I have, is that ulcers from patients treated with prostaglandins not only heal, but the mucosa endoscopically looks better. It often looks normal. Whereas in patients on H_2-receptor antagonists, even though the ulcer is gone, there are frequently red spots and erosions here and there. This is all impression, not evaluated in a prospective blinded fashion. And I do not know if better looking mucosa leads to a better patient, but if I were going to look for subpopulations for a specific indication for these drugs, I think this is where I would look.

SONTAG

I was going to say that, but our impressions of the beautifully normal mucosa seen on endoscopy are anecdotal. I do not feel as strongly as does Dr. Rachmilewitz about there being no indication for PGs as a first-line drug there. I think that the two classes of drugs are similar in duodenal ulcer healing rates. And I would have no problem with using them as a first-line drug in males, because they are relatively safe, if properly used. But I would not necessarily jump to using them as the first-line drug.

LANGMAN

Firstly, data are accumulating, including the Danish data and our own, that suggest H_2 blockers do tend to heal duodenal ulcers rather better than enprostil or misoprostol. Secondly, Australians have suggested that those with ulcers who continue to take salicylates do not seem to do any worse during ulcer healing treatment than those who stop taking them.

COHEN

I agree completely about the total lack of data to guide us as to which groups of patients would be appropriate for treatment with prostaglandin as the firs-line or even second-line therapy. I have two advantages which I would like to share. One is that I am a surgeon, and I see your treatment failures; the other is that we have available on the Canadian market a prostaglandin that we can use outside clinical trials. I do not have hard data, but I certainly have a number of experiences of patients with gastric ulceration on nonsteroïdal anti-inflammatory drugs, totally resistant to therapy with H_2 blockers, who are coming for surgery. At that point I have taken them off all therapy, except for the nonsteroidals and switched to prostaglandin. The ulcer promptly healed. Anecdotal, but I think it is a direction in which we might go with trials.

DOMSCHKE

I suppose these are the lines which should be followed in the future to define the patient groups who should be treated with prostaglandins as the second-line treatment modality.

SONTAG

I think we all have had similar experiences. Interestingly, cimetidine did not have to prove itself as thoroughly before it was released on to the market. Once cimetidine was released, further studies were very easy to do. But we are asking prostaglandins to do what the Almighty cannot do. And I think this is somewhat unfair since the drugs are safe when properly used, and they are effective. Once they are released, if they are released in the United States, the answer to your question, Dr. Domschke, will be forthcoming. But until released, the drug remains investigational and the real studies wil be very difficult to perform.

GRAHAM

The problem is not ulcer healing. Duodenal ulcers do heal. We know this from the past when we treated patients with milk or Maalox; Palmer treated his patients with gastric acid, chilly, and beans and their ulcers healed. When you look at every study shown, you always see the placebo rate never goes across or up, it goes down. So the problem is gastric ulcer, healing disease and ulcer recurrence, but it is not duodenal ulcer healing. And the slightly difference or slighty significant difference in healing rates does not mean much.

BIANCHI PORRO

I would like to comment on the problem of patients with gastric and duodenal ulcers on chronic administration of anti-inflammatory drugs. Because we have had the same impression as others, we treated in a double-blind fashion two groups of patients with gastric and duodenal ulcers during chronic administration of inflammatory drugs. And the healing rates obtained with both cimetidine and colloidal bismuth were not especially different from what we usually see in ordinary patients. This means healing rates of approximately 70%–75% after 4 weeks and a little higher, at 75%–80% after 8 weeks. Thus, under H_2 blocker therapy these patients seem to heal properly fast, inspite of the fact that they continue anti-inflammatory treatment. Interestingly enough, however, the patients who did not heal did not achieve healing after another 8 weeks of H_2-blocker therapy despite a withdrawal of anti-inflammatory drugs.

SZABO

My question is actually a follow-up to your attempt to define better the prostaglandin indication for treatment of ulcer disease and is question to both, Dr. Rachmilewitz and Dr. Sontag. Do any of these studies include a small subgroup of the so-called cimetidine-resistant ulcers? Do any of the studies deal with such a group of patients, and if so, was ist specifically tested whether these patients respond to any of the prostanoids?

SONTAG

These were not refractory studies at all. In fact, if patients had not responded to H_2 blockers, they were excluded from the studies.

SZABO

That is a pity, for this could be a good opportunity to compare PGs and H_2-receptor antagonists.

DOMSCHKE

Yes, and it could help in defining the appropriate indication for prostaglandin administration. Dr. Gitlin, e.g., presented a paper at the recent World Congress on Gastroenterology in São Paulo, describing H_2 blocker refractory duodenal ulceration being treated subsequently with misoprostol. Under these circumstances he could show a therapeutic success brought about by the prostaglandin analogue.

SONTAG

The problem with this study is that patients were deemed refractory if they had had only 4 or 8 weeks of treatment. The H_2 blocker was then stopped and the patients were randomized to placebo or misoprostol. Unfortunately the study did not really answer the question asked.

DOMSCHKE

So there might have been shortcomings in the study design; however, this is the first evidence in the right direction, I believe we can sum up by saying that studies of this kind are badly needed to define more precisely the indications for prostaglandin administration. This should be a challenge for future research.

Clinical Safety of Antiulcer Prostaglandins: An Overview

G. BIANCHI PORRO, and F. PARENTE

Introduction

The discovery that natural prostaglandins (PGs) of the E series inhibit gastric acid secretion [1] and prevent, at nonantisecretory dosage, experimentally induced ulcer caused by various noxious agents [2], suggested their potential usefulness as treatment for peptic ulcer. However, the progress toward the market for antiulcer PG has been hampered by some major disadvantages of natural PGE: first, a rapid metabolism which is responsible for the lack of activity after oral administration [3]; secondly, a wide variety of side effects due to their ubiquitous biological role in the human body [4]; and finally, a high chemical instability [5]. These problems have been to a great extend overcome by the development of PG synthetic analogues. At present, numerous PGE_1 and PGE_2 derivatives are under study as antiulcer agents; among these, four compounds have already reached phase III of pharmacological investigations: arbaprostil, misoprostol, enprostil, and rioprostil. Misoprostol and enprostil have proved to be effective in healing duodenal and gastric ulcer, both in placebo- and H_2 blocker-controlled studies [6] and they will soon be marketed in several countries.

To date, over 3000 patients from 20 countries and approximately 2500 patients from seven countries have completed participation in misoprostol- and enprostil-controlled clinical trials, respectively; thus data on their safety are available. The present article aims to establish the safety profile of antiulcer PGs by answering the following questions:

a) which are their most common unwanted effects;
b) what is the incidence of PG side effects compared to other antiulcer drugs (i. e., H_2 blockers);
c) how clinically relevant are these side effects?

Characterization of Unwanted Effects

The most common unwanted effects reported in placebo-controlled studies on misoprostol are summarized in Table 1. The drug was administered orally in doses ranging from 50 µg to 200 µg four times daily to 407 patients for the treatment of duodenal or gastric ulcers; placebo was given to 314 patients. The vast majority of recorded complaints was limited to the gastrointestinal tract and included diarrhea, nausea, vomiting, and abdominal pain; only occasional involvement of other organ systems was registered. These side effects correspond exactly to those observed among

Table 1. Most common unwanted effects observed in placebo-controlled studies on misoprostol in peptic ulcer treatment [7–9] (Adapted from [10])

Adverse effect	Misoprostol 50 μg q.i.d. (n = 101) (%)	Misoprostol 100 μg q.i.d. (n = 199) (%)	Misoprostol 200 μg q.i.d. (n = 107 (%)	Placebo (n = 314) (%)
Diarrhea	4.0	9.5	13.1	3.8
Nausea	3.0	5.0	2.8	4.1
Headaches	0	6.0	0.9	2.9
Vomiting	0	3.5	0.9	3.2
Abdominal pain	0	3.5	0	1.6
Aches/pain	2.0	2.0	0.9	2.5
Fatigue	4.0	1.0	0	1.6
Rash	1.0	2.0	0	1.9
Constipation	0	1.5	1.9	1.6

healthy volunteers in preclinical studies and they probably represent functional disturbances related to the physiological effect of PGE on the gastrointestinal system.

Diarrhea was the leading complaint occurring in this series with an overall prevalence of 9.1% ; it appeared, however, clearly dose-related with the lowest rate (4%) being observed on misoprostol 50 μg q.i.d. as compared to frequencies of 9.5% and 13.1% in patients who received 100 μg and 200 μg q.i.d., respectively. The latter rates were noticeably higher than the ones recorded in the placebo group (3.8%).

Similarly, in placebo-controlled studies on enprostil in peptic ulcer treatment the only adverse effect reported with significantly greater frequency than placebo was diarrhea; data from two clinical trials are available: in the one of Navert et al. [11] diarrhea occurred in 32% of patients receiving low doses of enprostil (35 μg b.i.d.) and in 51% of those receiving high doses (70 μg b.i.d.), in comparison to 17% of patients on placebo. In the study of Bright-Asare et al. [12] the incidence of diarrhea was 14% in patients on enprostil, 35 μg b.i.d, and 2% in those receiving placebo. As regards the behaviour of biochemical parameters monitored during short-term treatment, worldwide no clinically significant changes attributable to the drug have been observed with misoprostol [10], while the only change seen with enprostil was a lowering in serum cholesterol [13].

Comparative Evaluation of Unwanted Effects

The reported incidence of unwanted effects in comparative studies with H_2 blocker resembles those previously described. Pooled data from three double-blind comparisons of cimetidine and misoprostol in short-term treatment of 1094 patients with duodenal or gastric ulcer are presented in Table 2. The most common adverse effect secondary to the administration of misoprostol was abdominal pain, followed by diarrhea, dyspepsia, and nausea. Particularly, it must be noted that in comparison with cimetidine the overall incidence of gastrointestinal complaints with misoprostol was much higher, whereas for central nervous system effects the incidence was lower.

Table 2. Most common unwanted effects observed in cimetidine-controlled studies on misoprostol in peptic ulcer treatment. (Data from [14–16])

Adverse effect	Misoprostol 200 μg q.i.d. (*n* = 552) (%)	Cimetidine 300 mg q.i.d. (*n* = 542) (%)
Abdominal pain	17.4	12.0
Diarrhea	5.4	2.2
Dyspepsia	5.4	3.3
Nausea	5.1	3.3
Flatulence	3.1	1.3
Headache	2.5	4.1
Dizziness	0.5	1.1

A similar pattern has occurred in cimetidine-controlled clinical trials with enprostil as shown in Table 3. On the whole, the incidence of side effects with enprostil was roughly comparable to that with cimetidine, but digestive system complaints were much more frequently observed with enprostil, while central nervous system effects were approximately twice as frequent in the cimetidine group.

Table 3. Most common side effects registered in cimetidine-controlled studies on enprostil in peptic ulcer therapy. (Data from [17])

Adverse effect	Enprostil 35 μg b.i.d. (*n* = 180) (%)	Cimetidine 400 mg b.i.d. (*n* = 174) (%)
Diarrhea	8.3	2.3
Abdominal pain	3.3	0.6
Constipation	3.3	1.7
Nausea	2.2	1.1
Flatulence	2.2	0
Headache	1.7	2.9
Dizziness	1.6	2.3

If we specifically look at the complaint of diarrhea, we find a wide variation in its frequency from study to study, both with misoprostol and enprostil, which appears to be only partially related to the daily dosage of the drug. In fact, as it emerges from Fig. 1, the incidence of diarrhea for misoprostol, 200 μg q.i.d., in controlled trials was reported to range from 4% to 25%, while for enprostil, 35 μg b.i.d., it ranged from 5% to 32%. Such wide variability could probably be explainded by the lack of a narrow definition of the symptom in many studies, so that minor changes in bowel habits, such as soft or liquid stool, have been included and classified as diarrhea.

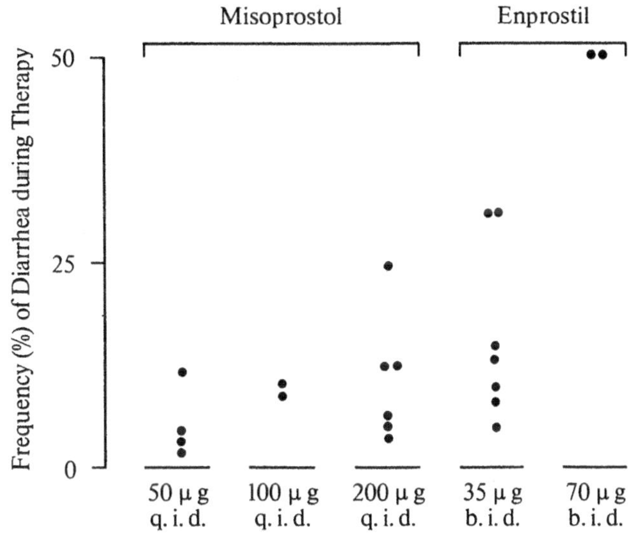

Fig. 1. Incidence of diarrhea in controlled studies with misoprostol 50–200 μg q.i.d. and enprostil 35–70 μg b.i.d. (Data from [7, 12, 14–22]).

Clinical Relevance of Unwanted Effects

The clinical relevance of the above-mentioned side effects seems to be fairly low since they did not significantly influence the patients' assessment of their overall response to the misoprostol and enprostil therapies. In fact, data from controlled clinical trials with misoprostol show that unwanted effects responsible for treatment suspension have seldom been observed; for instance, in the large multicenter study of Nicholson et al. [14], withdrawals for treatment-related reasons were 4.4% in 226 patients receiving misoprostol, 50 μg q. i. d., and 3% in the 231 treated with misoprostol, 200 μg, as compared to 2.1% in 236 patients receiving cimetidine 300 mg q. i. d.. Most of the treatment withdrawals, however, were not dependent on the drug; only one case in the misoprostol 50 μg group and two cases in the 200 μg group withdrew from the trial due to drug-related adverse effects.

Similarly, side effects occurring during the administration of enprostil appear to constitute a relatively minor problem. Pooled data from European multicenter studies [17] reveal that only 2.1% of 188 patients receiving enprostil, 35 μg b. i. d., discontinued therapy because of adverse effects in comparison with 1.1% of 181 patients treated with cimetidine, 400 mg b. i. d.

The most clinically significant PG side effect determining withdrawal from treatments was diarrhea; worldwide it accounts for approximately 0.4% and 0.9% of misoprostol and enprostil withdrawals, respectively [23, 13]. Although it occurs frequently, diarrhea is of mild or moderate severity, generally self-limiting, and of short duration; indeed, with enprostil diarrhea was reported only on 3.9% of the total number of days of drug administration [13].

An important problem which has given rise to the therapeutic use of antiulcer prostaglandin analogues is their reported effects on the pregnant uterus. The potential abortifacient properties of misoprostol were recently evaluated in two placebo-controlled studies conducted in first trimester pregnant women who were scheduled for legal abortion [10]. In the first study the administration of two 400 µg doses of misoprostol caused a significant increase in the uterine contractions and bleeding compared to placebo. In the second study, the administration of the same dose of misoprostol caused either partial or total expulsion of the uterine contents in 11% (6/56) of women in comparison with 0% (0/55) on placebo; even uterine bleeding was significantly more frequent after misoprostol 45% (25/56) than after placebo, 4% (2/55).

On the other hand, preliminary data suggest that enprostil is not abortifacient: clinical doses of the drug, in fact, did not cause expulsion of the uterine contents in 100 women who were in the first trimester of pregnancy and were seeking surgical termination; moreover, uterine bleeding was seen in only 4% of patients [13]. The aforesaid potential abortifacient properties raise concern about the use of these products for pregnancy termination and suggest a careful selection of patients eligible for this treatment as well as postmarketing surveillance studies.

In summary: the monitoring of clinical safety in short-term studies has shown that PGE analogues (misoprostol and enprostil) under study as antiulcer therapies are sufficiently safe. Their unwanted effects appear to be dose dependent and mainly restricted to the gastrointestinal system; although the drugs have been tested only in a limited number of patients, the frequency and the clinical relevance of their side effects seem to be relatively low even if, on average, they exceed that of H_2 blockers. It remains to be established whether the adverse side effects typically related to PGs are more relevant for the patient than those associate with H_2-antagonists.

References

1. Robert A, Nezamis JE, Lancaster C et al (1967) Inhibition of gastric secretion by prostaglandins. Am J Dig Dis 12: 1073–1076
2. Robert A, Nezamis JE, Lancaster C, Hanchar AJ (1979) Cytoprotection by prostaglandins in rat. Prevention of gastric necrosis produced by alcohol, HCl, NaOH, hypertonic NaCl, and thermal injury. Gastroenterology 77: 433–443
3. Wilson DE (1986) Therapeutic aspects of prostaglandins in the treatment of peptic ulcer disease. Dig Dis Sci 31 (Feb. Suppl.): 42–46
4. Hawkey CJ, Rampton DS (1985) Prostaglandins and the gastrointestinal mucosa: Are they important in its function, disease, or treatment? Gastroenterology 89: 1162–1188
5. Collins PW (1986) Development and therapeutic role of synthetic prostaglandins in peptic ulcer disease. J Med Chem 29: 437–443
6. Sontag SJ (1986) Prostaglandins in peptic ulcer disease. An overview of current status and future directions Drug 32: 445–457
7. Brand DL, Roufail WM, Thomson ABR, Tapper EJ (1985) Misoprostol, a synthetic PGE_1 analogue, in the treatment of duodenal ulcers: A multicentre double-blind study. Dig Dis Sci 30 (Nov. Suffl.): 147–158
8. Sontag SJ, Mazure PA, Pontes JF, Beker SG, Dajani EZ (1985) Misoprostol in the treatment of duodenal ulcer: A multicentre double-blind placebo-controlled study. Dig Dis Sci 30 (Nov. Suppl.): 159–163
9. Agrawal NM, Saffouri B, Kruss DM, Callison DA, Dajani EZ (1985) Healing of benign gastric ulcer: A placebo-controlled comparison of two regimens of misoprostol, a synthetic analogue of prostaglandin E_1. Dig Dis Sci 30 (Nov. Suppl.): 164–170

10. Herting RL, Clay GA (1985) Overview of clinical safety with misoprostol Dig Dis Sci 30 (Nov. Suppl.): 185-193
11. Navert H, Thomson ABR, Archambault A et al (1986) Treatment of gastric ulcer with enprostil. Am J Med 81 (Suppl.2A): 75-79
12. Bright-Asare P, Krejs GJ, Santangelo WC et al (1986) Treatment of duodenal ulcer with enprostil, a prostaglandin E_2 analog. Am J Med 81 (Suppl.2A): 64-68
13. Sevelius H (1985) Side effect data in 1850 patients document enprostil's safety. In: Protective and therapeutic effects of gastrointestinal prostaglandin. Enprostil: A new modality. Toronto, Canada, November 12-14 Abstracts, p. 23
14. Nicholson PA (1985) A multicentre international controlled comparison of two dosage regimens of misoprostol and cimetidine in the treatment of duodenal ulcer in outpatients. Dig Dis Sci 30 (Nov. Suppl.): 171-177
15. Shield MJ (1985) Interim results of a multicentre international comparison of misoprostol and cimetidine in the treatment of outpatients with benign gastric ulcers. Dig Dis Sci 30 (Nov. Suppl.): 178-184
16. Rachmilewitz D, Chapman JW, Nicholson PA et al (1986) A multicentre international controlled comparison of two dosage regimens of misoprostol with cimetidine in treatment of gastric ulcer in outpatients. Dig Dis Sci 31 (Feb. Suppl.): 75-80
17. Winters L, Willcox R, Ligny G et al (1986) Comparison of enprostil and cimetidine in active duodenal ulcer disease. Summary of pooled European studies. Am J Med 81 (Suppl. 2A): 69-74
18. Lam SK, Lau WY, Choi TK et al (1986) Prostaglandin E_1 (misoprostol) overcomes the adverse effect of chronic cigarette smoking on duodenal ulcer. Dig Dis Sci 31 (Feb. Suppl.): 68-74
19. Bardhan KD, Bose K, Hinchliffe RFC et al (1985) Enprostil (E) versus ranitidine (R) in duodenal ulcer. Gut 26: A 1149
20. Lauritsen K, Laursen SK, Havelund T et al (1986) Enprostil and ranitidine in duodenal ulcer healing: Double-blind comparative trial. Br J Med 292: 864-866
21. Dammann HG, Huttemann W, Kalek HD, Rohner HG, Simon B (1986) Comparative clinical trial of enprostil and ranitidine in treatment of gastric ulcer. Am J Med 81 (Suppl.2A): 80-84
22. Thomson ABR, Navert H, Halvorsen L et al (1986) Treatment of duodenal ulcer with enprostil, a synthetic prostaglandin E_2 analog. Am J Med 81 (Suppl.2A): 59-63
23. Herting RL, Nissen BA (1986) Overview of misoprostol clinical experiences. Dig Dis Sci 31 (Feb.Suppl.): 47-54

Discussion Following the Report of Prof. Bianchi Porro

PESKAR

Do synthetic prostaglandin analogues induce abortion in pregnant women? And if so, do you think that this might be a serious side effect and a problem particularly in countries without easy access to legal abortion?

BIANCHI PORRO

This is a point which I have not touched upon. There are recent studies, not yet published, of which probably most of you are aware, conducted especially with the aim of seeing whether prostaglandins are important here. I have been told that the results have been completely negative. I have not seen the results. I do not want to speak about my personal experience, but in the multicentered trials in which I have been involved I have been asked not to enroll women with the possibility of pregnancy. If there should be an effect of prostaglandins with regard to abortion, the road of these compounds as ulcer drugs will be very difficult.

COHEN

I think the study with misoprostol showed quite clearly that misoprostol given in standard therapeutic dose to first-trimester pregnant women caused abortion or uterine contraction in a significant number of the women, whereas the study with enprostil did not show any abortifacient effect when given to pregnant women in therapeutic doses. So I think there is a difference between these two analogues.

WEIHRAUCH

In your careful analysis of the incidence of diarrhea, which seems to be the major concern in various studies, you found that there were differences in the frequency reported by these studies. Did you have a chance to look into the definitions of diarrhea used? I believe, namely, that people sometimes consider one soft stool per day as diarrhea, and others do not. I think it would be a good point to define what we mean by diarrhea.

BIANCHI PORRO

Yes, it is important to define the symptom. Usually the symptom was considered important when it bothered the patient, independently of the number of movements and of fecal consistency.

SONTAG

In the original misoprostol studies the definition of diarrhea included anything greater than the usual pattern. Many of our patients had one bowel movement every third day before the study and then once or twice daily during the study. Many of them preferred it to their usual constipation. But the computer reported this as diarrhea by definition. My conclusion from the original misoprostol studies is that misoprostol is effective in relieving constipation.

4. Peskar BM, Holland A, Peskar BA (1976) Effect of carbenoxolone on prostaglandin synthesis and degradation. J Pharm Pharmac 28: 146-8
5. Peskar BM (1977) On the synthesis of prostaglandins by human gastric mucosa and its modification by drugs. Biochim Biophys Acta 487: 307-14
6. Peskar BM, Weiler H (1983) Carbenoxolone inhibits thromboxane B_2 synthesis by human gastric mucosa. Gut 24: A 480
7. Whittle BJR, Kauffman GL, Moncada S (1981) Vasoconstriction with thromboxane A_2 induces ulceration of the gastric mucosa. Nature 292: 472-82
8. Martin F, Farley A, Gagnon M, Bensemana D (1982) Comparison of the healing capacities of sucralfate and cimetidine in the short-term treatment of duodenal ulcer: a double-blind randomized trial. Gastroenterology 82: 401-5
9. Lahtinen J, Ankee S, Miettinen P (Suppl 83) Sucralfate and cimetidine for gastric ulcer. Scand J Gastroent 18: 49-51
10. Nagashima R (1981) Mechanism of action of sucralfate. J Clin Gastroenterol 3 (Suppl 2): 117-27
11. Nakazawa S, Nagashima R, Samloff IM (1981) Selective binding of sucralfate to gastric ulcer in man. Dig Dis Sci 26: 297-300
12. Tarnawski A, Hollander D, Krause WJ, Zipser Rd, Stachura J, Gergely H (1986) Does sucralfate affect the normal gastric mucosa? Histologic, ultrastructural, and functional assessment in the rat. Gastroenterology 90: 893-905
13. Ligumski M, Karmeli F, Rachmilewitz D (1984) Sucralfate stimulation of gastric PGE_2 synthesis – possible mechanism to explain its effective cytoprotective properties. Gastroenterology 86: 1146
14. Hollander D, Tarnawski A, Gergely H, Zipser RD (1984) Sucralfate protection of the gastric mucosa against ethanol-induced injury: a prostaglandin-mediated process? Scand J Gastroent 19 (Suppl 101): 97-102
15. Lanz R, Postius S, Szelenyi I, Brune K (1985) PGE_2 release from cultured macrophages induced by antacids and sucralfate. Gastroenterology 88: 1464
16. Quadros E, Ramsamooj E, Wilson DE (1985) Relationship between sucralfate, gastric cytoprotection and prostaglandin and mucus synthesis and secretion. Gastroenterology 88: 1548
17. Rachmilewitz D, Ligumsky M, Fich A, Goldin E, Eliakim A, Karmeli F (1986) Role of endogenous gastric prostanoids in the pathogenesis and therapy of duodenal ulcer. Gastroenterology 90: 963-9
18. Shea-Donohue T, Steel L, Montcalm E, Dubois A (1986) Gastric protection by sucralfate. Role of mucus and prostaglandins. Gastroenterology 91: 660-6
19. Hamilton I, Worsley BW, O'Connor HJ, Axon ATR (1983) The effect of tripotassium dicitrato bismuthate tablets or cimetidine in the treatment of duodenal ulcer. Gut 24: 1148-51
20. Hamilton I, O'Connor HJ, Wood NC, Bradbury I, Axon ATR (1986) Healing and recurrence of duodenal ulcer after treatment with tripotassium dicitrato bismuthate (TDB) tablets or cimetidine. Gut 27: 106-10
21. Capurso L, Koch MM, Tonon GC, Maladrino S (1983) Tripotassium dicitrato bismuthate (TDB): Cytoprotection in rats. Gastroenterology 86: 1040
22. Tarnawski A, Hollander D, Gergely H, Stachura J (1985) Comparison of antacid, sucralfate, cimetidine, and ranitidine in protection of the gastric mucosa against ethanol injury. Am J Med 79 (Suppl 2C) 19-23
23. Hollander D, Tarnawski A, Cummings D, Krause WJ, Gergely H, Zipser RD (1984) Cytoprotective action of antacids against alcohol-induced gastric mucosal injury. Morphologic, ultrastructural, and functional time sequence analysis. Gastroenterology 86: 1114
24. Hagel J, Renner H, Hirsch M, Weig G, Kaduk B, Ruppin H, Domschke W (1982) Gastric cytoprotection by antacids and papaverine in rats. Hepato-Gastroenterol 29: 271-4
25. Blum AL (1985) Stellung der Antacida in der modernen Ulcustherapie. Dtsch Med Wschr 110: 3-7
26. Halter F, Huber R, Häcki WJ, Varga L, Bachmann C (1982) Effect of food on antacid neutralizing capacity in man. Eur J Clin Invest 12: 209-17
27. Tarnawsky A, Hollander D, Cummings D, Krause WJ, Gergely H, Zipser RD (1984) Are antacids acid neutralizers only? Histologic, ultrastructural, and functional changes in normal gastric mucosa induced by antacids. Gastroenterology 86: 1276
28. Reimann H-J, Schmidt U, Wendt P, Dorsch W, von Sanden H, von der Ohe M, Lewin J, Ultsch B (1984) Die Wirkung von Antacida auf den Gehalt von Gewebshistamin und Prostaglandinen (PGE_2) in der Magenmucosa. Fortschr Med 102: 697/47-50/700

29. Robert A, Nezamis JE, Lancaster C, Davis JP, Field SO, Hanchar AJ (1983) Mild irritants prevent gastric necrosis through adaptive cytoprotection mediated by prostaglandins. Am J Physiol 245: G 113–21
30. Domschke W, Hagel J, Ruppin H, Kaduk B (1986) Antacids and gastric mucosal protection. Int. Symposium peptic ulcer research, Bellagio, April 16–17
31. Konturek SJ, Radecki T, Brzozowski T, Piastucki I, Dembinska-Kieć, Zmuda A (1981) Gastric cytoprotection by prostaglandins, ranitidine, and probanthin in rats. Scand J Gastroent 16: 7–12
32. Konturek SJ, Kwiecien N, Obtulowicz W, Polanski M (1983) Comparison of prostaglandin E_2 and ranitidine in prevention of gastric bleeding by aspirin in man. Gut 24: 89–93
33. Robert A, Hanchar AJ, Nezamis JE, Lancaster C (1979) Cytoprotection against acidified aspirin: comparison of prostaglandin, cimetidine, and probanthine. Gastroenterology 76: 1227
34. Robert A (1981) Prostaglandins and the gastrointestinal tract. In: Johnson LR: Physiology of the gastrointestinal tract. Raven press, New York, 1407–34
35. Branski D, Sharon P, Karmeli F, Rachmilewitz D (1984) Effect of cimetidine on human gastric and duodenal prostanoid synthesis. Scand J Gastroent 19: 457–60
36. Kobayashi K, Nakamura H, Arakawa T (1985) Cimetidine inhibits prostaglandin synthesis in rat gastric mucosa in vivo and in vitro Gastroenterology 88: 1450
37. Austin JE, Holroyde MJ (1985) Alterations in gastric prostaglandins may influence the ability of cimetidine to prevent stress ulcers. Gastroenterology 88: 1311
38. Levine RA, Schwartzel, EH (1984) Effect of indomethacin on basal and histamin stimulated human gastric acid secretion. Gut 25: 718–22
39. Konturek SJ, Mikos E, Pawlik W, Walus K (1979) Direct inhibitions of gastric secretion and mucosal blood flow by arachidonic acid. J Physiol (London) 286: 15–28
40. Robert A, Hanchar J, Lancaster C, Nezamis JE (1977) Antiulcer effect of aspirin. Gastroenterology 72: A-97/1120
41. Konturek SJ, Brzozowski T, Radecki T (1983) Protective actions of omeprazol, a benzimidazole derivative, on gastric mucosal damage by aspirin and ethanol in rats. Digestion 27: 159–64
42. Colton DG, Paige JB, Reiffenstein JC (1985) Inhibition of gastric ATPase by the cytoprotective/antiulcer agent SCH 28080. Gastroenterology 88: 1354
43. Foschi D, Ferrante F, Varin L, Del Soldato P, Rovati V (1986) Protection of gastric mucosa in rats. Differences between vagotomy, atropine, and PGE_2. Dig Dis Sci 31: 289–96
44. Konturek SJ, Brzozowski T, Radecki T, Piastucki I (1982) Gastric cytoprotection by pirenzepine: Role for endogenous prostaglandins. Scand J Gastroent 17 (Suppl 72): 855–60
45. Varin L, Del Soldato P, Foschi D, De Rosa M (1985) Further evidence of gastric cytoprotection exerted by pirenzepine. Pharmac Res Comm 16: 653
46. Somerville KW, Langman MJS (1983) Newer antisecretory agents for peptic ulcer. Drugs 25: 215–30
47. Bohmann T, Schrumpf E, Myren J (1977) The effect of trimipramine (Surmontil) on gastric secretion and the serum gastrin release in healthy young students. Scand J Gastroent 12 (Suppl. 43): 7–17
48. Deregnaucourt J (1979) Protection by trimipramine against gastric mucosal barrier dysfunction induced by ethanol in rats. Gastroenterology 76: 1119
49. Mangla JC (1985) Mucosal pepsinogens. Cytoprotective effects of doxepin (Dox) in rat experimental duodenal ulcer. Gastroenterology 88: 1488
50. Peskar BM, Lange K, Hoppe U, Peskar BA (1986) Ethanol stimulates formation of leukotriene C_4 in rat gastric mucosa. Prostaglandins 31: 283–92
51. Lange K, Hoppe U, Peskar BA, Rühl GH, Peskar BM (1986) Ethanol stimuliert die Leukotrien C_4 Synthese des Rattenmagens. Effekt gastroprotektiver Substanzen. Z. Gastroenterologie 24: 501
52. Samuelsson B (1983) Leukotrienes: mediators of immediate hypersensitivity reactions and inflammation. Science 220: 568–575
53. Malagelada J-R, Ahlquist DA, Moore C (1986) Defects in prostaglandin synthesis and metabolism in ulcer disease. Dig Dis Sci 31 (Suppl): 20S–7S

Discussion Following the Report of Dr. Ruppin

DOMSCHKE

From the clinician's point of view the question is whether or not via stimulation of endogenous prostaglandins by antacids, carbenoxolone, colloidal bismuth, or sucralfate the dilemma of side effects can be avoided, which arises with the administration of exogenous prostaglandins.

BEUBLER

As far as I know, aluminum ions do cause constipation, and I do not think that the potency of aluminum ions to release prostaglandins is relevant for the effect of aluminum ions on gastric ulcer, because aluminum does not cause diarrhea, even in very high doses. If it is potent to release prostaglandins, it should affect intestinal secretion as well.

RUPPIN

You are completely right. So far no study has shown that the release of enogenous prostaglandin by gastroprotective or gastric ulcer healing drugs causes diarrhea.

DOMSCHKE

This is another question, namely of the threshold concentrations of endogenous prostaglandins which may be responsible for gastric cytoprotection and for the stimulation of intestinal secretory processes, respectively.

PESKAR

Most probably prostaglandins, synthesized in increased amounts in response to the drug you have mentioned, are rapidly metabolized by the gastric mucosa. So we do not really expect that they reach distant organs such as the uterus, and they most probably do not even reach the small intestine. To my knowledge it has not been studied whether oral administration of carbenoxolone, sucralfate, or antacid stimulates prostaglandin formation in the small intestine. So, regardless of whether the mechanism of action of these drugs may be explained by their stimulatory action on gastric prostaglandin formation, it will most probably not induce side effects.

PELSTER

I am afraid your mouse macrophage model is not the best model to demonstrate prostaglandin biosynthesis in this special case, because macrophages produce prostaglandins after many stimuli. For instance, you can add zymosan to mouse macrophages, and you will have PGE liberation of more than 100% compared to untreated controls.

DOMSCHKE

I suspect Professor Peskar did direct determinations of endogenous prostaglandin levels in biopsy specimens not only in mouse macrophages. Would you like to comment on this?

PESKAR

Yes, it has been shown by my own group and by others that aluminum-containing antacids and sucralfate stimulate formation of prostaglandins by gastric mucosa tissue. It has also been shown that aluminum-containing antacids increase release of prostaglandins into the gastric juice. The same has been shown for carbenoxolone in man by Dr. Rask-Madsen's group. The mouse macrophage model was used to compare the effect of various antacids. It has been shown that not the size of the molecule but certain physicochemical properties of the compounds are important for their stimulatory action on prostaglandin formation. This physicochemical property has been found with aluminum-containing antacids and sucralfate. It has not been found with other antacids. This was the purpose of the mouse macrophage study.

DOMSCHKE

Just an extension of this question. I would be interested in whether you have comparative data available on the endogenous prostaglandin levels following administration of exogenous prostaglandins versus the levels following administration of antacids, sucralfate, and the other compounds which influence endogenous prostaglandin formation?

PESKAR

We saw some data on this topic yesterday, in the presentation given by Professor Halter. He showed that chronic administration of 16,16-dimethyl PGE_2 inhibited formation of endogenous PGE_2 by the gastric mucosa in rats. We have done similar studies with acute administration of synthetic prostaglandin E_2 and I_2 analogues in rats. We have not been able to show that these compounds, given 30 min prior to killing the animals, changed the synthesizing capacity of the gastric mucosa for prostaglandins.

RACHMILEWITZ

For the sake of completion I would like to add a few points. We have studied and published in *Gastroenterology* what happens to endogenous prostaglandins before and after various therapeutic modalities applied to patients with duodenal ulcer. We have shown that the two H_2 blockers cimetidine and ranitidine very effectively stimulate endogenous gastric prostaglandin production in duodenal ulcer patients following 4 weeks of therapy. In all the instances the ulcer also healed. Pirenzepine was not shown to have a similar effect. It did not affect endogenous prostaglandin. In this study we also determined the effect of the synthetic prostanoids, misoprostol and arbachet, on endogenous prostanoid production. We found that their administration for 4 weeks, which resulted in ulcer healing, was not accompanied by any change in endogenous gastric prostanoid production. Do not forget that ulcer disease is a disease of man. Therefore, I think that the studies here are very relevant because they were performed in humans. With regard to sucralfate in rats it was shown that sucralfate can stimulate endogenous prostanoids. In our study on DU patients we could not show this. It is still not 100% proven that the mechanism whereby sucralfate is effective is by stimulation of endogenous prostanoids.

DOMSCHKE

Just for completion of the data, what about the controls? That is to say, the ulcers of peptic ulcer patients healing under placebo treatment: What happens to their endogenous prostaglandin levels?

RACHMILEWITZ

No stimulation.

DOMSCHKE

So it might be really attributed to H_2 blocker administration?

RACHMILEWITZ

There may be another mechanism by which they exert their therapeutic effects. It definitely is not *the* mechanism, but maybe an additional mechanism.

DOMSCHKE

This should be kept in mind.

SZABO

Dr. Ruppin, you made an important point by stressing the dissociation between endogenous PG levels and sucralfate effect. I think even Dr. Hollander emphasized that he could not abolish the effect of sucralfate by indomethacin. The maximum decrease he got was 50%. And I just want to mention that there are new data now suggesting that the complex molecule of sucralfate can be dissociated into 3 components: sucrose, aluminum, and sulfate. And Dr. Orlando's and our studies are in agreement: the active principle seems to be the sulfate. The mechanism of action of sucralfate seems to be the preservation of microcirculation and this protection can be completely abolished by *N*-ethylmaleimide (NEM). I think the studies which you referred to were probably Dr. Szelenyi's, and he did not use sufficiently high doses of NEM, because if you give enough, it abolishes the sucralfate effect. The situation, however, is complex because I think Dr. Rees' study shows that the active principle in bicarbonate stimulation is aluminum. At least we now have data showing that the complex molecule of sucralfate can be dissected into three active components. Are there any data on the effect of sucralfate on leukotriene generation?

RUPPIN

No, I have not really seen any data dealing with this.

PESKAR

I think, if I understood the question correctly, you wanted to know whether sucralfate affects leukotriens. No, not in the rat.

RUPPIN

There was an increase in prostaglandin production in the rat stomach mucosa, but no change in LTC_4 generation.

RASK-MADSEN

Dr. Rachmilewitz' comments on conflicting results as regards the effect of drugs on local PG formation appear to distinguish between results obtained using different experimental designs. For example, Dr. Rachmilewitz told us that he had observed no change in the generation of prostanoids following pirenzepine administration. By contrast, we were told by Dr. Flemström yesterday that pirenzepine dose-dependently increased bicarbonate secretion – an effect which might be ascribed to the action of endogenous PGs. Actually, we have measured the release of endogenous prostaglandin E_2 into the gastric lumen in healthy volunteers during basal conditions and following modified sham feeding. We observed an increase in basal and stimulated PGE_2 values, in addition to an increased response to luminal acid. These findings suggest that neural reflexes via, for instances, afferent nerves in the gastric lumen or some receptor at the mucosal border of the gastric epithelium may respond to luminal acid by stimulating mucosal PG formation. If this is the case with pirenzepine, we would not expect an effect in vitro using mucosal biopsies or homogenates but – as you observed – no effect.

BIANCHI PORRO

During the International Conference on Prostaglandins in Florence this year Japanese authors claimed that histamine exerts a prostaglandin-mediated cytoprotection through H_2-receptor stimulation. Consequently, H_2-receptor blockers would reduce the mucosal content of prostaglandins which could possibly favor the occurrence of peptic ulcer relapse at the end of treatment. What is the experts' opinion regarding this point?

DOMSCHKE

Very obviously this remains controversial, and I think that we cannot deal with this at the present moment.

SONTAG

We are only talking about drugs which stimulate endogenous prostaglandins, but there are three articles in the literature, two in the surgical literature and one in the *Journal of Clinical Investigation*, which show that polyunsaturated fats increase endogenous synthesis of prostaglandins. And milk prevents the gastric erosions in stressed rats. And feeding linoleic acid increases urinary metabolites of prostaglandins. And recently there was an editorial in *Gut* about the higher intake of polyunsaturated fats in the United States and the decrease in the incidence of ulcer disease. So maybe we should start eating more vegetables.

DOMSCHKE

Obviously, there are prostanoid precursors naturally occurring in the food which might be able to stimulate endogenous prostaglandin synthesis. Admittedly, this point needs further clarification.

Smoking and Ulcer Healing – Role for Prostaglandins?

E. J. S. BOYD, and K. G. WORMSLEY

Introduction

Cigarette smoking is causally related to duodenal ulcer (DU) and gastric ulcer (GU) disease: there is an increased incidence of DU [1] and GU [2] in patients who are smokers compared with non-smokers; there is a dose-response, in that the greater the number of cigarettes a patient smokes and the longer the history of smoking, the greater the relative risk of developing an ulcer [3]; and cigarette smoking is associated with pathophysiological abnormalities which may predispose to or aggravate duodenal or gastric ulcer disease (Table 1). In addition, cigarette smoking is associated with a slower rate of healing of duodenal and gastric ulcers during treatment with a variety of non-prostaglandin ulcer-healing drugs or placebo [4].

Table 1. Possible adverse effects of smoking in ulcer disease

↑ Gastric acid secretion	[16]
↑ Gastric pepsin secretion	[17]
↑ rate of gastric emptying	[11]
↓ pancreatic and duodenal HCO_3 secretion	[18, 19]
↑ duodeno-gastric reflux	[20]
↓ gastric mucus secretion	[21]
↓ mucosal blood flow	[22, 23]

In a therapeutic trial comparing 15(R)-15-methyl prostaglandin E_2 (arbaprostil) with placebo in the treatment of duodenal ulcer, healing rates at 4 weeks were significantly lower in smokers than non-smokers who were receiving placebo (28% v. 65% respectively $p < 0.05$), while there was no significant difference in healing rates between smokers and non-smokers receiving 15(R)-15-methyl PGE_2 (65% and 79%, respectively) [5]. The occurrence of similar findings in some of the more recent studies using prostaglandin (PG) analogues has lead to claims that PG analogues have a specific beneficial therapeutic effect in patients with DU or GU who smoke.

In order to provide a rational basis for the use of PG analogues in the treatment of DU or GU in patients who smoke, we have attempted to answer four questions:

Is there Abnormal Prostaglandin Metabolism in the Upper Gastrointestinal Tract of Patients with Duodenal or Gastric Ulcer Disease?

In patients with DU there have been several studies in which PG "content" or "synthesis" has been measured in the mucosae of the upper gastrointestinal tract. Results are difficult to interpret because in some studies patients had active ulcers, while in others the ulcers had healed; different PGs were measured (often using differing or unsatisfactory assay techniques); and biopsies were obtained from different sites. The findings for gastric antral and fundic mucosal, and duodenal bulbar mucosal PG_2), 6-keto-$PGF_{1\alpha}$ (the stable metabolite of prostacyclin PGI_2, and TXB_2 (the stable metabolite of thromboxane A_2) "synthesis" from the most important studies are summarized in Table 2. The most consistent finding in active DU disease has been a reduction in PGE_2 in the gastric antral mucosa. Duodenal mucosal PGs, particularly PGE_2 and $PGF_{2\alpha}$, may be reduced during active ulceration. However, one study showed that fasting synthesis of major PGs or their metabolites in patients with healed DU was higher than in healthy controls, although the increase in PG synthesis in response to a meal-stimulated acid load was proportionatel less than in healthy controls [6].

Less information is available for GU. Two studies have shown a reduction in mucosal PGE [7], or PGE_2, 6-keto-$PGF_{1\alpha}$, and TXB_2 [8] during active ulceration and in one study this was related to therapeutic outcome – non-healers had lower mucosal PGE than patients who healed. One other study, which used a crude assay for PGE- plus PGA-like, and PGF-like immunoreactivity showed an increase in the mucosal content of these PGs in patients with active GU (but not in patients with acitve DU) which was attributed to gastritis [9]. PGA- plus PGE-like immunoreactivity was normal in patients with healed GU, but PGF-like immunoreactivity remained raised.

Thus in both active DU and GU there appears to be a reduction in gastric mucosal production or content of cytoprotective PGs, and possibly a reduction in prostacyclin (as assessed by accumulation of 6-keto-$PGF_{1\alpha}$) relative to thromboxane A_2 (as assessed by accumulation of TXB_2).

Table 2. Abnormalities of mucosal prostaglandin synthesis in duodenal ulcer. [6, 8, 13, 24, 25, 26]

		Active DU	Healed DU
PGE_2	Antrum	↓	–
	Fundus	↓	→
	Duodenum	↓ or →	↑
6-keto-$PGF_{1\alpha}$	Antrum	↓	–
	Fundus	↓	→
	Duodenum	↓	↑
TXB_2	Antrum	↓	–
	Fundus	–	→
	Duodenum	→	↑

↑ increased
↓ decreased
→ unchanged
– no satisfactory data

Does Smoking cause Abnormalities of Prostaglandin Metabolism in the Upper Gastrointestinal Tract?

Two recent studies indicate that smoking may alter PG metabolism in the upper gastrointestinal tract. Prostaglandin E_2 output into gastric juice during maximal stimulation with pentagastrin (6 μcg kg^{-1} h^{-1})was measured once when cigarettes were smoked, and again during sham smoking [10]. The output of PGE_2 during smoking decreased by 46%. However, the volume of gastric juice recovered during cigarette smoking was also reduced by 29%. Since marker recovery was not used, and because cigarette smoking may increase the rate of gastric emptying [11], it may be that much of the reduction in PGE_2 output was caused by transpyloric loss. In habitual smokers, active smoking reduced production of PGE_2 and 6-keto-$PGF_{1\alpha}$ in gastric antral mucosa to values which were significantly lower than those from non-smoking controls [12]. However, antral mucosal levels of PGE_2 and 6-keto-$PGF_{1\alpha}$ in the habitual smokers, when cigarettes had been prohibited for 12 hours, were significantly higher than those in non-smoking controls! If this study is confirmed it means that most of the previously published work on mucosal PGs in patients with DU and GU is uninterpretable, since in few of the studies has any attempt been made to separate smokers from non-smokers, and in none of the studies has time of smoking pre-biopsy been controlled.

Are there Abnormalities of Prostaglandin Metabolism in Patients with Duodenal or Gastric Ulcer who Smoke?

Gastric mucosal PGs were similar in non-smoking DU patients, and in DU patients who smoked either from 11–20 cigarettes daily or >20 cigarettes daily [13]. This finding severely weakens the hypothesis that cigarette smoking causes a specific abnormality of PG metabolism in patients with DU.

Is there a Specific Beneficial Therapeutic Effect of Prostaglandin Analogues in Patients with Duodenal or Gastric Ulcers who Smoke?

As indicated above, one of the early reported trials of a PG analogue in the treatment of DU showed that there was no difference in healing rates between smokers and non-smokers in the PG-treated group [5]. However, the authors of this study themselves pointed out that this effect was not unique to 15(R)-15-methyl PGE_2 and had also been observed in trials with high-dose antacids [14] and with cimetidine [15]. We have analysed studies in which a PG analogue has been compared either with placebo or with a histamine H_2-receptor antagonist, and in which information on relative healing rates in smokers and non-smokers has been provided. We have divided these studies into those in which the difference in healing rates among smokers in the PG-treated group has been greater than that in the comparative group ("positive PG effect"), and those in which the difference in healing rates between smokers and non-smokers has been similar to, or less than, that in the comparative group ("negative PG effect"). An example of an individual trial demonstrating each effect is given in Table 3 and a sum-

Table 3a. Example of a "postive PG effect" in smokers with DU [5]

	Arbaprostil 100 μcg q.i.d.	Placebo
Numbers	82	91
Smokers (%)	56	59
Healing in smokers (%)	65	28*
heaing in non-smokers (%) at 4 weeks	79	65

* $P < 0.05$ v. non-smokers

Table 3b. Example of a "negative PG effect" in smokers with DU – healing rates are proportionately higher in placebo-treated smokers than in enprostil-treated smokers [27]

	Enprostil 35 μcg bd	Placebo
Numbers	33	37
Smokers (%)	58	57
Healing in smokers (%)	58	48
Healing in non-smokers (%) at 4 weeks	86	50

Table 4a. Trials showing positive prostaglandin effect

Duodenal Ulcer		
Vantrappen et al., 1982	[5]	Arbaprostil (100 μcg q.i.d) v. Placebo
Lam et al., 1986	[28]	Misoporostol (200 μcg or 400 μcg bd) v. Placebo
Gastric Ulcer		
None		

Table 4b. Trials showing negative prostaglandin effect

Duodenal Ulcer		
Thomson et al., 1986	[29]	Enprostil (35μcg or 70 μcg bd) v. Placebo
Lauritsen et al., 1986	[30]	Enprostil (35μg bd) v. Ranitidine (150 μcg bd)
Bright-Asare et al., 1986	[31]	Misoprostol (200 μcg or 400 μcg bd) v. Placebo
Bright-Asare et al., 1986	[27]	Enprostil (35 μcg bd) v. Placebo
Gastric Ulcer		
Rachmilewitz et al., 1986	[32]	Misoprostol (50 μcg or 200 μcg q.i.d) v. Cimetidine (300 mg q.i.d)
Dammann et al., 1986	[33]	Enprostil (35 μcg bd) v. Ranitidine (150 mg bd)

mary of published trials is given in Table 4. The majority of studies shows no specific beneficial effect of PG analogues in smokers.

Conclusions

There is evidence that PG metabolism may be abnormal in patients with DU or GU, particularly PGE_2 "synthesis" in the gastric antrum of patients with active ulcers. However, although smoking does appear to alter the metabolism of PG in the gastric mucosa in acute studies, it has not been possible to relate smoking to specific abnormalities of PG metabolism in DU patients who smoke. There is no evidence that PG analogues are of specific or special therapeutic benefit in smokers compared with non-smokers with ulcer disease.

References

1. Friedman GD, Siegelaub AB, Seltzer CC (1974) Cigarettes, alcohol, coffee, and peptic ulcer, New Eng J Med 290: 469-473
2. Doll R, Jones FA, Pygott F (1958) Effect of smoking on the production and maintenance of gastric and duodenal ulcers, Lancet 1: 657-662
3. Ainley CC, Forgacs IC, Keeling PWN, Thompson RPH (1986) Outpatient endoscopic survey of smoking and peptic ulcer, Gut 27: 648-651
4. Kikendall JW, Evbaul J, Johnson LF (1984) Effect of cigarette smoking on gastrointestinal physiology and non-neoplastic digestive desease, J Clin Gastroenterol 6: 65-78
5. Vantrappen G, Janssens J, Popiela T, et al (1982) Effect of 15(R)-15-methyl prostaglandin E_2 (Arbaprostil) on the healing of duodenal ulcer, Gastroenterol 83: 357-363
6. Ahlquist DA, Dozois RR, Zinsmeister AR, Malagelada J-R (1983) Duodenal prostaglandin synthesis and acid load in health and in duodenal ulcer disease, Gastroenterol 82: 522-528
7. Wright JP, Young GO, Klaff LJ, Weers LA, Price SK, Marks IN (1982) Gastric mucosal prostaglandin E levels in patients with gastric ulcer disease and carcinoma, Gastroenterol 82: 263-267
8. Konturek SJ, Obtulowicz W, Kwiecien N, Oleksy J (1984) Generation of prostaglandins in gastric mucosa of patients with peptic ulcer disease: effects on non-steroidal anti-inflammatory compounds, Scand J Gastroenterol 19 (Suppl 101): 75-77
9. Schlegel W, Wenk K, Dollinger HC, Raptis S (1977) Concentrations of prostaglandin A-, E- and F-like substances in gastric mucosa of normal subjects and of patients with various gastric diseases, Clin Sci Mol Med 52: 255-258
10. McCready DR, Clark L, Cohen M (1985) Cigarette smoking reduces human gastric luminal prostaglandin E_2, Gut 26: 1192-1196
11. Grimes DS, Goddard J (1978) Effect of smoking on gastric emptying, Br Med J 2: 460-461
12. Quimby GF, Bonnice CA, Burstein SH, Eastwood GL (1986) Active smoking depresses prostaglandin synthesis in human gastric mucosa, Ann Int Med 104: 616-619
13. Rachmilewitz D, Ligumsky M, Fich A, Goldin E, Eliakim A, Karmeli F (1986) Role of endogenous gastric prostanoids in the pathogenesis and therapy of duodenal ulcer. Gastroenterol 90: 963-969
14. Peterson WL, Sturdevant RAL, Franke HD, et al (1977) Healing of duodenal ulcer with an antacid regimen, N Eng J Med 297: 341-345
15. Bardhan KD, Saul DM, Edwards JL et al (1979) Comparison of two doses of cimetidine and placebo in the treatment of duodenal ulcer: a multicentre trial, Gut 20: 68-74
16. Parente F, Lazzaroni M, Sangaletti O, Baroni S, Bianchi Porro G (1986) Cigarette smoking, gastric acid secretion, and serum pepsinogen 1 concentrations in duodenal ulcer patients, Gut 26: 1327-1332
17. Walker V, Taylor WH (1979) Cigarette smoking, chronic peptic ulceration, and pepsin 1 secretion, Gut 20: 971-976

18. Bocheneck WJ, Koronczewski R (1973) Effect of cigarette smoking on bicarbonate and volume of duodenal contents, Am J Dig Dis 729–733
19. Bynum TE, Solomon TE, Johnson LR, Jacobsen ED (1972) Inhibition of pancreatic function in man by cigarette smoking, Gut 13: 361–365
20. Read NW, Grech P (1973) Effect of cigarette smoking on competence of the pylorus: preliminary study, Br Med J 2: 313–316
21. Yeomans ND, Millar SJ (1980) Effect of tobacco smoke condensate on mucus, protein, and DNA synthesis in cultured antral mucosa. Aust NZ J Med 10: 590
22. Sonnenberg A, Husmert N (1982) Effect of nicotine on gastric mucosal blood flow and acid secretion, Gut 23: 532–535
23. Fletcher DR, Shulkes A, Hardy KJ (1985) The effect of cigarette smoking on gastric acid secretion and gastric mucosal blood flow, Aust NZ J Med 15: 417–420
24. Hillier K, Smith CL, Jewell R, Arthur MJP, Ross G (1985) Duodenal mucosa synthesis of prostaglandins in duodenal ulcer disease, Gut 26: 237–240
25. Sharon P, Cohen F, Zifroni A, Karmeli F, Ligumsky M, Rachmilewitz D (1983) Prostanoid synthesis by cultured gastric and duodenal mucosa: possible role in the pathogenesis of duodenal ulcer, Scand J Gastroenterol 18: 1045–1049
26. Branski D, Sharon P, Karmeli F, Rachmilewitz D (1984) Effect of cimetidine on human gastric and duodenal prostanoid synthesis, Scand J Gastroenterol 19: 457–460
27. Bright-Asare P, Krejs GJ, Santangelo W, et al (1986) Treatment of duodenal ulcer with enprostil, a prostaglandin E_2 analog, Am J Med 81(2A): 59–63
28. Lam S-K, Lau W-Y, Choi T-K, et al (1986) Prostaglandin E_1 (Misoporostol) overcomes the adverse effect of chronic cigarette smoking on duodenal ulcer healing, Dig Dis Sci 31: 68S–74S
29. Thomson ABR, Navert H, Halvorsen L et al (1986) Treatment of duodenal ulcer with enprostil, a prostaglandin E_2 analog, Am J Dig Dis 81(2A): 59–63
30. Lauritsen K, Laursen LS, Havelund T, Bytzer P, Svendsen LB, Rask-Madsen J (1986) Enprostil and ranitidine in duodenal ulcer healing : double-blind comparative trial, Br Med J 292: 864–866
31. Bright-Asare P, Sontag SJ, Gould RJ et al (1986) Efficacy of misoprostol (twice daily dosage) in acute healing of duodenal ulcer: a multicentre double-blind controlled trial, Dig Dis Sci 31: 63S–67S
32. Rachmilewitz D, Chapman JW, Nicholson PA (1986) A multicentre international controlled comparison of two dosage regimens of misoprostol with cimetidine in treatment of gastric ulcer in outpatients, Dig Dis Sci 31: 75S–80S
33. Dammann H-G, Hüttemann W, Kalek HD, Rohner HG, Simon B (1986) Comparative clinical trial of enprostil and ranitidine in the treatment of gastric ulcer, Am J Dig Dis 81(2A): 80–84

Discussion Following the Report of Dr. Boyd

DOMSCHKE

Would you tell us what your favorite ulcer drug is for heavily smoking patients?

BOYD

Ranitidine. And if they do not respond, we increase the dosage.

DOMSCHKE

That is a diplomatic answer.

PESKAR

Discussing the possibility that peptic ulcer disease is related to a deficiency of gastric or duodenal mucosa to synthesize prostaglandins we have to bear in mind that it is difficult to assess the activity of the prostaglandin system in vivo. Most studies have measured the synthesizing capacity of the mucosa ex vivo, and this is not necessarily related to what actually happens in vivo. I refer particularly to the study of Malagelada's group which you have cited, showing that patients with duodenal ulcer disease synthesize less 6-keto-prostaglandin $F_1\alpha$ in response to a specific acid load than do normal persons. In this study mucosal tissue was homogenized, and excess amounts of exogenous substrate and cofactors were added to the incubation mixture. I doubt, whether the in vivo reaction of the duodenal mucosa to a physiological stimulus such as acid load can be evaluated using such a complex in vitro system. The notion that peptic ulcer disease is due to decreased formation of endogenous prostaglandins is an interesting hypothesis, but in my opinion it has not been established unequivocally.

BOYD

My reply to this is that I fully agree with you; this was the point of the last slide. I think that we really do not know what we are measuring, and if, for example, the effects of smoking and abstaining are true, again, it makes everything even less interpretable.

RASK-MADSEN

There is no reason to be suspicious about the handling of the results although we gave figures on healing rates in smokers and nonsmokers only at 2 weeks. We did so because medication was stopped if the ulcer was shown to be healed upon endoscopy at 2 or 4 weeks. Thus, only at 2 weeks it appeared reasonable to analyze the influence of smoking on healing rates.

BOYD

I'm glad to hear that. I was just a bit curious that all the other data apart from the smoking data were given also at 4, 6, and 8 weeks. There is something rather unusual about that.

RAMPTON

I would like to ask what you may consider to be an unfair question. Smoking is apparently good for ulcerative colitis, but do you or does anybody else here know any data on the effects of smoking on colonic arachidonic-acid metabolism?

BOYD

I am not aware of any data. And I think I would be very sceptical about encouraging patients with ulcerative colitis to smoke in the belief that it may be helpful to them.

DOMSCHKE

Professor Peskar, are you aware of any data connecting ulcerative colitis and smoking habits of patients?

PESKAR

To my knowledge effects of smoking on the intestinal prostaglandin system in patients with ulcerative colitis have not been studied so far.

DOMSCHKE

All in all, if I should sum up, there is no convincing argument that smokers may be defined as a special subpopulaion of peptic ulcer patients who should be treated preferentially with prostaglandin analogues. Do you agree?

BOYD

Yes. I did not make the conclusion clear and I am glad that you have. I agree with this conclusion.

Ulcer Healing by Prostaglandins – Due to Decreased Acidity or Enhanced Mucosal Defense?

H. G. DAMMANN, TH. A. WALTER, M. DREYER, B. DAU, P. MÜLLER, and B. SIMON

Introduction

During the last few years numerous prostaglandin analogs, mainly of the E_1 and E_2 series, have been developed for the treatment of peptic ulcer disease. Prostaglandins are characterized by two mechanisms of action. In man they reduce acid secretion substantially and are believed to enhance mucosal resistance, as has been shown impressively in animal studies. This combination of the major principles of ulcer therapy – decrease of aggressive and strengthening of defensive mechanisms – should make them ideally suited for the treatment of peptic ulcers (Table 1).

Table 1. Characeristics of prostaglandins PGE_1 and PGE_2

Inhibition of gastric acid secretion
Enhancement of mucosal defense mechanism against injury
Stimulation of gastric and duodenal bicarbonate secretion
Effects on gastroduodenal blood flow
Effects on mucosal repair and regeneration

It was to be expected that this unique combination of antiulcer properties should lead to higher healing rates of peptic ulcers, especially of gastric ulcers. The mucosa-protecting actions, i.e., cytoprotection, should lower ulcer relapse rate without disturbing circadian acid secretion.

Today, worldwide experience with a number of prostaglandin analogs allows a critical statement on their clinical efficacy in peptic ulcer treatment (Table 2). At present, in some Western countries two of them, misoprostol (Cytotec) and rosaprostol (Rosal), are already on the market. Enprostil has been recently submitted for approval.

Cytoprotection and Ulcer Healing

The term "cytoprotection" is derived from acute experiments in rats showing that pretreatment with low-dose nonantisecretory prostaglandin analogs protects gastric mucosa against a variety of noxious agents like acetylsalicylic acid, bile acid, boiling

Table 2. Prostaglandin analogs

	Type of analog	Dose
On the market		
Misoprostol	PGE_1	200 μg q.i.d., 400 μg b.i.d.
Rosaprostol	PGE_2	500 mg q.i.d.
Submitted for approval		
Enprostil	PGE_2	35μg b.i.d., 70 μg at night
Currently undergoing clinical trials		
Rioprostil	PGE_1	300 μg b.i.d., 600 μg at night
Mexiprostil	PGE_1	800 or 1200 μg q.i.d.
Nocloprost	PGE_2	not yet known
Dinoprost	PGE_2	5 mg q.i.d.
Arbaprostil	PGE_2	10 μg q.i.d., 25 μg q.i.d., 50 μg q.i.d., 100 μg q.i.d.
Tiprostanid	PGE_1	250 μg b.i.d.
Withdrawn from further clinical trials		
Trimoprostril	PGE_2	125 μg q.i.d., 0,75 mg q.i.d., 3 mg b.i.d.
FCE 20700	PGE_1	250 μg t.i.d., 750 μg t.i.d.

water, etc. [6, 20, 27]. Cytoprotection appeared to be a promising new therapeutic modality counteracting the pathogenetic principle of decreased mucosal defense. Consequently, the first step in the further clinical development of these drugs was characterized by a number of therapeutic studies using nonantisecretory cytoprotective doses in peptic ulcer patients.

In these doses the antiulcer potency of trimoprostil, arbaprostil, and tiprostanid was compared to either placebo or histamine H_2-receptor antagonists (cimetidine, ranitidine) (Table 3). All these trials, however, show that cytoprotective doses do not speed ulcer healing. Prostaglandin healing rates in duodenal and gastric ulcer disease did not surpass that of placebo. The same applies to alleviation of ulcer symptoms. In the comparative trials the H_2-receptor blockade by cimetidine and ranitidine proved to be by far superior to the cytoprotective approach (Dammann, unpublished).

Acid Inhibition by Prostaglandins and Ulcer Healing

The failure of this promising cytoprotective approach prompted a basic change in the concept of how to use prostaglandins effectively in peptic ulcer disease. Thereafter, prostaglandins were administered exclusively in antisecretory doses (Table 4). Since higher doses of prostaglandins induce "enteropooling effects" causing various degrees of diarrhea and abdominal cramps, the final therapeutic antiulcer dose had to be literally titrated against the side effect rate.

Table 3. Duodenal ulcer and gastric ulcer healing by "cytoprotective" doses of prostaglandin analogs

Author	Patients (n)	Comparator drug or Prostaglandin	Dose	Cumulative percentage of healing 2 weeks	6 weeks	8 weeks	Significance
Duodenal ulcer							
Unpublished	54	Placebo			47		
		Trimoprostil	125 μg q.i.d. a.c.		41		NS
		Trimoprostil	125 μg q.i.d. p.c.		44		
Unpublished	70	Cimetidine	400 mg b.i.d.		57		
		Trimoprostil	125 μg q.i.d. a.c.		33		$P < 0.05$
		Trimoprostil	125 μg q.i.d. p.c.		36		
Unpublished	82	Placebo		24	45		NS
		Arbaprostil	10 μg q.i.d.	26	50		
Dammann	45	Ranitidine	150 mg b.i.d.		67		$P < 0.05$
		Tiprostanid	250 μg b.i.d.		47		
Gastric ulcer							
unpublished	137	Placebo			31	62	
		Trimoprostil	125 μg q.i.d. a.c.		33	42	NS
		Trimoprostil	125 μg q.i.d. p.c.		46	69	

Table 4. Prostaglandin analogs used in peptic ulcer disease

	Therapeutic dose	Acid supression
Misoprostol	200 μg q.i.d. 400 μg b.i.d.	+
Rosaprostol	500 mg q.i.d.	no data
Enprostil	35 μg b.i.d. 70 μg at night	+
Rioprostil	300 μg b.i.d. 600 μg at night	+
Mexiprostil	800-1200 μg q.i.d.	+
Dinoprost	5 mg q.i.d.	no data
Trimoprostil	0.75 mg q.i.d.	+
	1.50 mg q.i.d.	+
	3.00 mg b.i.d.	+
Arbaprostil	25 μg q.i.d.	+
	50 μg q.i.d.	+
	100 μg q.i.d.	+
Tiprostanid	250 μg b.i.d.	–

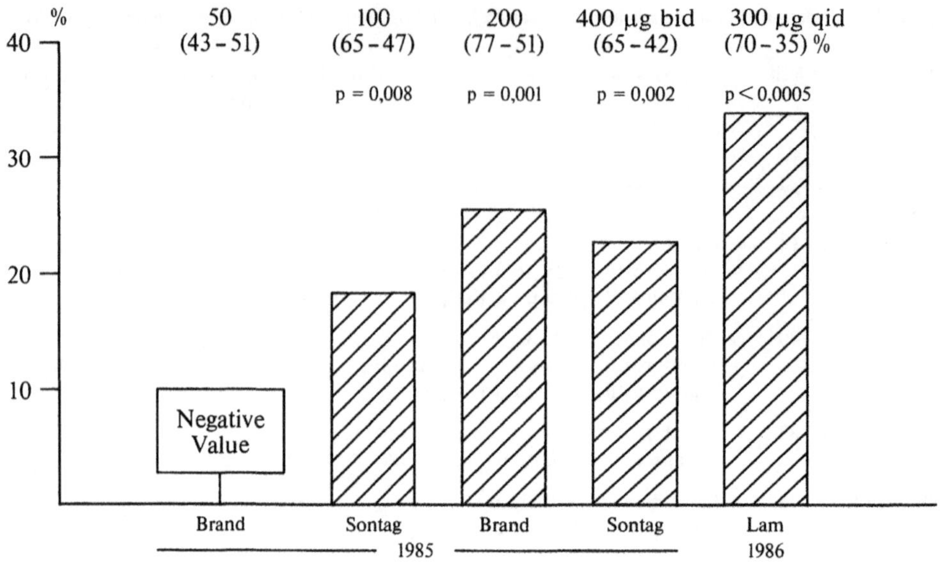

Fig. 1. Percentage increment in 4-week healing rates misoprostol vs. Placebo

Most data about dose finding are available for misoprostol [7, 21, 30]. Fig. 1 shows that misoprostol has virtually no antiulcer effect when given in a low acid inhibitory dose. A dose of 50 μg q.i.d. did not differ significantly from placebo. A substantial increment in 4-week healing rates was only observed with doses higher than 100 μg q.i.d.. A dose of 800 μg daily either in a q.i.d. or b.i.d. regimen showed a comparable increase of 26% and 23%, respectively. The 300 μg q.i.d. administration form proved to be the most effective (plus 35%). Thus, the efficacy of misoprostol as an ulcer-healing agent is clearly dose-dependent.

Unfortunately, however, an increase in dose is paralleled by a higher incidence of unwanted gastrointestinal effects (Fig. 2) [2, 5, 21, 23, 26, 29, 30]. There was, in particular, a dramatic rise in the frequency of diarrhea after 300 μg q.i.d, which made this dose impractical in peptic ulcer therapy [21].

Ulcer Healing Rates Prostaglandins Versus H_2-receptor Antagonists

Duodenal Ulcer

Although the side effects typically associated with prostaglandins prevent the application of the full antisecretory dose, misoprostol, enprostil, and rioprostil reached cimetidine duodenal ulcer-healing, rates (Table 5). Relief of duodenal ulcer pain was equal with enprostil and rioprostil, but significantly less with misoprostol compared to cimetidine [3, 4, 11, 17, 22, 23, 32, 33].

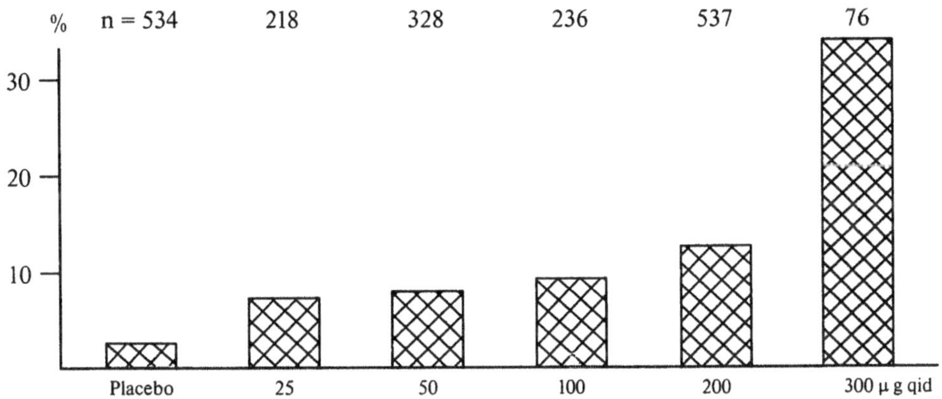

Fig. 2. Percentage of diarrhea with increasing misoprostol doses

Table 5. Duodenal ulcer healing by prostaglandin analogs versus H_2-blockers

Author	Patients (n)	Comparator drug or Prostaglandin	Dose	Cumulative percentage of healing 2 weeks	4 weeks	6 weeks	Significance
Nicholson [23]	475	Cimetidine	300 mg q.i.d.		67		NS
		Misoprostol	200 μg q.i.d.		60		
Winters [33]	346	Cimetidine	400 mg b.i.d.	42	77		NS
		Enprostil	35 μg b.i.d.	40	75		
unpublished	243	Cimetidine	400 mg b.i.d.		60	78	NS
		Rioprostil	300 μg b.i.d.		55	83	
Bardhan et al. [3]		Cimetidine	200 mg t.i.d. plus 400 mg at night		62		$P < 0.02$
		Trimoprostil	750 μg q.i.d.		90		
Hentschel et al. [17]	174	Cimetidine	200 mg t.i.d. plus 400 mg at night		78		$P < 0.0008$
		Trimoprostil	750 μg q.i.d.		54		
Bardhan et al. [4]	85	Ranitidine	150 mg b.i.d.		93	97	$P < 0.05$
		Enprostil	35 μg b.i.d.		46	82	
Lauritsen et al. [22]	180	Ranitidine	150 mg b.i.d.	64	87	94	$P < 0.05$
		Enprostil	35 μg b.i.d.	47	69	79	
Walt et al. [32]	102	Ranitidine	300 mg at night		76		$P < 0.05$
		Enprostil	70 μg at night	51			
unpublished	319	Ranitidine	150 mg b.i.d.		72	94	NS
		Rioprostil	300 μg b.i.d.		63	86	
Dammann et al. [11]	208	Ranitidine	300 mg at night	54	90		NS
		Rioprostil	600 μg at night	50	84		

In contrast to enprostil and rioprostil, misoprostol was not tried against the more potent H_2 blocker ranitidine. Compared to ranitidine, enprostil showed both, a significantly lower antiulcer effect and inferior relief of duodenal ulcer pain, while rioprostil turned out to be equally effective [4, 11, 22, 32].

Today H_2 blockers are used successfully in a convenient single bedtime dose both in duodenal and gastric ulcer disease. This follows the concept of nocturnal acid secretion as a major factor in the pathogenesis of duodenal ulcer. Large multicenter trials have shown that H_2-receptor antagonists in a single night-time dose are as effective in duodenal ulcer therapy as a twice-daily administration.

Most trials with prostaglandin analogs, however, used q.i.d. or b.i.d. dosage regimens. Since enprostil and rioprostil have a longer half-life than the other prostaglandin analogs, once-daily dosage seems to be rational and might reduce side effect rates. Consequently, both enprostil and rioprostil were tried in single nocturnal doses against ranitidine in duodenal ulcer disease [11, 32]. Again, enprostil healing rates were significantly lower, while rioprostil was almost as good as ranitidine. Pain relief with enprostil, but not with rioprostil, was also worse than with ranitidine.

Table 6. Decrease of nocturnal acid secretion

Author		Drug	Dose	Inhibition (%)
Prostaglandin analogs				
Akdamar et al.	[1]	Misoprostol	200 μg q.i.d. plus 10 mg diazepam	58
Dammann et al.			400 μg b.i.d.	30
unpublished		Arbaprostil	10 μg q.i.d.	0
			25 μg q.i.d.	no data
			50 μg q.i.d.	
			100 μg q.i.d.	
Santana et al.	[28]	Enprostil	35 μg b.i.d.	45
Deakin et al.	[13]		70 μg at night	50
Dammann et al.	[13]	Rioprostil	300 μg b.i.d.	52
			600 μg at night	74
		Mexiprostil	800–1200 μg q.i.d.	no data
Dammann et al.	[7]	Trimoprostil	125 μg q.i.d.	0
			1.5 mg q.i.d. a.c.	20
			1.5 mg q.i.d. p.c.	60
			3.0 mg b.i.d.	30
unpublished		Tiprostanid	250 μg b.i.d.	0
H_2-Receptor antagonists				
Dammann et al.	[9]	Ranitidine	150 mg b.i.d.	75
Walt et al.	[31]		300 mg at night	95
Pounder et al.	[25]	Cimetidine	400 mg b.i.d.	50
Gledhill et al.	[14]		800 mg at night	70

Since the antisecretory effect at night seems to be directly related to healing rates at 4 weeks, the differences in antiulcer efficacy between enprostil and ranitidine is not surprising. Enprostil (70 μg at night) reduced nocturnal acidity only by about 50%, ranitidine by 95% (Table 6). In contrast, rioprostil is much more similar to ranitidine with respect to night-time acid suppression (Dammann, unpublished) [7, 8, 9, 13, 14, 25, 28, 31].

Gastric Ulcer

In gastric ulcer, comparative trials with H_2 blockers (cimetidine, ranitidine) and prostaglandins revealed no marked differences in 4- and 6-week healing rates (Table 7). Prostaglandins seemed to be equipotent in gastric ulcer pain relief. These good results in gastric ulcer treatment contrast with the duodenal ulcer studies. Thus, misoprostol 200 μg q.i.d., enprostil 35 μg b.i.d., and rioprostil 300 μg b.i.d. provide effective means of treating acute benign gastric ulcers [12, 26, 29]. With trimoprostil healing rates were significantly lower than with cimetidine, although the trimoprostil dose used (750 μg q.i.d.) has a comparable antisecretory activity. A dose of 750 μg trimoprostil given orally reduces basal acid output by 67% over a 6-h period.

Table 7. Gastric ulcer healing by prostaglandin analogs versus H_2-blockers

Author	Patients	Comparator drug or Prostaglandin (*n*)	Dose	Cumulative percentage of healing 2 weeks	4 weeks	6 weeks	Significance
Shield [29]	280	Cimetidine	300 mg q.i.d.		60		NS
		Misoprostol	200 μg q.i.d.		58		
Rachmilewitz et al. [26]	447	Cimetidine	300 mg q.i.d.		60		NS
		Misoprostol	200 μg q.i.d.		53		
Dammann et al. [12]	93	Ranitidine	150 mg b.i.d.		66	84	NS
		Enprostil	35 μg b.i.d.		58	80	
unpublished	182	Ranitidine	150 mg b.i.d.		54	81	NS
		Rioprostil	300 μg b.i.d.		47	76 (8 weeks)	
unpublished	59	Cimetidine	200 mg t.i.d. plus 400 mg at night			93	$P < 0.001$
		Trimoprostil	750 μg q.i.d.			43	

Prostaglandins and Duodenal Ulcer Relapse Rates

It has been speculated that successful acute treatment of duodenal ulcers with prostaglandin analogues would be followed by later relapses than with H_2 blockers. Three studies in patients with duodenal ulcers healed by cimetidine or trimoprostil and

Table 8. Relapse rates in patients with healed ulcers after 4 weeks of therapy

Author	Patients (*n*)	Comparator drug or Prostaglandin	Dose	Median time for relapse (days)	6 month recurrence rates (%)
Barakat, unpublished	81	Cimetidine	400 mg b.i.d.	102	71
		Trimoprostil	3 mg b.i.d.	104	59
			3 mg at night	180	61
Bardhan et al. [3]	33	Cimetidine	200 mg b.i.d. plus 400 mg at night	–	64
		Trimoprostil	750 µg q.i.d.	–	64
Änishänslin et al. [2]	83	Cimetidine	300 mg q.i.d.	–	38
		Misoprostol	50 µg q.i.d.	–	39
			200 µg q.i.d.	–	39
O'Keefe et al. [24]	48	Cimetidine	300 mg q.i.d.	–	85
		Misoprostol	50 µg q.i.d.	–	50
			200 µg q.i.d.	–	38

misoprostol did not confirm this speculation. Six months after the end of treatment, relapse rates were not significantly different in either treatment group (Barakab, unpiblished; (Table 8) [2, 3, 24].

Enprostil 35 µg at night, was inferior to ranitidine in maintenance therapy. Three-, 6-, and 12-month recurrence rates with enprostil and ranitidine (150 mg at night) were 37%, 58%, and 68% versus 9%, 19%, and 30% ($P < 0.0002-0.0004$). The number of relapses with enprostil very similar to placebo recurrence rates seen in numerous long-term studies (Rask-Madson, personal communication).

Comment

Although prostaglandins probably combine both acid inhibition and mucosal protection, they are effective, but not outstanding ulcer-healing drugs. Until now the cytoprotective properties of prostaglandins have been exclusively demonstrated in rats. Obviously, none of the prostaglandins available today shows cytoprotective actions in man. Even if cytoprotection could be demonstrated definitely in man, its clinical relevance would still remain to be proven. At present any connection between cytoprotection and ulcer healing is speculative. The prostaglandin doses used in peptic ulcer disease substantially inhibit gastric acid secretion and therapeutic benefit is explicable solely by this effect. As a rule, healing rates with prostaglandins reflect their antisecretory potency.

References

1. Akdamar K, Agrawal N, Ertan A (1982) Inhibition of nocturnal gastric secretion in normal human volunteers by misoprostol: a synthetic prostaglandin E_1 methyl ester analog. Am J Gastroenterol 77: 902
2. Änishänslin W, Bärlocher C, Bernoulli R, Egger G, Eissner M, Fumagalli T, Güller R, Leuthold E, Osterkorn K, Pelloni S, Plancherel P, Seiler P, Stocker H, Blum AL (1985) Misoprostol und Cimetidin bei der Behandlung des Ulcus duoden. Eine multizentrische Schweizer Doppelblindstudie. Schweiz med Wschr 115: 1225
3. Bardhan KD, Whitaker K, Hinchliffe RFC, Cleur K, Bose K (1984) Trimoprostil vs. cimetidine in duodenal ulcer. Brit Soc Gastroenterol Gut 25: 1580
4. Bardhan KD, Bose K, Hinchliffe RFC, Whitaker L, Morris P, Massey H, Thomson M (1985) Enprostil (E) versus ranitidine (R) in duodenal ulcer (DU). Gut 26: 1149
5. Brand DL, Roufail WM, Thomson ABR, Tapper EJ (1985) Misoprostol, a synthetic PGE_1 analogue, in the treatment of duodenal ulcers. A multicentre double-blind study. Dig Dis Sci 30: 147S
6. Charlet N, Gallo-Torres HE (1985) Prostaglandins and the protection of the gastroduodenal mucosa in humans: A critical review. J Clin Pharmacol 8: 564
7. Dammann HG, Walter Th A, Wolf N, Müller P, Simon B (1986) Die intragastrale Säurekonzentration unter dem Prostaglandin E_2-Analogon Trimoprostil. Arzneim.-Forsch. /Drug Res 36: 500
8. Dammann HG, Palmer M, Walter Th A, Müller P, Simon B (1986) Rioprostil 600 μg nocte: Ausgeprägte Hemmung der nächtlichen intragastralen Azidität des Menschen. Z Gastroenterologie 24: 245
9. Dammann HG, Müller P, Simon B (1983) 24-hour intragastric acidity and single night-time dose of three H_2-blockers. Lancet II: 1078
10. Dammann HG, Müller P, Simon B (1983) Hemmung der Nüchtersekretion durch Trimethyldesoxyprostaglandin E_2 beim Menschen. Arzneim Forsch / Drug Res 33: 905
11. Dammann HG, Walter Th A, Müller P, Simon B (1986) Night-time rioprostil versus ranitidine in duodenal ulcer healing. Lancet II: 335
12. Dammann, HG, Hüttemann W, Kalek HD, Rohner HG, Simon B (1986) comparative clinical trial of enprostil and ranitidine in the treatment of gastric ulcer. Am J Med 81: 80
13. Deakin M, Ramage J, Paul A, Gray SP, Billings J, Williams JG (1986) Effect of enprostil, a synthetic prostaglandin E_2, on 24-hour intragastric acidity, nocturnal acid, and pepsin secretion. Gut 27: 1054
14. Gledhill T, Howard OM, Buck M et al (1983) Single nocturnal dose of an H_2-receptor antagonist for the treatment of duodenal ulcer. Gut 24: 904
15. Hawkey CJ, Rampton DS (1985) Prostaglandins and the gastrointestinal mucosa; are they important in its function, disease or treatment? Gastroenterology 89: 1162
16. Hawkey CJ, Walt RP (1986) Prostaglandins for peptic ulcer: A promise unfulfilled. Lancet II: 1084
17. Hentschel E, Bounameaux Y, Kratochvil P, Koch H, Ottenjann R, Ongevalle P van (1985) Behandlung des Ulcus duodeni mit Trimoprostil oder Cimetidin. Z Gastroenterologie 23: 445
18. Howden CW, Jones DB, Burget DW, Kerr GD, Hunt RH (1986) Acid suppression in healing duodenal ulcer: How much is enough? Gut 27: A 611.
19. Howden CW, Jones DB, Burget DW, Hunt RH (1986) Comparison of the effects of gastric antisecretory agents in healthy volunteers and patients with duodenal ulcer. Gut 27: 1058
20. Konturek SJ, Piastucki I, Brzozowski T et al (1982) Role of locally generated prostaglandins in adaptive gastric cytoprotection. Dig Dis Sci 27: 967
21. Lam SK, Lau WY, Choi TK, Lai CL, Lok ASF, Hui WM, Matthew MT, Choi KY (1986) Prostaglandin E_1 (misoprostol) overcomes the adverse effect of chronic cigarette smoking on duodenal ulcer healing. Dig Dis Sci 31: 68S
22. Lauritsen K, Larsen LS, Havelund T, Byther P, Svendsen LB, Rask-Madsen J (1986) Enprostil and ranitidine in duodenal ulcer healing: double-blind comparative trial. Br Med J 292: 864
23. Nicholson PA (1985) A multicentre international controlled comparison of two dosage regimens of misoprostol and cimetidine in the treatment of duodenal ulcer in outpatients. Dig Dis Sci 11: 171S
24. O'Keefe SJD, Spitaels JM, Mannion G, Naicer N (1985) Misoprostol, a synthetic prostaglandin E_1 analog in the treatment of duodenal ulcers. South A.M.J. 67: 321

25. Pounder RE, Hunt RH, Vincent SH, Milton-Thompson GJ, Misiewicz JJ (1977) 24-hour intragastric acidity and nocturnal acid secretion in patients with duodenal ulcer during oral administration of cimetidine and atropine. Gut 18: 85
26. Rachmilewitz D, Chapman JW, Nicholson PA (1986) A multicentre international controlled comparison of two dosage regimens of misoprostol with cimetidine in treatment of gastric ulcer in outpatients. Dig Dis Sci 31: 75S
27. Robert A, Nezamis JE, Lancaster C, Davis JP, Field SO, Hanchar AJ (1983) Mild irritants prevent gastric necrosis through "adaptive cytoprotection" mediated by prostaglandins. Am J Physiol 245: G113
28. Santana IA, Sharma BK, Orchard K, Pounder RE (1985) Twenty-four-hour intragastric acidity before and during treatment with enprostil. Gut 26: A545
29. Shield MJ (1985) Interim results of a multicentre international comparison of misoprostol and cimetidine in the treatment of outpatients with benign gastric ulcers. Dig Dis Sci 30: 178S
30. Sontag SJ, Mazure PA, Pontes JF, Beker SG, Dajani EZ (1985) Misoprostol in the treatment of duodenal ulcer. A multicentre double-blind placebo-controlled study. Dig Dis Sci 30: 159S
31. Walt RP, Male P-J, Rawlings JRA, Hunt R, Milton-Thompson GJ, Misiewicz JJ (1981) Comparison of the effects of ranitidine, cimetidine, and placebo on the 24-hour intragastric acidity and nocturnal acid secretion in patients with duodenal ulcer. Gut 22: 49
32. Walt RP, Long RG, Logan RFA, Somerville KW, Langman MJS, Hawkey DJ (1986) Double-blind clinical trial comparing night-time enprostil with ranitidine in duodenal ulcer. Gut 27: A 608
33. Winters L (1986) Comparison of enprostil and cimetidine in active duodenal ulcer disease. Summary of pooled European studies. Am J Med 81: 69

Discussion Following the Report of Prof. Dammann

BIANCHI PORRO

Professor Dammann, can you give a further comment on this last point: Did you say that our colleague, Dr. Rask-Madsen, has performed maintenance treatment with enprostil?

DAMMANN

Yes.

BIANCHI PORRO

Dr. Rask-Madsen, can you please give us details?

RASK-MADSEN

Enprostil (35 μg) or ranitidine (150 mg) were given at bedtime to 142 patients with duodenal ulcer disease, healed on one of the named drugs. Endoscopy was performed at 3, 6, and 12 month. Relapse rates were significantly higher in the enprostil group (values were less than 0.005 in all cases). And the relapse rates observed in patients treated with enprostil were not different from placebo relapse rates observed in other studies on the same population.

DOMSCHKE

But this does not necessarily mean that cytoprotectin or lack of cytoprotection have no meaning in ulcer pathogenesis. Perhaps the amounts of prostaglandins given must be higher to induce cytoprotective effects. Are you aware of any data in man on increasing prostaglandin dosages and cytoprotective actions with gastric-acid secretion held constant?

DAMMANN

No, but there are protective effects of prostaglandin analogues when given in antisecretory doses. And this makes the problem very difficult to differentiate. The question is, what is due to the antisecretory effect, and what is due to the hypothetical cytoprotective effect in man.

DOMSCHKE

But I suppose it could be done by the use of the intragastric titration technique to keep the intragastric pH constant, and then higher dosages of prostaglandins could be administered just to show their cytoprotective effects. All in all, your data show some kind of differentiation between clinically relevant cytoprotective and antisecretory actions of prostaglandins, and this is that which counts for us clinicians. I would like to sum up quite briefly what we have dealt with this morning concerning the potential therapy of peptic ulceration by prostaglandins. If I have understood correctly, the presently available data in ordinary peptic ulceration do not suggest an advantage of prostaglandins and prostaglandin analogues as compared with conventional ulcer drugs such as H_2 blockers. And secondly, specific target groups of peptic ulcer patients who might benefit from prostaglandin therapy remain to be defined.

Diarrheagenic Syndromes Sensitive to Prostaglandin Synthetase Inhibitors

J. RASK-MADSEN, E. BEUBLER, and K. BUKHAVE

Introduction

Diarrhea may be defined as an increase in frequency, fluidity, or volume of bowel movements relative to the usual habit of each individual [1]. Transposed into pathophysiological terms, diarrhea results from the passage of stools containing excess of water. The mechanisms of diarrhea vary with the underlying disorder, and often more than one mechanism is involved, and their effects may be additive. Active electrolyte secretion, decreased electrolyte absorption, luminal hyperosmolality, changes in mucosal morphology and permeability characteristics, and disordered motor activity are among the mechanisms responsible for the production of diarrhea.

One of the most intriguing aspects of the pathogenesis of diarrheal disease involves the cyclooxygenase products of arachidonic acid metabolism, i.e., the prostanoids, among which particularly prostaglandins (PGs) of the E type have potent effects on intestinal fluid and electrolyte secretion both in animals and in man [2, 3,]. These effects are also considered to be responsible for the diarrhea accompanying the therapeutic use of PGs and their analogues, but the processes governing the regulation of electrolyte transport by PGs, although extensively addressed, are not clearly understood. However, in the last few years important new findings have enhanced our understanding of their significance in secretory diarrhea.

Functional role of PGs

As regards the functional role of PGs, it could be speculated that they reinforce or synergize normal homeostatic mechanisms that could proceed in their absence, but occur more efficiently in their presence [3]. This may have a dramatic impact on the diseased organism. For example, indomethacin, which inhibits synthesis of prostanoids, enhances spontaneous fluid absorption in the small intestine and reduces luminal fluid accumulation caused by cholera toxin, heat-stable *Escherichia coli* enterotoxin, and invasive Salmonella and Shigella. Secretion will also occur after administration of a PG synthetase inhibitor (e.g., indomethacin) when appropriately stimulated, but the epithelium is much more responsive to the same secretagogue in the presence of PG production [3]. Thus the importance of PGs for intestinal secretion is well recognized, but attention has been focused in the past on the effects of supraphysiologic doses on experimental animals, with only little regard to the influence of endogenous PGs in human diarrheal disease.

Increased PG Synthesis

Evidence of increased PG synthesis has been demonstrated for virtually every recognized category of diarrheal disease [2], but it remains to be established whether stimulation of PG synthesis is causally connected with the primary stimulus causing diarrhea. Exploring the role of endogenous prostaglandins in diarrheagenic syndromes has, however, been associated with fundamental problems of methodology and interpretation. Most important are the analytical difficulties associated with determination of PGs in biological material and the difficulties inherent in the choice of an experimental design which prevents nonspecific stimulation of PG formation (e.g., during the sampling procedure). To demonstrate the involvement of PGs in the genesis of a particular diarrhea, it is also necessary to provide evidence that inhibition of an abnormally increased PG synthesis will reduce or abolish the diarrhea. The use of aspirin or indomethacin for this purpose has been doubted because these drugs may affect intestinal transport by PG-independent actions [4, 5]. It should be emphasized, however, that the concentrations of aspirin (10 m*M*) and indomethacin (1 m*M*) used in such studies are some orders of magnitude above their potency to inhibit PG synthesis – a consideration that weakens the objection.

PGs may be involved physiologically, pathophysiologically, and as mediators of pharmacologic agents in the regulation or disturbance of intestinal ion transport, and different secretagogues may use different pathways, each of which ends up with stimulation of PG synthesis and ultimately intestinal secretion [3].

Bacterial Toxins

Infectious diarrheas are generally secretory in nature and the endotoxins of many bacteria that cause diarrhea have been demonstrated to stimulate PG synthesis [2, 3]. Noninvasive, toxin-producing bacteria, such as *Vibrio cholerae* or certain strains of *Escherichia coli,* form the most common etiology of secretory diarrhea associated with increased PG formation. Intestinal secretion, evoked by *Shigella Flexneri* and *Salmonella* as *Vibrio cholerae thyphimurium* infection, in addition to Salmonella and Escherichia coli enterotoxins, is virtually abolished by indomethacin in animal experiments.

Much work has been done to elucidate the role of PGs in cholera, which has traditionally served as a model for intestinal secretion in experimental work. Recently it has also been demonstrated that human cholera is associated with a markedly increased "overflow" of PGE_2 from the intestinal mucosa into the gut lumen [6], but neither aspirin, indomethacin [7], nor ibuprofen [2] are capable of reducing the high purging rates observed in the acute phase. This lack of effect of PG synthetase inhibitors might be explained by a rise in local PG synthesis, which is so extreme that even a 40%–70% inhibition of the cyclooxygenase, obtained by conventional doses of indomethacin, would result in a near maximum secretory response. This is illustrated in Fig. 1 by comparing the dose-response curve for effect of exogenous PGE_2 on ion transport in the isolated human jejunum with the relative values for jejunal PGE_2 release obtained in acute cholera and late convalescence [8]. The transformation of data was made on the assumption that the concentration of PGE_2 at mucosal "receptor sites" is at k_m, i.e.,

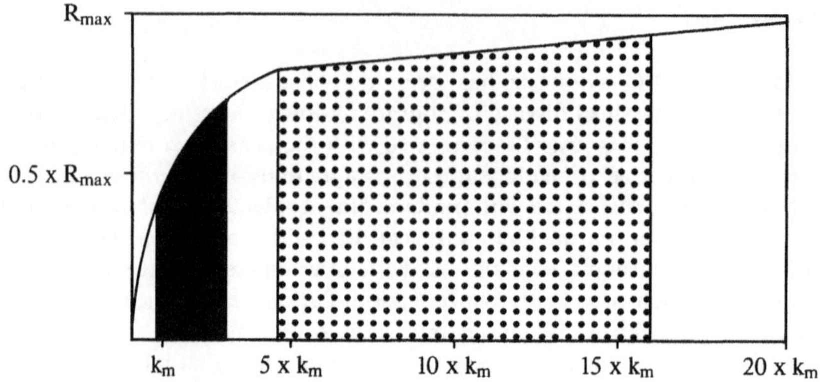

Fig. 1. Comparison of the dose-response curve for effect of exogenous PGE_2 on ion transport in the isolated human jejunum (in vitro formation of PGE_2 blocked by indomethacin 2.9×10^{-5} M) and fasting jejunal flow rate of PGE_2 in patients with acute cholera (*clotted area*) and convalescent patients (*black area*). (From [8])

10^{-9} *M*, during basal conditions. Although correlative in nature, the above-mentioned results also support the notion that PGs, in addition to cyclic AMP, may play a primary role in human cholera.

In a recent animal study we have demonstrated that pure cholera toxin stimulates intestinal 5-hydroxytryptamine (5-HT) and PGE_2 formation and that indomethacin, as well as the $5\text{-}HT_2$ receptor antagonist, ketanserin, shifted the dose-response curve of cholera toxin to the right. This observation also indicates that at least part of the cholera toxin-induced fluid secretion is caused by PGE_2 using 5-HT as a primary mediator [9]. The hypothesis corresponds with that of Lundgren and coworkers, who have provided a considerable body of evidence that cholera toxin stimulates secretion in vivo, also through an indirect mechanism involving enteric neural reflexes and release of 5-HT. That indomethacin reduces cholera toxin-induced fluid accumulation, without reducing elevated mucosal cyclic AMP levels [10], also supports the view that PG synthesis is not involved in cholera toxin-induced stimulation of the adenylate cyclase, but may be responsible for part of the secretory response. Together with our recent observation that PG-induced fluid secretion is inhibited by the calcium channel-blocking agent, verapamil [11], the findings indicate that PGs, at physiologically low concentrations, may act by facilitating calcium entry, rather than by increasing intracellular calcium through activation of the adenylate cyclase [12]. This concept is further substantiated by the finding that fluid secretion occurring in morphine withdrawal diarrhea uses a similar mechanism, i. e., 5-HT-stimulated PGE_2 formation, which causes fluid secretion without involving cyclic AMP [13].

Chemical Stimulants

Laxative abuse is probably the most common cause of chronic PG-mediated secretory diarrhea and bisacodyl, phenolphthalein, ricinoleic acid, dioctyl sodium sulfosuccinate, and anthraquinones may increase the luminal contents of PGE, probably because they are capable of damaging the intestinal epithelium [14, 15]. Indomethacin partially reduces fluid secretion caused by some laxatives. The reason may be the same as in human cholera, i.e., that mucosal PGE_2 levels are abnormally raised, in spite of the presence of anti-inflammatory drugs [16]. However, other mechanisms, beside PG-induced active secretion, may be involved [14].

The secretagogues responsible for the named diarrheal diseases are all present in the intestinal lumen and act from the mucosal border of the epithelium. In other known cases of PG-mediated secretory diarrhea, hormones or neurotransmitters, present on the contraluminal border of the epithelium, are produced in excess into the circulation by endocrine tumors derived from the neural crest. For example, in patients with carcinoid syndrome, ketanserin, in addition to indomethacin, may alleviate gastrointestinal symptoms [12]. The diarrhea associated with medullary carcinoma of the thyroid and observed in carcinoid syndrome appears to result from elaboration by the tumor of agents, such as calcitonin, bradykinin, histamine, and 5-HT that cause secretion of fluid and electrolytes by activating local intestinal PG formation [3, 12]. By contrast, a villous adenoma of rectum has been shown to release large amounts of PGE_2 produced locally by the neoplastic cells [17]. Finally, secretory diarrhea associated with increased intestinal PG formation may occur in response to increased intestinal reflex activity (irritable bowel syndrome), hypoxia (intestinal ischemia, collagen colitis), and physical damage to the epithelial membranes (irradiation syndrome) [12, 18].

Summary

In summary, PGs mediate, at least to some extent, the diarrhea associated with a large number of clinical conditions and administration of various pharmacologic agents. Several types of diarrhea respond, at least partially, to drugs which inhibit PG biosynthesis, but mechanisms other than stimulation of PG synthesis may be involved. On the other hand, some potent secretagogues, such as for example, vasoactive intestinal peptide, do not involve PG biosynthesis and are not affected by PG synthetase inhibitors. Determination of the luminal "overflow" of PGs, which is not "flow dependent", appears most appropriate for clinical use because it avoids nonspecific stimulation of PG synthesis [19].

References

1. Phillips SF (1975) Diarrhea: pathogenesis and diagnostic techniques. Postgrad Med 57: 65–72
2. Hawkey CJ, Rampton DS (1985) Prostaglandins and the gastrointestinal mucosa: Are they important in its function, disease or treatment? Gastroenterology 89: 1162–88
3. Rask-Madsen J (1986) Eicosanoids and their role in the pathogenesis of diarrhoeal diseases. Clin Gastroenterol 15: 545–66
4. Farris RK, Tapper EJ, Powell DW, Morris SM (1976) Effect of aspirin on normal and cholera toxin stimulated intestinal electrolyte transport. J Clin Invest 57: 916–24
5. Smith PL, Blumberg JB, Stoff JS, Field M (1981) Antisecretory effects of indomethacin on rabbit ileal mucosa in vitro Gastroenterology 80: 356–65
6. Speelman P, Rabbani GH, Bukhave K, Rask-Madsen J (1985) Increased jejunal PGE_2 concentrations in patients with acute cholera. Gut 26: 188–93

7. Rabbani GH, Butler T (1985) Indomethacin and chloroquine fail to inhibit fluid loss in cholera. Gastroenterology 89: 1035–7
8. Rask-Madsen J, Bukhave K, Bytzer P, Lauritsen K (1984) Prostaglandins in the gastrointestinal tract. Acta Med Scand (Suppl 685): 30–46
9. Beubler E, Kollar G, Saria A, Bukhave K, Rask-Madsen J (1987) The Role of 5-hydroxytryptamine and prostaglandin E_2 in cholera toxin-induced fluid secretion in the small intestine of the rat in vivo. Gastroenterology 92: 1315
10. Wald A, Gotterer GS, Rajendra GR, Turjman NA, Hendrix TR (1977) Effect of indomethacin on cholera-induced fluid movement, unidirectional sodium fluxes, and intestinal cAMP. Gastroenterology 72: 106–10
11. Beubler E, Bukhave K, Rask-Madsen J (1986) The Significance of calcium for the prostaglandin E_2 mediated secretory response to 5-hydroxytryptamine in the small intestine of the rat in vivo. Gastroenterology 90: 1972–7
12. Rask-Madsen J, Bukhave K (1983) Prostaglandins and intestinal secretion. In: Turnberg, ed. Intestinal secretion. Proceedings of the third BSG/SK&F international workshop 1982. Oxford: Knapp, Drewitt & Sons Ltd., 76–83
13. Beubler E, Bukhave K, Rask-Madsen J (1984) Colonic secretion mediated by prostaglandin E_2 and 5-hydroxytryptamine may contribute to diarrhea due to morphine withdrawal in the rat. Gastroenterology 87: 1042–8
14. Beubler E (1983) Laxatives: how they work. In: Barbara L, Miglioli M, Phillips SF, eds. New trends in pathophysiology and therapy of the large bowel. New York, Elsevier 119–26
15. Beubler E, Kollar G (1985) Stimulation of PGE_2 synthesis and water and electrolyte secretion by senna anthraquinones is inhibited by indomethacin. J Pharm Pharmacol 37: 248–51
16. Beubler E, Juan H (1979) Effect of ricinoleic acid and other laxatives on net water and prostaglandin E release by the rat colon. J Pharm Pharmacol 31: 681–3
17. Steven K. Lange P, Bukhave K, Rask-Madsen J (1981) Prostaglandin E_2 mediated secretory diarrhea in villous adenoma of rectum: effect of treatment with indomethacin. Gastroenterology 80: 1562–4
18. Rask-Madsen J, Bukhave K (1984) The irritable bowel syndrome: The role of intestinal secretion. In: Read NW, ed. Irritable bowel syndrome. London: Academic Press Inc. Ltd., 111–23
19. Rask-Madsen J, Bukhave K (1984) The difficulties of establishing the pathophysiologic role of prostaglandins in secretion. In: Skadhauge E, Heintze K, eds. Intestinal absorption and secretion. Lancaster: MTP Press Ltd., 453–68

Discussion Following the Report of Prof. Rask-Madsen

DOMSCHKE

Would you be kind enough as to give us some hints as how to establish the diagnosis of a secretory diarrhea?

RASK-MADSEN

For the clinician to establish the diagnosis of secretory diarrhea, I would suggest that the patient be kept fasting for at least 24 h while on parenteral fluid and electrolyte administration. If diarrhea continues, the patient has secretory diarrhea. You could also make analysis of stool water, i.e., concentrations of sodium and potassium, in addition to osmolality and pH. If the observed osmolality equals that calculated from the sum of sodium and potassium concentrations times two and does not deviate significantly from 290 mosmol, you may define a state of secretory diarrhea.

DOMSCHKE

Yes, diagnostically it is most important that upon fasting secretory diarrheas will not stop.

RASK-MADSEN

This approach is simple and relatively inexpensive, but should be applied only in chronic diarrhea, i.e., upon duration of at least 2 weeks.

DOMSCHKE

And then, one has to differentiate between the various causes of secretory diarrheal states, as you have pointed out, that is to say, to differentiate between infectious diarrheas and diarrheal states which might be due to endocrine tumors, etc.. And at the end, with a definitely negative diagnostic workup, we are accustomed to establishing the diagnosis of irritable bowel syndrome. In most cases, secretory diarrheas can be treated specifically, e.g., by antibiotics. If, however, patients do not respond appropriately, do you think that for symptomatic therapy they should be treated additionally with prostaglandin-synthesis inhibitors?

RASK-MADSEN

I would emphasize that I am not impressed by the clinical response following the administration of indomethacin or aspirin, and I do not think that these drugs add very much to our treatment. I think that those studies I have shown, and those studies I have made in patients are more for exploring pathogenesis of diarrhea. However, some patients with villous adenomas of the colon may benefit from indomethacin treatment, which may reduce bowel discharge by about 50%. Thus, the preoperative mangement of body fluid and electrolytes can be alleviated.

DOMSCHKE

So in most cases specific therapy is preferred, and in some cases with tumors prostaglandin synthesis inhibitors may serve just as a preoperative therapeutic means. But what about the clinical condition of irritable bowel syndrome? How should we manage these patients when they suffer from secretory diarrheas? You showed us a column representing the cases of two patients who did respond to the administration of prostaglandin-synthesis inhibitors.

RASK-MADSEN

The two patients with chronic "nervous diarrhea" that you refer to responded in the same way, i.e., by reducing the frequency of bowel movements and the diarrheal volume by roughly 40%–50%, which was insufficient to normalize bowel habits and should not be characterized as a clinically successful treatment. However, by making an intensive double-blind study of the efficacy in single patients we were able to prove statistically that the treatment really had an effect over a long period, because the patients were able to define those 3 periods during which active drug was given from the 9 periods during which they received placebo capsules. But although the patients were able to define the periods of active treatment they considered the effect insufficient to permit "normal life".

DOMSCHKE

Professor Rask-Madsen, from a clinical point of view it may be important to try to treat appropriately the secretory states in patients suffering from irritable bowel syndrome. When viewing the therapeutic means available at present, including opioid drugs, pectin preparations, loperamide, and prostaglandin-synthesis inhibitors, which sequence of administration seems most reasonable to you? Or, in other words, what is the first-line drug that you would choose in this clinical condition?

RASK-MADSEN

In those clinical situations in which the patient has chronic secretory diarrhea that ultimately may be classified as irritable bowel syndrome, I would suggest that controlled clinical trials of the effect of verapamil, ketanserin, and clonidine be carried out. This way of avoiding the influence of increased PG formation in the noninflamed gut appears more promising than the use of cyclooxygenase inhibitors. I would certainly use indomethacin only in cases of proven increase in local prostaglandin formation.

DOMSCHKE

Is it meaningful to send samples of intestinal perfusions, for instance, those harvested during double-contrast radiologic examination of the small intestine to your laboratory in Copenhagen for prostaglandin measurement?

RASK-MADSEN

Until now we have only measured PGs for scientific purposes, and I am afraid we cannot deliver results in due time for the clinician, and I would advise not contaminating the small intestinal fluid with hyperosmotic contrast medium. It is only feasible to make analysis in samples of fasting secretion.

DOMSCHKE

But nevertheless it may be a good idea to send samples to your laboratory, as this might give you an appropiate argument to expand your facilities.

RASK-MADSEN

This is correct; I find that a good argument.

COHEN

I was intrigued by your observation about the use of cyclooxygenase inhibitors in the treatment of radiation enteritis. I think Mennie reported in the *Lancet* about 10 years ago that aspirin was effective in this situation. This is not really a clinically important problem – while it is common, it is self-limiting. The clinically important problem, which of course occurs only in a small number of patients, is chronic radiation enteritis, which is progressive and is really intractable to treatment. Is there any evidence that prostaglandins are involved in the pathogenesis of this condition, and does it respond to cyclooxygenase inhibitors?

RASK-MADSEN

To my knowledge this has not been studied, and I would not suggest that cyclooxygenase inhibitors are of clinical value since this condition is the result of previous damage to the epithelium, the absorptive surface area of which is reduced, maybe with chronic inflammatory changes and raised levels of leukotrienes as well. I was referring strictly to the short period in which the patient is discomforted by diarrhea during high-voltage irradiation. If you want to emphasize the clinical aspects, I would recommend that patients irradiated for malignancies are not given milk products until their brush-border enzymes are normalized several weeks later. Aspirin has been shown to be effective only in the acute phase.

DOMSCHKE

So, at present, with regard to the small intestine the clinical application of prostaglandin-synthesis inhibitors is a rare occasion. In the future, the indications for the administration of compounds of this kind should be checked in prospective controlled trials, considering all the various clinical conditions. At present, it seems to me that it is quite interesting to learn more about the basic secretory processes, but the direct transfer to clinical practice has not yet been fully accomplished, is this correct?

RASK-MADSEN

I agree with your views, but would still suggest that clinical trials with verapamil, clonidine, and ketanserin be carried out in patients with proven increased luminal release of PGE_2.

DOMSCHKE

So we are witnessing the beginning of a new era in the treatment of diarrheal states originating from the small intestine.

Colitis and Non-Steroidal Anti-Inflammatory Drugs

D. S. RAMPTON

Introduction

Elsewhere in this symposium evidence is presented that non-steroidal anti-inflammatory drugs (NSAIDs), acting as inhibitors of cyclo-oxygenase, may be of therapeutic value in certain diarrhoeal syndromes in which enhanced prostaglandin (PG) synthesis is thought to be of pathogenic significance. It is clear on the other hand, however, that the same group of drugs has a deleterious effect on the upper gastrointestinal tract [1, 2]. This review outlines the emerging body of data indicating that NSAIDs also at times damage the lower bowel; it concentrates in particular on their adverse effects in patients with ulcerative colitis (UC), whether active or inactive, and on their propensity to induce a colitis in patients with a previously normal large intestine.

Active Ulcerative Colitis

Assays of eiconsanoids in faeces, in vivo rectal and faecal dialysate, venous blood, urine, and the colorectal mucosa itself [3], all point to increased synthesis of PGs, thromboxanes, and leukotrienes (LTs) in the large bowel of patients with active UC. Regrettably, however, several small studies have shown that, rather than benefitting colitis in relapse by inhibiting synthesis of putatively pathogenic PGs, NSAIDs given either orally or as enemas tend to cause deterioration, whether assessed clinically [4–6] or in terms of rectal mucosal transport function [4, 7].

Inactive Ulcerative Colitis

A number of patients has been described in whom taking NSAIDs for short periods appeared to provoke relapse of their previously quiescent colitis [8–10]; in one individual, each of four different NSAIDs prescribed for ankylosing spondylitis precipitated recurrence of his bloody diarrhoea within a few days [8]. These observations provoked a prospective survey of patients with UC [11]. Recent ingestion of analgesics in general was found to be twice as common in patients presenting with active disease (76%) as in those attending in remission (39%, $P < 0.01$), paracetamol being the drug most frequently used; 29% of the patients in relapse against 18% of those in remission had been taking NSAIDs, a difference which in this small survey did not reach statistical significance. The limitations of this study suggest that it should be repeated on a larger scale, but the presently available information indicates that NSAIDs should be used with caution in patients with pre-existing inflammatory bowel disease.

NSAIDs and the Previously Normal Colon

The increasing evidence that NSAIDs damage the normal large intestine can be classified as anecdotal, epidemiological, and experimental, the untoward effects including haemorrhage, perforation, ulceration, diarrhoea, and clinically occult mucosal dysfunction as well as a frank colitis.

Anecdotal Evidence

Case-reports describing colonic disorders attributed to NSAIDs are summarized in Table 1. The most convincing of these are the re-challenge data. In 1975 Levy and Gaspar described a patient who, while on indomethacin suppositories, developed rectal bleeding due to a proctitis, which resolved on stopping treatment only to recur with dose-related intensity after resumption of the NSAID [13]. More recently, several patients have been described, in whom re-challenge confirmed oral mefenamic acid, flufenamic acid and naproxen as the cause of bloody diarrhoea due to an acute enterocolitis closely resembling UC, except in its rapid reversibility on withdrawing the drug

Table 1. Case reports of colonic disorders attributed to NSAIDs

Drug	No of patients	Effect	Reference
Re-challenge data:			
Phenylbutazone	1	Sigmoid colon ulcers	12
Indomethacin suppos.	1	Proctitis	13
Mefenamic acid	4	Enterocolitis	14–16
Flufenamic acid	1	Colitis	16
Naproxen	1	Colitis	16
Physical association:			
Indomethacin (Osmosin)	2	Perforated ileal and colonic ulceration	17
Temporal association only:			
Oxyphenbutazone	1	Perforated caecal ulcer	18
Indomethacin	1	Perforated colonic diverticula	19
Indomethacin	1	Perforated colon	20
Indomethacin	13	Necrotising enterocolitis (infants)	21
Indomethacin suppos.	1	Bleeding rectal ulcer	22
Mefenamic acid	6	Enterocolitis	15, 23–25
Ibuprofen	1	Caecal ulcer	26
Ibuprofen	1	Proctitis	16

[14–16]. It is worth adding that anecdotal reports, albeit describing only a temporal association between taking the drug and its putative side effect, indicate that NSAIDs may also occasionally damage the small bowel, producing ulceration, haemorrhage, perforation, stricture formation, and steatorrhoea; in several instances the clinical (but not histological) features have resembled Crohn's disease [17, 20, 27–32].

Epidemiological Evidence

Langman et al in a major case-controlled survey published in 1985 [33] showed that intake of NSAIDs was more than twice as common in patients presenting to hospital with small or large bowel perforation or haemorrhage as in controls presenting with uncomplicated lower bowel disease. Patients with UC and Crohn's disease were unfortunately excluded from the study and, as mentioned earlier, a similar survey in relation to inflammatory bowel disease is needed.

Experimental Evidence

High doses of indomethacin produce an enterocolitis with ulceration in the large bowel of the rat [34] and dog [35]; local instillation of various NSAIDs increases rectal mucosal permeability in at least three species [36, 37]. An uncontrolled study showed that withdrawal of treatment with indomethacin suppositories in patients with various musculoskeletal disorders was associated with significant improvement in rectal mucosal appearance and function as indicated by measurement of potential difference and ion transport using rectal dialysis [38]. More recently, in patients with rheumatoid and osteo-arthritis, several NSAIDs have been shown to increase small and possibly large intestinal permeability to 51 Cr-EDTA [39]. 111 Indium-labelled leucocyte scans indicated that these drugs also cause ileocaecal inflammation [39], a conclusion supported by the subsequent demonstration by further isotopic techniques of increased intestinal loss of blood and protein in patients on NSAIDs [40].

Mechanism of NSAID-Induced Colitis

While this anecdotal, epidemiological, and experimental evidence implicates NSAIDs as toxic to the colon, whether previously inflamed or normal, the mechanism of this effect, like its incidence, remains uncertain.

Inhibition of PG synthesis leading to a loss of mucosal "cytoprotection" [41] is an obvious candidate, for which there is some experimental support as well as a theoretical basis. In the rat small bowel, as in the stomach, prior administration of exogenous PGs prevents the noxious effects of NSAIDs [41, 42]. Furthermore, 16,16-dimethyl PGE_2 appears to prevent ethanol-induced damage in the rat colon [43] and clindamycin-induced colitis in the hamster [44]: in the latter instance, however, the PG's benefical effect may be due to inhibition of toxin release from Clostridium difficile rather than any direct effect on the gut mucosa itself [45]. In any event, there is no evidence yet that PGs are necessary for the maintenance of the integrity of the mucosa of the human large bowel. Indeed, Goldin and Rachmilewitz [46] found that 15(R), 15-dimethyl PGE_2 did not prevent relapse in patients with inactive UC, but their conclusions were compromised by the selection of a pro-inflammatory diarrhoeagenic PG for the study, in which, in addition, the PG-treated patients had recently had their sulphasalazine withdrawn.

As well as reducing synthesis of PGs, cyclo-oxygenase inhibition by NSAIDs may divert arachidonic acid metabolism towards the lipoxygenase pathway [47], with consequent bowel damage by LTs and free radicals. Alternatively, the toxicity of NSAIDs could be quite unrelated to their influence on arachidonic acid metabolism. Fenamates, for example, have a direct cytolytic action [48] which could explain their effects on gut mucosa. Animal studies, furthermore, suggest that bacterial flora [34], food [49], and the enterohepatic circulation [50] play some role in the pathogenesis of NSAID-induced lesions, at least in the small intestine.

Conclusions

There seems to be little doubt that in some patients NSAIDs may provoke a colitis de novo; in others they may re-activate previously quiescent UC or exacerbate pre-existing relapse. Although the incidence and mechanism of these occasionally very serious adverse effects are unknown, doctors should be aware of them. Clearly, a detailed drug history should be elicited from patients presenting with diarrhoea with or without rectal bleeding. Furthermore, special care should be exercised when prescribing NSAIDs to patients with established inflammatory bowel disease.

References

1. Somerville KW, Faulkner G, Langman MJS (1986) Non-steroidal anti-inflammatory drugs and bleeding peptic ulcer. Lancet 1: 462–4
2. Walt RP, Katschinski B, Logan R, Ashley J, Langman MJS (1986) Rising frequency of ulcer perforation in elderly people in the United Kingdom. Lancet 1: 489–92
3. Rampton DS, Hawkey CJ (1984) Prostaglandins and ulcerative colitis. Gut 25: 1399–1413
4. Rampton DS, Sladen GE (1981) Prostaglandin synthesis inhibitors in ulcerative colitis: Flurbiprofen compared with conventional treatment. Prostaglandins 21: 417–25
5. Campieri M, Lanfranchi GA, Bazzochi G et al (1980) Prostaglandins, indomethacin and ulcerative colitis. Gastroenterology 78: 193
6. Gould SR, Brash AR, Conolly ME, Lennard-Jones JE (1981) Studies of prostaglandins and sulphasalazine in ulcerative colitis. Prostaglandins Med 6: 165–82
7. Rampton DS, Sladen GE (1984) Relationship between rectal mucosal prostaglandin production and water and electrolyte transport in ulcerative colitis. Digestion 30: 13–22
8. Rampton DS, Sladen GE (1981) Relapse of ulcerative proctocolitis during treatment with non-steroidal anti-inflammatory drugs. Postgrad Med J 57: 297–9

8a. Kaufmann HJ, Taubin HL (1987). Nonsteroidal anti-inflammatory drugs activate quiescent inflammatory bowed disease. Ann Int Med 107: 513–6

9. Schwartz HA (1981) Lower gastrointestinal side effects of non-steroidal anti-inflammatory drugs. J Rheumatol 8: 952–4
10. Walt RP, Hawkey CJ, Langman MJS (1984) Colitis associated with non-steroidal anti-inflammatory drugs. Brit Med J 288: 238
11. Rampton DS, McNeil NI, Sarner M (1983) Analgesic ingestion and other factors preceding relapse in ulcerative colitis. Gut 24: 187–9

12. Bravo AJ, Lowman RM (1968) Benign ulcer of the sigmoid colon. An unusual lesion that can simulate carcinoma. Radiology 90: 113–5
13. Levy N, Gaspar E (1975) Rectal bleeding and indomethacin suppositories. Lancet 1: 577
14. Hall RI, Petty AH, Cobden I, Lendrum R (1983) Enteritis and colitis associated with mefenamic acid. Br Med J 287: 1182
15. Phillips MS, Fehilly B, Stewart S, Dronfield MW (1983) Enteritis and colitis associated with mefenamic acid. Br Med J 287: 1626
16. Ravi S, Keat AC, Keat ECB (1986) Colitis caused by non-steroidal anti-inflammatory drugs. Postgrad Med J 62: 773–6
17. Day TK (1983) Intestinal perforation associated with osmotic release indomethacin capsules. Br Med J 287: 1671–2
18. Debenham GP (1966) Ulcer of the cecum during oxyphenbutazone (Tanderil) therapy. Can Med Ass J 94: 1182–4
19. Coutrot S, Roland D, Barbier J, van der Marq P, Alcalay M, Matuchansky C (1978) Acute perforation of colonic diverticula associated with short-term indomethacin. Lancet 2: 1055–6
20. Stewart JT, Pennington CR, Pringle R (1985) Anti-inflammatory drugs and bowel perforations and haemorrhage. Br Med J 290: 787–8
21. Nagaraj HS, Sandhu AS, Cook LN, Buchino JJ, Groff DB (1981) Gastrointestinal perforation following indomethacin therapy in very low birth weight infants. J Pediatr Surg 16: 1003–7
22. Walls J, Bell D, Schorr W (1968) Rectal bleeding and indomethacin. Br Med J 1: 52
23. Edwards AL, Heagerty AM, Bing RF (1983) Enteritis and colitis associated with mefenamic acid. Br Med J 287: 1626–7
24. Rampton DS, Tapping PJ (1983) Enteritis and colitis associated with mefenamic acid. Br Med J 287: 1627
25. Williams R, Glazer G (1983) Enteritis and colitis associated with mefenamic acid. Br Med J 287: 1627
26. Charuzi I, Ovnat A, Zirkin H, Peiser J, Sukenik S (1985) Ibuprofen and benign caecal ulcer. J Rheumatol 12: 188–9
27. Sturges HF, Krone CL (1973) Ulceration and stricture of the jejunum in a patient on long-term indomethacin. Am J Gastroenterol 59: 162–9
28. Madhok R, MacKenzie JA, Lee FD, Bruckner FE, Terry TR, Sturrock RD (1986) Small bowel ulceration in patients receiving non-steroidal anti-inflammatory drugs for rheumatoid arthritis. Quart J Med 58: 53–8
29. Bjarnason I, Lang J, Gumpel JM, Levi AJ, Price AB (1986) Non-steroidal anti-inflammatory drugs (NSAIDs) and intestinal pathology. Gastroenterology 90: 1347
30. Saverymuttu SH, Thomas A, Grundy A, Maxwell JD (1986) Ileal stricturing after long-term indomethacin. Postgrad Med J 62: 967–70
31. Marks JS, Gleeson MH (1975) Steatorrhoea complicating therapy with mefenamic acid. Br Med J 4: 442
32. Chadwick RG, Hossenbocus A, Colin-Jones DG (1976) Steatorrhoea complicating therapy with mefenamic acid. Br Med J 1: 397
33. Langman MJS, Morgan L, Worrall A (1985) Use of anti-inflammatory drugs by patients admitted with small or large bowel perforations and haemorrhage. Br Med J 290: 347–9
34. Kent TH, Cardelli RM, Stamler FW (1969) Small intestinal ulcers and intestinal flora in rats given indomethacin. Am J Pathol 53: 237–49
35. Stewart THM, Hetenyi C, Rowsell H, Orizaga M (1980) Ulcerative enterocolitis in dogs induced by drugs. J Pathol 131: 363–78
36. Yaginuma H, Nakata T, Toya H, Murakami T, Yamazaki M, Kamada A (1981) Rectal delivery of anti-inflammatory drugs. I. The influence of anti-inflammatory drugs on rectal absorption of β-lactam antibiotics. Chem Pharm Bull 29: 2974–82
37. Nakanishi K, Ogata A, Masada M, Nadai T (1984) Effect of non-steroidal anti-inflammatory drugs on the permeability of the rectal mucosa. Chem Pharm Bull 32: 1956–66
38. Rampton DS, Barton TP (1984) Are prostaglandins cytoprotective in the human large intestine? The effect of indomethacin on rectal mucosal function and prostaglandin E_2 release in vivo. Agents Actions 14: 715–8
39. Bjarnason I, Williams PL, So A, Ansell BM, Peters TJ (1984) Intestinal permeability and inflammation in rheumatoid arthritis: effects of nonsteroidal anti-inflammatory drugs. Lancet 2: 1171–5

40. Bjarnason I, Zanelli G, Prouse P, Smethurst P, Smith T, Levi S, Gumpel MJ, Levi AJ (1987) Blood and protein loss via small-intestinal inflammation induced by non-steroidal anti-inflammatory drugs. Lancet 2: 711-5
41. Robert A (1979) Cytoprotection by prostaglandins. Gastroenterology 77: 761-7
42. Robert A (1974) Intestinal disease produced experimentally by prostaglandin deficiency. Gastroenterology 69: 1045-7
43. Wallace JL, Whittle BJR, Boughton-Smith NK (1985) Prostaglandin protection of rat colonic mucosa from damage induced by ethanol. Dig Dis Sci 30: 866-76
44. Robert A, Nezamis JE, Lancaster C, Hanchar AF (1980) Prevention, through cytoprotection, of clindamycin-induced colitis in hamster with 16,16-dimethyl PGE_2. Gastroenterology 78: 1245
45. Ruwart MJ, Renis HE, Erwandson AL et al (1983) 16,16-dimethyl prostaglandin E_2 inhibits toxin release from Clostridium difficile. Adv PG Thrombox Leucotriene Res 12: 93-8
46. Goldin E, Rachmilewitz D (1983) Prostanoids cytoprotection for maintaining remission in ulcerative colitis. Failure of 15(R), 15-methyl prostaglandin E_2. Dig Dis Sci 28: 807-11
47. DeRubertis FR, Craven PA, Saito R (1984) Bile salt stimulation of colonic epithelial proliferation. Evidence for involvement of lipoxygenase products. J Clin Invest 74: 1614-24
48. Gullikson GW, Sender M, Bass P (1982) Laxative-like effects of non-steroidal anti-inflammatory drugs on intestinal fluid movement and membrane integrity. J Pharmacol Exp Therap 220: 236-42
49. Satoh H, Guth PH, Grossman MI (1982) Role of food in gastrointestinal ulceration produced by indomethacin in the rat. Gastroenterology 83: 210-5
50. Brodie DA, Cook PG, Bauer BJ, Dagie GE (1970) Indomethacin induced intestinal lesions in the rat. Toxicol Appl Pharmacol 17: 615-24

Discussion Following the Report of Dr. Rampton

LANGMAN

Am I right in thinking that the data about paracetamol are based upon the 21 people who had relapses?

RAMPTON

They are based on a comparison between the 21 who had relapses and the 62 who did not.

LANGMAN

Did you think it was worth perhaps giving paracetamol enemas to volunteers, to see whether this had any effect on the bowel?

RAMPTON

Yes, but we have not yet done this. Does anyone else have information on the effects of paracetamol on colonic mucosal prostaglandin synthesis?

PESKAR

I just wanted to continue on this line. Generally it is supposed that paracetamol inhibits prostaglandin formation in the central nervous system only. We have been able to show that paracetamol does not inhibit formation of prostaglandins by the gastric mucosa in vitro, and similar findings have been reported by Konturek's group after in vivo treatment of healthy volunteers and of gastroduodenal ulcer patients.

RAMPTON

Has anyone looked at the colon?

PESKAR

No.

RAMPTON

The effect of paracetamol on prostaglandin synthesis is organ-specific, is it not?

PESKAR

Yes; the question arises as to whether it does inhibit prostaglandin formation in the colon.

RAMPTON

I do not know. And one way to look at this would be to give paracetamol enemas or, indeed, tablets orally, and assess prostaglandin metabolism with rectal dialysis before and after treatment.

SZABO

Dr. Rampton, these agents affect mostly the functions of the colon and cause diarrhea. But do any of these cause ulcers? One of the reasons that we know so little about these agents is because there is no good animal model of colitis. Can you produce morphological changes with any of the nonsteroidal anti-inflammatory drugs in the colon?

RAMPTON

Yes, there are a number of anecdotal reports with and without rechallenge, indicating major morphological changes, including frank perforation, which you do not need a microscope to detect. And, of course, a more diffuse colitis in the case of mefenamic acid.

SZABO

I am aware of this happening in rodents. But has anyone systematically investigated this to develop an animal model, in which we can study the sequence of events?

RAMPTON

There are various models, as you know, of colitis. I do not know of any systematic testing of nonsteroidal anti-inflammatories in this context. I am not very keen on animal models in general, and certainly there is no animal model which in any way resembles human ulcerative colitis.

SZABO

Let me defend the animal models. They certainly may have major limitations, but certain things such as what comes first can only be studied in animals models, because patients have developed lesions, so you never know where and how the lesions start.

RAMPTON

I think one of the things we must to try to avoid in the lower bowel is going through the same rather tortured sequence that has been gone through in relation to the stomach when investigating adverse effects of NSAIDs, which may be even rarer in the lower than they are in the upper gastrointestinal tract.

BOMELAER

Excuse me for this very simple question, but how do you explain the benefit of aminosalicylate in ulcerative colitis with respect to your presentation?

RAMPTON

I hesitate going into this question before the next two talks, particularly as the next two speakers are much greater experts than I am on the subject. All I would say is, I do not think we know how 5-aminosalicylic acid works in ulcerative colitis. We do not know whether its effect is in any way related to arachidonic acid metabolism. I know there are data compatible with the idea that it works as a prostaglandin-synthesis inhibitor, a prostaglandin-degradation inhibitor, or a lipoxygenase inhibitor. As to whether any of these effects have a relation to its therapeutic action in ulcerative colitis, I am extremely uncertain. So I do not have to relate them to these observations with NSAIDs.

DOMSCHKE

All in all, one can say that in ulcerative colitis patients either in the active state or in the quiescent state non-steroidal anti-inflammatory drugs obviously do more harm than good. This could be due to a prostaglandin deficiency following the inhibition of prostaglandin synthesis. Therefore, Professor Rachmilewitz is now going to talk about the potential cytoprotective effects of prostaglandins in ulcerative colitis. As an alternative pathogenetic explanation it might be discussed that following inhibition of the cyclooxygenase pathway by administration of NSA compounds, shunting of the metabolism may occur from the cyclooxygenase pathway to the lipoxygenase pathway, resulting in increased formation of leukotrienes. Consequently, it would seem reasonable that a patient with ulcerative colitis in remission who is to take nonsteroidal anti-inflammatory drugs should simultaneously take an inhibitor of the lipoxygenase pathway, e. g. sulfasalazine. Do you think this could help prevent the occurrence of the 40% of relapses which you have found in patients within 4 weeks following ingestion of NSA compounds?

RAMPTON

I think this is a perfectly reasonable recommendation in theory. The majority of our patients who turned up in relapse after taking these drugs were, of course, on maintenance sulfasalazine already. This is another instance of our not having the information in practice to back up a sensible theoretical suggestion. I would hope that in due course it might be possible to give them an even more specific lipoxygenase inhibitor, whether they have active or inactive disease.

PELSTER

Am I right, that you said fenamates harm the cell membrane?

RAMPTON

Yes, there is evidence which was produced in about 1982 by Gullikson and others in the United States. They showed a direct cytolytic effect of fenamates on human red cells, which correlated well with their enteropooling effect in hamster small intestine but had no relation to prostaglandin-synthesis inhibition.

PELSTER

But on the other hand you possibly know that the fenamates are lipoxygenase inhibitors in the same range as BW 755C.

WHITTLE

Many compounds that have been claimed to be selective 5-lipoxygenase inhibitors based on in vitro data, have not shown in vivo lipoxygenase inhibition. Therefore we must be very cautious before saying that we already have clinically useful lipoxygenase inhibitors. The chairman mentioned sulfasalazine, and we will be hearing about this later. We must, of course, distinguish between cause and effect, and whether the reduction in leukotrienes by sulfasalazine in vivo is simply a consequence of reducing the inflammatory response.

RAMPTON

Perhaps I could just add something on those drugs. Benoxaprofen, when it was available, was said to be a lipoxygenase inhibitor. I did a study with Chris Hawkey in Nottingham, giving it orally to patients with active ulcerative colitis for 2.5 weeks, and it made not the slightest difference to them.

WHITTLE

That is an exact case in point. That compound was claimed to be a lipoxygenase inhibitor based on in vitro data, but when the compound was studied in vivo, it was clear that it was not a selective lipoxygenase inhibitor.

RAMPTON

I quite agree. Our benoxaprofen trial in no way precludes further lipoxygenase inhibition studies in the future.

PESKAR

An additional comment to Dr. Whittle's remarks. I do believe that sulfasalazine and 5-aminosalicylic acid inhibit release of both LTB_4 and the sulfidopeptide leukotrienes, and that this effect is not secondary to an anti-inflammatory effect as it is observed in vitro in human colonic mucosa within a 10–20 min incubation period. This could not be the consequence of an anti-inflammatory action. Furthermore, Bachand and his associates have shown an inhibitory action on 5-lipoxygenase and glutathione transferase purified from rat basophil leukemia cells. And, again, this could not be due to an anti-inflammatory action.

WHITTLE

I agree; we have also published data showing that sulfasalazine will inhibit the formation of lipoxygenase products in vitro. All I am saying is that demonstration of activity in vitro does not necessarily mean the therapeutic effect one sees with the compound is directly dependent on that biochemical effect. We should perhaps be somewhat cautious until we have selective 5-lipoxygenase inhibitors that we can use in man to test the hypothesis.

RAMPTON

Are we ever going to get such drugs? Will we ever know they are entirely selective and are not doing something else as well?

WHITTLE

All one can say from a pharmacological point of view is that you can achieve a certain degree of selectivity, and such 5-lipoxygenase inhibitors should be available for clinical use in the next few years.

DOMSCHKE

Needless to say, it is highly desirable to have commercially available the selective inhibitors of the lipoxygenase pathway for the treatment of inflammatory bowel disease.

Therapeutic Role for Prostaglandins in Ulcerative Colitis?

D. RACHMILEWITZ

Introduction

Prostanoids exert cytoprotective properties in the upper gastrointestinal tract of both experimental animals and human subjects. "Cytoprotection" is the term used to describe their capacity to prevent mucosal damage induced by various injurious agents as well as by nonsteroidal anti-inflammatory drugs (NSAIDs). Prostanoids prevent gastric damage induced by agents such as strong alkali, acid, and 100% ethanol, and prevent mucosal ulceration induced by cyclooxygenase inhibitors such as indomethacin [1]. In addition, endogenous gastric prostanoid synthesis was shown to be decreased in patients with peptic ulcer disease [2], whereas prostanoid-induced cytoprotection may be one of the mechanisms contributing to the acceleration of peptic ulcer healing [3]

It is therefore natural to expect that prostanoids may have also cytoprotective effects in the large bowel. Robert et al. [4] were the first to show that the synthetic prostanoid 16,16-dimethyl-PGE_2 prevents clindamycin-associated cecitis in hamsters. Both subcutaneous and oral administration of this prostanoid prevented cecitis induced by this broad-spectrum antibiotic, the pathogenesis of which involves overgrowth of clostridium difficile. In addition, PGE_2 was shown to protect rat colonic mucosa against ethanol-induced damage [5].

In human subjects, indirect evidence suggests that prostanoids have an important role in maintaining colorectal integrity. This property is reflected by the damage to colonic mucosa induced by cyclooxygenase inhibitors. Inhibition of prostanoid synthesis may be detrimental to healthy as well as to previously diseased colorectal mucosa: high incidence of rectal irritation is found in patients with rheumatoid disorders treated with suppositories of indomethacin and naproxen [6]. Rectal side effects in these patients include tenesmus and bleeding, whereas sigmoidoscopy reveals the presence of edema and erythema.

However, it has to be stressed that a direct causal relationship between decrease in colonic prostanoids on the one hand and damage to colonic mucosa on the other has not yet been proven. Moreover, NSAIDs affect other enzymes in addition to their inhibition of cyclooxygenase activity. Indomethacin, for instance, inhibits phosphodiesterase, oxidative phosphorylation, histidine decarboxylase, and collagenase, all of which may contribute to the pathogenesis of colonic damage [7].

Ulcerative colitis is a disease in which mucosal ulceration and inflammation are the predominant features. In view of the above, it is worthwhile exploring the question whether synthetic prostanoids may be beneficial for the treatment of active ulcerative colitis – a possibility which so far has never been investigated. On the other hand, it has been repeatedly shown that in active ulcerative colitis, colonic prostanoid synthesis is enhanced. This observation was confirmed by various methods such as organ culture [8–9], rectal dialysis [10], determination of colonic cyclooxygenase activity [11], and of prostanoid metabolites in stool and urine [12]. As in other organs and disease states, this enhanced prostanoid production may mediate certain disease features such as mucosal vasodilation and fever, may also mediate the immune response and the pathogenesis of diarrhea. Moreover, steroids, sulfasalazine, and 5-amino-salicylic acid inhibit colonic prostanoid synthesis [17, 21] and this may be the, or one of the mechanisms responsible for their therapeutic effect in ulcerative colitis.

Inhibition of Colonic Prostanoids

The facts mentioned above thus suggest that inhibition of colonic prostanoids may be beneficial and may contribute to the healing of active colitis. It was therefore logical to anticipate that cyclooxygenase inhibitors would also be beneficial. However, several small trials, all of which were not controlled, demonstrated the opposite: indomethacin [13], flurbiprofen [14], and enemas of flufenamic acid were all found to have no efficacy in the treatment of the active stages of the disease. In contrast, it was suggested that these agents may provoke or exacerbate the disease [15]. These latters studies indicate that prostanoids are important in maintaining mucosal integrity, that inhibition of their synthesis is harmful and definitely of no benefit to actively inflammed colorectal mucosa, further supporting the concept that their exogenous administration may be of benefit in active ulcerative colitis.

However, these arguments do not take into consideration the fact that NSAIDs may induce mucosal damage irrespective of their inhibition of the cyclooxygenase pathway. Moreover, their induced inhibition of the cyclooxygenase pathway directs more substrate-arachidonic acid to be metabolized via the lipoxygenase pathway and thus to enhanced leukotriene synthesis [15]. Leukotrienes are important mediators of the inflammatory response and their enhanced synthesis may definitely contribute to the pathogenesis of the disease.

Can this be regarded as indicating that prostanoids are cytoprotective in ulcerative colitis? Their possible importance in maintaining, the remission was advocated by Hoult et al. who showed that sulfasalazine was also a potent inhibitor of prostanoid catabolism [17] and could stimulate PGI_2 synthesis. In that study, sulfasalazine was found to inhibit the activity of PG 15-hydroxydehydrogenase, the first and most important enzyme in the degradation pathway of prostanoids. It was suggested that potentiation of colonic prostanoids consequent to their reduced degradation was the mechanism whereby sulfasalazine maintains the remission. Unfortunately, this concept is not consistent with the fact that in ulcerative colitis patients in remission maintained by sulfasalazine, colonic prostanoid synthesis is not enhanced and is even suppressed [8].

Efficacity of Prostanoids

The only direct study published which was designed to assess the efficacy of prostanoids for maintaining remission in ulcerative colitis was conducted by Goldin et al. [18]. In this study, 24 patients with ulcerative colitis in remission maintained by sulfasalazine were randomly assigned to either continue with sulfasalazine or to receive instead 15-(R)-15-methyl-PGE_2 (200 μg/day; Upjohn, Kalamazoo) for 28 weeks. 15-(R)-15-Methyl-PGE_2 was shown to induce duodenal ulcer healing when administered at a dose of 400 μg/day for 4 weeks [18]. Of the 12 patients who discontinued sulfasalazine and were allocated to receive the synthetic prostanoid, five flared up within the 1 month of the trial and three others had to stop the trial because of severe diarrhea. Because of the high incidence of flare-up, the study was brought to an end before its scheduled termination. In contrast, only two of the 12 sulfasalazine-treated patients flared up and the other ten concluded the trial symptom free. This trial revealed that 15-(R)-15-methyl-PGE_2 at the dose and mode of administration was not effective in maintaining remission in ulcerative colitis.

There are several possibilities to explain the failure of 15-(R)-15-methyl-PGE_2 to maintain the remission. All the prostanoid-treated participants discontinued sulfasalazine, which by itself may have been responsible for the flare-up. It is also possible that the diarrhea which preceded the flare-up in most of the subjects was responsible for its induction. 15-(R)-15-methyl-PGE_2 has secretory properties. One third of the duodenal ulcer patients treated with 400 μg/day had diarrhea [18]. Although duodenal ulcer patients treated with 100 μg/day did not have significant diarrhea [19], ulcerative colitis patients may be more sensitive. It is still intriguing why a prostanoid which has been shown to exert cytoprotective properties in the upper gut [20] did not have a similar effect in the lower gut. It is therefore possible that the various prostanoids differ in their effects in different organs.

The disappointing results with 15-(R)-15-methyl-PGE_2 should not discourage more trials with other synthetic prostanoids now available commercially. A trial with synthetic prostanoids such as misoprostol and enprostil, whose secretory effects are less pronounced, is to be recommended. It would be advisable to test the potential cytoprotective effects of smaller doses since a cytoprotective dose may be smaller than the one which induces intestinal accumulation of electrolytes and water. The latter possibility is analogous to the upper gut where the cytoprotective doses are much smaller than the antisecretory doses of the same prostanoid [1]. It is also advisable to test the effect of prostanoids administered locally as enema preparations instead of being administered orally.

Conclusion

In conclusion, it is evident that at present there is conflicting direct and indirect evidence about the possible cytoprotective properties of prostanoids in the colon and rectum. So far, in the upper gut, no study has shown efficacy of any prostanoid when administered in a small cytoprotective dose for any therapeutic indication. In spite of this, it would be worthwhile to explore further the possible potency of several prostanoids as cytoprotective agents in the large bowel in order to maintain remission in ulcerative colitis or, on the contrary, to induce remission in patients who have flared up.

References

1. Robert A (1979) Cytoprotection by prostaglandins. Gastroenterology 77: 761-7
2. Rachmilewitz D, Ligumsky M, Fich A, Goldin E, Eliakim A, Karmeli F (1986) Role of endogenous gastric prostanoids in the pathogenesis and therapy of duodenal ulcer. Gastroenterology 90: 963-9
3. Fich A, Goldin E, Zimmerman J, Ligumsky M, Rachmilewitz D (1985) Comparison of misoprostol and cimetidine in the treatment of duodenal ulcer. Isr J Med Sci 21: 102-6
4. Robert A, Bundy GL, Field SO, Nezamis JE, Davis JP, Hanchar AJ, Lancaster C, Ruwart MJ (1985) Prevention of cecitis in hamsters by certain prostaglandins. Prostaglandins 29: 960-80
5. Jones IRG, Psaila JV (1982) Cytoprotection by PGE_2 in the rat colon. Scand J Gastroenterol 78: 416 (abstract)
6. Berry H, Swinson D, Jones J, Hamilton EBD (1978) Indomethacin and naproxen suppositories in the treatment of rheumatoid arthritis. Ann Rheumatol Dis 37: 370-2
7. Flower RJ (1974) Drugs which inhibit prostaglandin biosynthesis. Pharmacol Rev 26: 33-67
8. Sharon P, Ligumsky M, Rachmilewitz D, Zor U (1978) Role of prostaglandins in ulcerative colitis. Enhanced production during active disease and inhibition by sulfasalazine. Gastroenterology 75: 638-40
9. Ligumsky M, Karmeli F, Sharon P, Zor U, Cohen F, Rachmilewitz D (1981) Enhanced thromboxane A_2 and prostacyclin production by cultured rectal mucosa in ulcerative colitis and its inhibition by steroids and sulfasalazine. Gastroenterology 81: 444-9
10. Rampton DS, Sladen GE, Youlten LY (1980) Rectal mucosal prostaglandin E_2 release and its relation to disease activity, electrical potential difference, and treatment in ulcerative colitis. Gut 21: 591-6
11. Harris DW, Smith PR, Swan CHJ. Determination of prostaglandins synthetase activity in rectal biopsy material and its significance in colonic disease. Gut 19: 875-7
12. Gould SR, Brash AR, Conolly ME, Lennard-Jones JE (1981) Studies of prostaglandins and sulfasalazine in ulcerative colitis. Prostaglandins Med 6: 165-82
13. Gilat T, Ratan J, Rosen P, Peled Y (1979) Prostaglandins and ulcerative colitis (lett). Gastroenterology 76: 1083
14. Rampton DS, Sladen GE (1981) Prostaglandin synthesis inhibitors in ulcerative colitis: Flurbiprofen compared with conventional treatment. Prostaglandins 21: 417-25
15. Rampton DS, Sladen GE (1981) Relapse of ulcerative proctocolitis during treatment with nonsteroidal anti-inflammatory drugs. Postgrad Med J 57: 297-9
16. Donowitz M (1985) Arachidonic acid metabolites and their role in inflammatory bowel disease. An update requiring addition of a pathway. Gastroenterology 88: 580-7
17. Hoult JRS, Moore PK (1978) Sulfasalazine is a potent inhibitor of prostaglandin 15 hydroxy dehydrogenase: Possible basis for therapeutic action in ulcerative colitis. Br J Pharmacol 64: 6-8
18. Goldin E, Rachmilewitz D (1983) Prostanoids cytoprotection for maintaining remission in ulcerative colitis. Failure of 15(R), 15-methylprostaglandin E_2. Dig Dis Sci 28: 807-11
19. Vantrappen G, Janssens J, Popiela T, et al (1982) Effect of 15(R)-15 methyl prostaglandin E_2 (Arbaprostil) on the healing of duodenal ulcers. A double-blind multicenter study. Gastroenterology 83: 357-63
20. Wengrower D, Fich A, Goldin E, Eliakim A, Ligumsky M, Rachmilewitz D Cytoprotective doses of arbacet with minimal antisecretory properties are not effective in duodenal ulcer healing. Dig Dis Sci, in press
21. Glbert DA, Surawicz CM, Silverstein FE et al (1984) Prevention of acute aspirin-induced gastric mucosal injury by 15(R)-15-methyl prostaglandin E_2: An endoscopic study. Gastroenterology 86: 339-45

Discussion Following the Report of Prof. Rachmilewitz

DOMSCHKE

All in all it seems clear that prostaglandins are not miracle drugs in the treatment of inflammatory bowel disease according to the experience you have reported this afternoon. Who has personal experience in this field?

SZABO

I do not have personal experience, but I would like to follow up your comment. First, prostaglandins are, indeed, not miracles, and some people use this as a criticism against cytoprotection, which infers a general protection. It is better to speak about gastroprotection and to refer to the stomach and not to all organs. But Dr. Rachmilewitz, I was really not surprised that this flare-up occurred because, if you think pathogenetically, this is what we would expect. Both in esophagitis and in colitis the inflammation is the major pathogenetic component, and PGs are well-known mediators of the inflammation. There are more and more people criticizing Vane's 1971 *Nature* article, but I think the basic fact is true: PGs are mediators of inflammation. So if we introduce PGs, we exacerbate the inflammation.

RACHMILEWITZ

That is one side of the coin. The other side is that when you administer prostanoids in the upper gut, they are very effective.

SZABO

They are protective in the stomach but not against esophagitis. The results are contradictory.

RACHMILEWITZ

It may vary from organ to organ. The crucial thing really is to decide what is the role of prostanoids in the pathogenesis of the disease events in ulcerative colitis and, if you want, also in Crohn's disease. Are they really responsible for the inflammation? Are they really responsible for the diarrhea? There are pro's and con's for each argument. I do not know the anser.

SZABO

You had a nice study design using ulcerative colitis and Crohn's disease in parallel. Now, by classic definition ulcerative colitis is superficial lesion while Crohn's disease is usually more severe, although there are skip lesions. But most of the products you examined showed no difference between the two lesions; sometimes ulcerative colitis produced an increase, sometimes Crohn's disease. What is your prediction? Would this not indicate that these are perhaps not the major mediators of inflammation, since Crohn's disease is usually more severe? Or is there something else which is involved?

RACHMILEWITZ

It is evident that you are not a clinician. We are clinicians.

SZABO

I am a pathologist, and I see things closely and not at distance or through endoscope.

RACHMILEWITZ

It was obvious from the way you presented the question. For us clinicians these are two inflammatory diseases of the bowel. All that you have said about therm is true. In principle, they are similar. But there are also differences. Ulcerative colitis is superficial, Crohn's disease involves the whole thickness of the bowel. Ulcerative colitis involves only the colon. Crohn's disease can involve any part of the gut. Unfortunately, we do not know the etiologies of them, so we tend to regard them as two nonspecific inflammatory diseases of the bowel, and I think as long as we do not know the etiology, all that has to do with the pathogenesis should be regarded by us in a similar fashion. I agree that we are limited.

SZABO

Did you not try to measure leukotrienes?

RACHMILEWITZ

No, we did not, but Dr. Sharon will talk about this.

PESKAR

I should like to add a comment to the question of Dr. Szabo. Prostaglandins are not only pro-inflammatory; it has been shown that in chronic inflammation prostaglandins may have anti-inflammatory actions. Thus, the role of endogenous prostaglandins or the therapeutic action of exogenous prostaglandin may differ in the acute stage of colonic inflammation and in remission. We have been able to show that sulfasalazine can both inhibit and increase formation of prostaglandins E_2 by colonic mucosa in vitro, depending on the experimental conditions used. Sulfasalazine increases release of prostaglandin E_2 from the tissue, resulting from both stimulation of synthesis and inhibition of metabolism, when a short incubation period is used. During prolonged incubation as in the experiments of Dr. Rachmilewitz, who used a 24-h organ-culture technique, sulfasalazine inhibits release of prostaglandins. This differential effect may be due to the fact that sulfasalazine stimulates prostaglandin synthesis at high concentrations of the substrate arachidonic acid, but inhibits prostaglandin formation at low substrate concentrations. During the initial phase of an in vitro incubation more arachidonic acid may be released, leading to higher concentrations at the site of cyclooxygenase than during prolonged incubations. Due to the complex and variable effects of sulfasalazine on the enzymes of prostaglandin synthesis and metabolism it is difficult to predict from in vitro studies, whether sulfasalazine in vivo may increase or inhibit prostaglandin release.

RACHMILEWITZ

I agree with all you have said. One should keep in mind the point that when tissue was obtained from patients with ulcerative colitis in remission, maintained by sulfasalazine, prostanoid production was as in normal subjects. We did not in this instance add sulfasalazine to the culture medium; this was an in vivo experiment in which the patients were taking the sulfasalazine, and their disease was in remission.

PESKAR

This does not exclude the possibility that in vivo patients under treatment with sulfasalazine may act in a different way to a stimulus of prostaglandin formation than nontreated patients do.

DOMSCHKE

That cannot be excluded. With regard to the potential therapeutic use of prostaglandins I do have indirect evidence which might be able to militate against the potentially beneficial effect of prostaglandins in inflammatory bowel disease. We have tried enemas containing carbenoxolone, which is capable of inhibiting the prostaglandin catabolism, thus increasing endogenous prostaglandin levels. And as a consequence dramatic clinical deterioration occured in the patiens treated in this way.

RACHMILEWITZ

I think that we will not be able to say the last word in this regard until someone treats locally with a different prostanoid preparation which has less or minimal secretory effects. This must be done if we really want a clear answer to this question.

DOMSCHKE

What I have presented is only indirect evidence.

RAMPTON

Can I just ask the chairman directly whether he measured colonic prostaglandin production in patients given carbenoxolone?

DOMSCHKE

No, we did not.

RAMPTON

So you do not actually know whether it inhibited prostaglandin catabolism or not?

DOMSCHKE

Yes, you are right.

COHEN

Dr. Rachmilewitz, I think your enthusiasm is admirable, but I find it very difficult, based on the evidence that you have presented, to share it. You seem to be saying that because prostaglandins have been shown to protect against acute injury in the stomach, they are therefore "cyto- or gastro-protective", and that they therefore are an appropriate treatment of inflammatory conditions. To me, this makes no sense at all. Where is the clinical evidence that prostaglandin is effective in the treatment of any acute inflammatory or chronic inflammatory condition? Where is the evidence that they are effective in esophagitis? Is there evidence that they are effective in the treatment even of gastritis? What is the evidence that they are effective in the treatment of pancreatitis, for example? Why do you still want to try them in colitis despite your disastrous results with arbacet?

RACHMILEWITZ

First, I am surprised: you know me long enough to know that I do not sound enthusiastic about it at all. At the time we were really forced to do that kind of an experiment or clinical trial, and we did not know much about leukotrienes – hardly anything. All information was about prostanoids. Viewing the emerging information about the positive effects of PGs in the upper gut, we got the courage to do that trial. The lower gut and the upper gut including the esophagus are embryologically derived from the same root. This was the only idea behind the trial. I still think that it may be possible that prostanoids will share properties in the upper and lower gut. I agree with all that you have said. As far as we know, prostanoids may mediate inflammatory conditions. You introduce them to the joint and induce inflammation; you introduce them to the eye and induce uveitis. But this still does not explain why nonsteroidals are not effective in ulcerative colitis.

COHEN

So why do you even want to try it again?

RACHMILEWITZ

Why are nonsteroidals not effective? Why do you give indomethacin to patients with active colitis and see a tragedy?

COHEN

But they do other things than inhibit cyclooxygenase.

RACHMILEWITZ

I think that many things intervene here and share effects. I do not feel strongly about this issue, and I was just saying that because of the results of our study, I would not give up the whole possibility.

COHEN

I suppose what I am asking is: How many more disasters do we need before we drop it?

RACHMILEWITZ

If you administer locally, say, misoprostol to 12 subjects and they do not do well. I will drop it. But until this is done. I think there is a small niche which one should still try.

SZABO

Actually I am just encouraged by Dr. Cohen's statement. What I tried to put mildly, as a pathologist he said with the surgeon's aggressiveness, with sharp questions. And actually this is what I wanted to ask Professor Peskar, since I take her word, and because she is a respected authority. You mentioned that there are data showing that prostaglandins have anti-inflammatory actions in chronic conditions. I am not aware of any such data. Are these your studies or others' published data?

PESKAR

These are mainly data by two groups. Morley has shown that prostaglandin E_1 inhibits lymphokiene secretion by human lymphocytes, and work by Bonta's group has demonstrated that in experimental models of chronic inflammation prostaglandins exert anti-inflammatory effects.

WHITTLE

We know that prostaglandins can protect against luminal challenging agents in the gastric mucosa and, indeed, in the colon. Is there any evidence that ulcerative colitis or Crohn's disease is a disease that is mediated by luminal injurious agents. If there is such evidence, then perhaps this would be a rationale for using prostaglandins in maintenance.

RACHMILEWITZ

Both ulcerative colitis and Crohn's disease are obscure diseases, and there is no indication for any contributing factor to their etiology. Therefore we strike in the dark. We had a probe, and if someone suggests something that may be beneficial, people may try it. By the way, it would be worthwhile to see whether if one administers synthetic prostanoids to normal subjects with normal colonic mucosa, one induces colonic inflammation. This is a question by itself; I am not so sure it would.

WHITTLE

Prostaglandins themselves may be only weak inflammatory mediators, but potentiate the actions of other mediators. These pro-inflammatory effects of prostaglandins are largely attributed to their local vasodilator effects. Many of the other inflammatory properties that were described early in the literature such as chemotactic properties are usually achieved at relatively high concentrations.

Inflammatory Bowel Disease: Treatment Modalities and Mucosal Prostaglandin/Leukotriene Formation

P. SHARON

Introduction

Ulcerative colitis (UC) and Crohn's disease are inflammatory diseases of unknown etiology. Not only are the etiologies unknown, but the soluble mediators that amplify and modulate the inflammatory response have not been fully explored. Our studies have focused on delineating the soluble mediators of inflammation in inflammatory bowel disease (IBD) with emphasis on the role played by arachidonic acid metabolitis via the cyclooxygenase pathway, prostaglandin E_2 (PGE_2), thromboxane A_2 (TXA_2), prostacyclin I_2 (PGI_2), and the lipoxygenase product leukotriene B_4 (LTB_4) and 5-hydroxy-6,8,11,14-eicosatetraenoic acid (5-HETE). Some early events in inflammation, such as vascular dilatation and increased vascular permeability with gaps between vascular endothelial cells, are common to all organ systems. Monocytes and neutrophils adhere to the surface of venule endothelial cells and subsequently migrate from the bloodstream into injured tissue through the process of diapedesis.

Soluble mediators of inflammation like bradykinia, histamine, platelet activating factor, and arachidonic acid metabolites share certain biologic effects. Several of these compounds increase vascular permeability, vasodilatation, edema, and fever and some, including a number of arachidonate metabolites, are neutrophil chemotactic agents. A combination of these mediators is involved in most inflammatory processes, making it difficult to assign responsibility for any portion of the inflammatory process to a particular mediator. The large number of potentially important mediators complicates therapy, in that pharmacologic agents directed against one mediator may have no effect upon the others.

Production of Eicosanoids in Patients with IBD

There are two major pathways of arachidonic acid metabolism in mammalian cells (Fig. 1). The cyclooxygenase pathway leads to the production of PGE_2, TXA_2, and PGI_2 which is present in all mammalian cells, including the cells of the gastrointestinal tract. The lipoxygenase pathway, the second major pathway of arachidonic metabolism, is found in only a few mammalian cells including neutrophils and monocytes. The lipoxygenase pathway leads to the production of leukotriene and monohydroxy fatty acids.

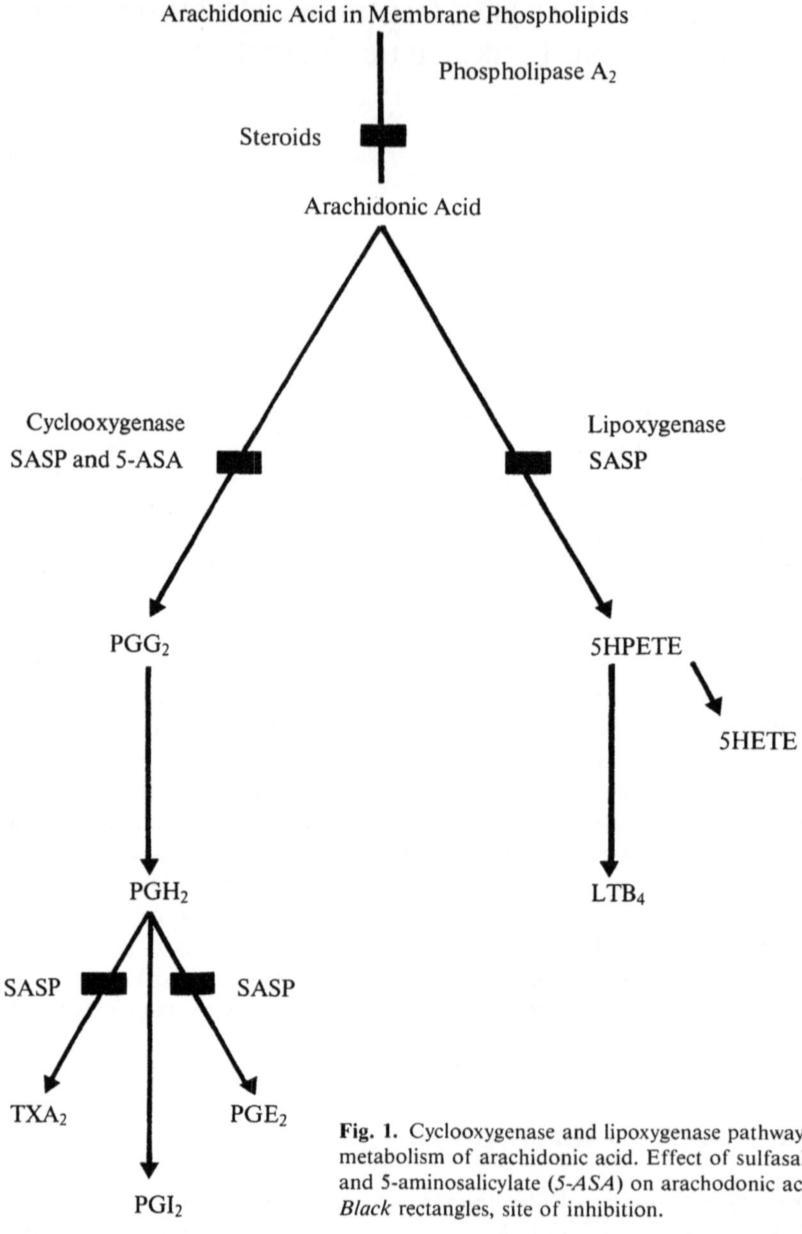

Fig. 1. Cyclooxygenase and lipoxygenase pathways of metabolism of arachidonic acid. Effect of sulfasalazine *(SASP)* and 5-aminosalicylate (*5-ASA*) on arachodonic acid metabolism. *Black* rectangles, site of inhibition.

Prostaglandins

Colonic mucosa of patients with active IBD produces increased quantities of prostanoids, whether assessed in vitro or in vivo by assay of feces, rectal dialysate, or urine [1–4]. We have demonstrated an increase in prostanoid synthesis by cultured rectal mucosa obtained from patients with active UC. The accumulation in the medium of PGE_2, TXA_2, and PGI_2 by cultured rectal mucosa obtained from patients with active UC was significantly higher than their respective accumulation by cultured biopsy specimens obtained from normal subjects. Moreover, the accumulation of the different prostanoids by rectal mucosa of UC patients in remission was not enhanced [5].

The cell type responsible for the increase in prostanoid production in active IBD is uncertain; intestinal epithelial cells, leukocytes, mononuclear cells, and endothelial cells are all capable of prostanoid synthesis. The enhanced intestinal prostanoid synthesis in active Crohn's disease is probably derived from stimulated local mononuclear cells [6]. Of more clinical relevance is whether the observed alteration in prostanoid metabolism in IBD has any role in the pathophysiology of the disease. There is much experimental evidence suggesting that prostaglandins are involved in mediation of inflammation. They produce vascular permeability vasodilatation, and alteration in the absorption and motility of intestinal electrolyte [2–3]. Prostaglandin levels decline when patients with IBD are treated with either corticosteroids or sulfasalazine. However, prostaglandin levels also decline when patients with IBD are treated with cyclooxygenase inhibitors like indomethacin, but patients do not show clinical improvement. There is, in fact, some evidence that nonsteroidal anti-inflammatory drugs may increase the severity of IBD. This last finding suggests that PGE_2 may not be an important mediator in IBD and that the mechanism of action of corticosteroids and sulfasalazine may not relate to the inhibition of prostaglandin synthesis.

Leukotriene B_4 and Monohydroxy Fatty Acids

LTB_4 and 5-HETE are products of the lipoxygenase pathway and are the major arachidonate metabolites in neutrophils. LTB_4 and, to a lesser extent, 5-HETE exert significant biologic effects. In addition to being a potent neutrophil chemotactic agent, LTB_4 also increases vascular permeability and induces aggregation and degranulation of neutrophils [7]. A less potent chemotactic agent, 5-HETE, also causes neutrophils to degranulate and, at high concentrations, increases colonic chloride secretion [8]. There are at least two points of correlation between BD and the biologic effects of these compounds: the mucosa in IBD is infiltrated with neutrophils, suggesting the presence of a neutrophil chemotactic factor, and there is edema in the mucosa in IBD suggesting increased vascular permeability.

To investigate the role played by lipoxygenase metabolites of arachidonic acid as mediators of inflammation in IBD, mucosa scraped from colonic surgical specimens from patients with IBD or normal mucosa from uninvolved areas of colonic resections for adenocarcinoma was incubated with radiolabeled arachidonic acid. In mucosa from normal subjects, some of the arachidonic acid was incorporated into phospholipids and triglycerides, but the vast majority was not metabolized. In contrast, in mucosa from patients with IBD, either Crohn's disease or UC, much of the arachidonic acid was converted through the lipoxygenase pathway to LTB_4 or to monohydroxy fatty acids, including 5-HETE. The same effects were observed whether the lipids were separated by thin-layer chromatography or by reverse-phase high-pressure liquid chromatography (HPLC). The amount of arachidonic acid converted to the lipoxygenase products was several times higher than the amount converted to cyclooxygenase products. These data may shed some light on the role of prostaglandins in IBD [9].

Lipids were extracted from the colonic mucosa and separated by HPLC in order to determine whether these lipoxygenase products exist in the tissue endogenously. LTB_4, 12-HETE, 15-HETE, and 5-HETE were present endogenously in the IBD mucosa. The LTB_4 contents of IBD mucosa averaged 254 ng per gram of mucosa, whereas normal mucosa contains less than 5 ng of LTB_4 per gram of mucosa (which was the lower limits of sensitivity of our assay). If this concentration of LTB_4 in IBD mucosa were in solution, it would be well within the biologically active range for LTB_4.

Other groups have investigated the lipoxygenase pathway in IBD.

Broughton-Smith et al. found increased synthesis of mono-HETEs by IBD mucosa incubated with ^{14}C arachidonic acid [10]. Peskar et al. incubated rectal biopsies from normal patients and patients with IBD in the presence and absence of A23187. They found increased synthesis of both LTB_4 and sulphidopeptide-leukotrienes by biopsies from IBD patients [11]. Finally, Lauritsen et al. studied PGE_2 and LTB_4 production in vivo in UC. They placed bags of dialysis tubing in the rectums of normal patients and patients with UC. After 4-h the bags were removed, and the concentrations of LTB_4 and PGE_2 were measured.

The concentrations of LTB_4 and PGE_2 were much higher in the rectal dialysates from the UC patients than from the controls. Moreover, the concentrations of LTB_4 and PGE_2 declined markedly when the UC patients were treated with a short course of prednisolone [12].

The Acetic Acid Colitis Model

The absence of a good animal model has plagued research in IBD. All animal models are deficient in varying degrees in their similarities to human IBD. We used a simple toxic model of inflammation to examine the synthesis of arachidonic metabolites. Diluted acetic acid was injected into rat colon an effects were observed after 24–48h [13]. Histologic analysis of this model of intestinal inflammation showed the formation of ulcers and profound neutrophil infiltration. Arachidonic acid metabolism in colonic mucosa from acetic acid-treated rat was compared with that from normal rat. The normal rat mucosa metabolized only a very small portion of the exogenous arachidonic acid, whereas the colonic mucosa from acetic acid-treated rat converted a significant portion of exogenous arachidonate to lipoxygenase products LTB_4, 5-HETE, 12-HETE, and 15-HETE, and a small portion of the arachidonate to PGE_2 and TXA_2. When the endogenous mucosal lipids of the normal and acetic acid-treated rats were compared, the acetic acid-treated colonic mucosa was found to have significant amounts of LTB_4, 5-HETE, 12-HETE, and 15-HETE. These compounds were not present in the normal mucosa. Moreover, arachidonic acid metabolism in acetic acid-treated mucosa clearly resembles that in human IBD (Fig. 2).

The precise cellular origin of gastrointestinal arachidonic acid metabolites is not certain. While colonic and ileal epithelial cells are capable of producing prostanoids, the enhanced intestinal prostanoid synthesis in IBD is derived from stimulated local mononuclear cells [6]. The acuteness of the inflammatory response correlates with the

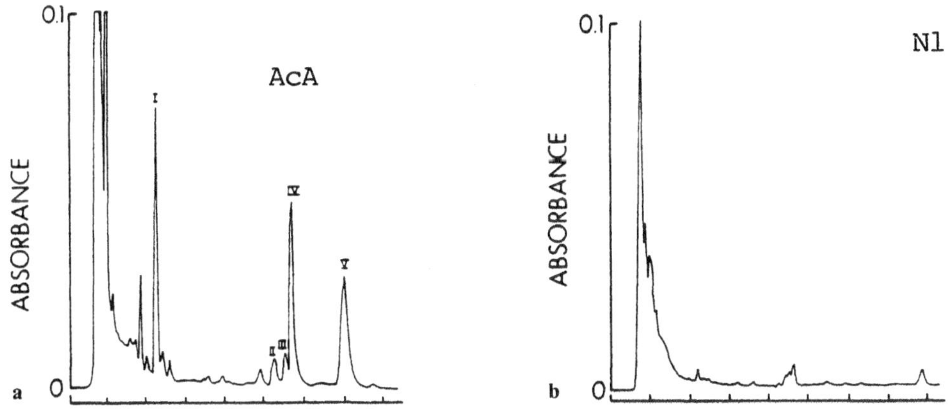

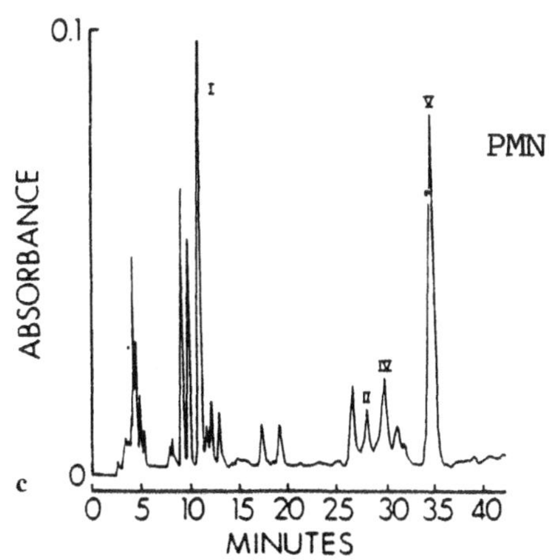

Fig. 2a–c. Metabolism of exogenous arachidonic acid by acetic acid-treated and normal rat mucosa and rat neutrophils. Colonic mucosa (500 mg) or neutrophils ($5x10^7$/ml) were incubated for 5 min at 37 °C with arachidonic acid (100 μ*M*) and A23187 (2 μ*M*). The incubation was terminated, the mucosa was homogenized, and the lipids were extracted. The extracted lipids were subjected to reverse-phase PLC. The chromatogram was developed isocoitically with methanol/water/acetic acid (75 :25 :0.04) at 1 ml/min. Absorbance was measured at 270 nm for 20 min and then at 235 nm. **a** Acetic acid-treated rat colonic mucosa. **b** Normal rat colonic mucosa. **c** Rat peritoneal exudate neutrophils. *Peak I*, LTB_4; *peak II*, 15-HETE; *peak III*, 11-HETE; *peak IV*, 12-HETE; *peak V*, 5-HETE

presence of numerous neutrophils in the mucosa. The pattern of the lipoxygenase arachidonic acid metabolites in acetic acid colitis closely resembles that of stimulated peripheral blood neutrophils [14], with LTB_4 and 5-HETE being the most prominent products (Fig. 2). To determine if the neutrophils that infiltrate the mucosa in acid colitis are the main source of arachidonate metabolites, we performed an experiment with neutrophil-depleted rats. Rats were treated with antineutrophil serum raised in rabbits. The antineutrophil serum caused a fall of 80% in the blood neutrophils. The neutrophil-depleted rats were then treated with acetic acid. The rats were sacrificed 24h later, and the colonic mucosa was incubated with arachidonic acid in the presence of ionophore A23187. The mucosa from undepleted rats produced LTB_4 and 5-HETE, in addition to 12-HETE, 11-HETE, and 15-HETE. The mucosa from the neutrophil-depleted rats produced similar amounts of 12-HETE, 11-HETE, and 15-HETE, but only 15% of LTB_4 or 5-HETE compared to undepleted rats. These results suggest that in the acetic acid colitis mucosa, the major source of LTB_4 and 5-HETE ist the neutrophils that infiltrate the mucosa. In conclusion, the lipoxygenase metabolites of arachidonic acid in both IBD an acetic acid colitis are formed primarily by components of acute rather than chronic phase of the inflammatory response. The most important cellular component appear to be the neutrophils. The pattern of arachidonate metabolism seen in IBD mucosa is not specific to IBD and is probably common to all forms of intestinal inflammation with an acute component.

Chemotactic Activity in IBD

Having established the presence of LTB_4 in the mucosa of patients with IBD, we next studied the role of LTB_4 as a chemotactic agent responsible for the heavy neutrophil infiltration in the colonic mucosa in IBD. These functional studies involved primarily assays of chemotaxis, the movement of neutrophils through a chemical gradient in the direction of the highest concentration. Among the soluble mediators of inflammation that are important neutrophil chemotactic agents are C5a, which is a part of the complement cascade, bacterially derived peptides including formylmethionyllenicyphenylalamine (FMLP), and the arachidonate metabolites LTB_4 and, to a lesser extent, 5-HETE. Colonic mucosa from two normal patients and nine patients with IBD was assayed for chemotactic activity for human neutrophils in vitro in a Boyden chamber [15]. The chemotactic response to UC mucosa (fife patients) was about 20-fold higher than normal mucosa and the response to Crohn's colitis mucosa was more than 20 times as much compared to normal mucosa. Analysis of the chemotactic activity in the IBD mucosa revealed that most was lipid extract. Moreover, when the lipid extract was fractionated by reverse-phase HPLC, the only fraction with significant chemotactic activity was the fraction that coeluded with LTB_4. The chemotactic response to IBD mucosa was blocked by anti-LTB_4 antisera. The amount of chemotactic activity in lipid extracts of different IBD specimens correlates well with the concentration of LTB_4 in the mucosa (250 ng/g of mucosa). These data suggest that LTB_4 is an important stimulus to neutrophil chemotaxis in IBD and may thus play a major role in the amplification of the inflammatory response in this condition.

Treatment Modalities

One major potential benefit from the increased understanding of the metabolism of arachidonic acid in IBD is the chance to understand how drugs known to be useful in the treatment of IBD work, with the intention of developing even more effective, safer therapy. Most drugs that are used in IBD have more than a simple effect, and just because a drug alters arachidonic acid metabolism in a certain way does not indicate that it is acting to alter the course of IBD via that mechanism. Glucocorticoids, which are the most effective drugs in the treatment of IBD, prevent formation of free arachidonic acid from arachidonic acid bound into membrane phospholipids by inhibiting phospholipase A_2 and thus block both the cyclooxygenase and lipoxygenase pathways. Sulfasalazine (SASP), which is also effective in the treatment of IBD, is metabolized in the colon to 5-aminosalicylic acid (5-ASA) and sulfapyridine.

While it is thought that SASP and 5-ASA is the therapeutic agent, there is substantial evidence that the parent compound, SASP, possesses pharmacologic properties distinct from those of 5-ASA. One of the difficulties in determining therapeutically relevant pharmacologic effects is determining the appropriate concentrations of these compounds for study. In treated patients the concentrations of these compounds in stool are enormous: 2 m*M* for SASP and 10 m*M* for 5-ASA. However, they are poorly absorbed, and the serum concentrations are quite low. Thus, high concentrations of these agents are observed on the lumenal side of the inflamed mucosa, while concentrations in the capillaries are minimal. The concentration of drugs to which relevant cells in the mucosa are exposed is unclear. When tested in in vitro assay systems at concentrations found in the colonic lumen, these compounds exert many pharmacologic effects, including inhibition of arachidonic metabolism, whereas when tested at concentrations found in the serum, their pharmacologic effects are relatively minimal.

SASP and 5-ASA in concentrations of 1,5 m*M* and 2,5 m*M* respectively, inhibit the accumulation of PGE_2, TXA_2, and PGI_2 by cultured rectal mucosa obtained from active UC patients [5]. SASP also decreased the products of the lipoxygenase pathway in a colonic mucosa of IBD patients by 60% [10]. The effects of SASP and 5-ASA on arachidonic acid metabolism in acetic acid colitis rat are what would be predicted, based on studies in other systems [13]. SASP blocked both the cyclooxygenase and lipoxygenase pathways in a manner consistent with previous studies in periferal blood neutrophils [14], while 5-ASA blocked the cyclooxygenase but not the lipoxygenase pathway (Fig. 1). Sulfapyridine had no effect on arachidonate metabolism. Determining which of the wide range of pharmacologic effects of these agents is relevant to their mechanisms of action in treating IBD is yet to be resolved. Presently there is no selective inhibitor of 5-lipoxygenase available for clinical use. If such a compound were identified, it might be interesting to observe its effects on the production of chemical mediators in animal models of intestinal inflammation. One may be able to predict their efficacy in the treatment of IBD.

Conclusion

Conclusions that can be drawn from this study are:

1. Arachidonic acid is metabolized by the inflamed colinic mucosa into the cyclo-oxygenase pathway and the lipoxygenase pathway.
2. The major arachidonic acid metabolites of human IBD mucosa are the lipoxygenase products (LTB_4 and 5-HETE), rather than the cyclooxygenase products (PGE_2, TXB_2, and PGI_2).
3. These products are present at much higher concentration in IBD mucosa than in normal mucosa.
4. There is significantly more chemotactic activity in IBD mucosa than in normal mucosa, mostly attributable to LTB_4.
5. The inflammatory infiltrate, mainly with neutrophils, in the mucosa of IBD patients may be responsible for the production of arachidonic acid metabolites. While it is unlikely that LTB_4 plays a role in the initiation of the inflammatory response or the recruitment of the first neutrophils out of the bloodstream in the mucosa, it appears to be responsible for the promulgation of the chemotactiv response and the subsequent attraction of other circulating neutrophils into the mucosa. Thus, the enhanced synthesis of LTB_4 may account, in part, for the preservation and amplification of the inflammatory response in IBD.

6. The mechanistic basis for future therapy for IBD may be based on selective inhibitors of the lipoxygenase pathway.

References

1. Gould SR, Brash AR, Connolly ME, Lennard-Jones JE (1981) Studies of Prostaglandins and Sulfasalazine in Ulcerative Colitis. Prostaglandins and Medicine 6: 165–185
2. Donowitz M (1985) Arachidonic Acid Metabolites and Their Role in Inflammatory Bowel Disease. Gastroenterology 88: 580–587
3. Rampton DS, Hawkey CJ (1984) Prostaglandins and Ulcerative Colitis. Gut 25: 1399–1413
4. Sharon P, Ligumsky M, Rachmilewitz D, Zor U (1978) Role of Prostaglandins in Ulcerative Colitis. Enhanced Production During Active Disease and Inhibition by Sulfasalazine. Gastroenterology 75: 638–640
5. Ligumsky M, Karmali F, Sharon P, Zor U, Cohen F, Rachmilewitz D (1981) Enhanced Thromboxane A_2 and Prostaglandin Production by Cultured Rectal Mucosa in Ulcerative Colitis and Its Inhibition by Steroids and Sulfasalazine. Gastroenterology 81: 444–449
6. Zifroni A, Treves AJ, Sachar DB, Rachmilewitz D (1983) Prostanoid Synthesis by Cultured Intestinal Epithelial and Mononuclear Cells in Inflammatory Bowel Disease. Gut 24: 659–664
7. Ford-Hutchinson AW, Bray MA, Doig MV, Shipley ME, Smith JF (1984) Leukotriene B, a Potent Chemotactic and Aggregating Substance Released from Polymorphonuclear Leukocytes. Nature 266: 264–265
8. Musch MW, Kachur JF, Miller RJ, Field M (1983) Bradykinin Stimulates Electrolyte Secretion in Rabbit and Guinea Pig Intestine: Involvement of Arachidonic Acid Metabolites. Journal of Clinical Investigation 71: 1073–1083
9. Sharon P, Stenson WF (1984) Enhanced Synthesis of Leukotriene B_4 by Colonic Mucosa in Inflammatory Bowel Disease. Gastroenterology 86: 453–460
10. Broughton-Smith NK, Hawkey CJ, Whittle BJR (1983) Biosynthesis of Lipoxygenase and Cyclooxygenase Products from ^{14}C-Arachidonic Acid by Human Colinic Mucosa. Gut 24: 1176–1182
11. Peskar BM, Dreyling KW, May B, Thieves M, Morgenroth K, Goebell H, Peskar BA (1985) Increased Formation of Leukotriene B_4 and Sulphidopeptide-Leukotrienes by Rectal Mucosa of Patients with Crohn's Disease and Ulcerative Colitis. (Abstract) Gut 26: A542–A543
12. Lauritsen K, Laursen LS, Bukhave K, Rash-Madsen J (1985) Effects of Systemic Prednisolone on Arachidonic Acid Metabolites Determined by Equilibrium In Vivo Dialysis of Rectum in Severe Relapsing Ulcerative Colitis. (Abstract) Gastroenterology 88: 1466
13. Sharon P, Stenson WF (1985) Metabolism of Arachidonic Acid in Acetic Acid Colitis Rats: Similarity to Human Inflammatory Bowel Disease. Gastroenterology 88: 55–63
14. Stenson WF, Lobos EA (1982) Sulfasalazine Inhibits the Synthesis of Chemotactic Lipids by Neutrophils. Journal of Clinical Investigation 69: 494–497
15. Lobos EA, Sharon P, Stenson WF Chemotactic Activity in Inflammatory Bowel Disease: Role of Leukotriene B_4. Dig Dis and Sci (in press)

Discussion Following the Report of Prof. Sharon

HAMMARSTRÖM

I have two questions. One relates to the methodology: When you incubated the tissues and measured leukotriene levels, did you add some stimuli?

SHARON

Yes, we did. We added, ionophore to most of the experiments; on the TLC studies in half the cases we used ionophore, and in half we did not.

HAMMARSTRÖM

The second question is: You did not say anything about the cysteine-containing leukotrienes, LTC_4, LTD_4, LTE_4?

SHARON

We did not test any of the other leukotrienes, neither LTC_4 not the other leukotrienes.

HAMMARSTRÖM

What was the reason? Were they not picked up by your assay?

SHARON

The time was short, and we ran into a difficult problem getting them in the HPLC system; this is basically why we did not check them.

PELSTER

Have you ever tested nafazatrom in your animal model? Nafazatrom is a selective lipoxygenase inhibitor.

SHARON

No, we did not. In the beginning we tried to use the BW755, that in a very low dose looked like a selective lipoxygenase inhibitor but not so at higher doses.

PELSTER

BW755C is a duodenal inhibitor, but nafazatrom is a selective lipoxygenase inhibitor. You should try it if you are searching for a selective 5-lipoxygenase inhibitor.

SZABO

My question is related to Dr. Hammarström's remark, because I was also impressed that there were no increases in cysteinyl leukotrienes. We picked up with Dr. O'Brien that in most of your data the so-called "other" group was the major group of compounds. LTB_4 and thromboxane were in the range 0.3, whatever the units were, and the so-called "other" category was usually around 3.0. So you have quite a lot of other compounds in that category. But I think you are lucky, and you had a good design because even the so-called "other" category was increased 3-fold, both in the samples from the patients and from acetic-acid colitis.

SHARON

The "others" are mainly phospholipids and equivalents.

SZABO

Are the cysteinyl leukotrienes included, or are they separated?

SHARON

No, this system is not able to separate LTC_4.

PESKAR

We studied the release of cysteinyl-containing leukotrienes in patients with ulcerative colitis and Crohn's disease and found a significantly increases synthesizing capacity of the mucosa for this type of leukotrienes. We also studied the effect of 5-aminosalycylic acid on formation of both LTB_4 and on cysteinyl-containing leukotrienes by noninflamed human colonic mucosa and inflamed colonic mucosa from patients with Crohn's disease. In this tissue 5-aminosalicylic acis dose-dependently inhibits formation of prostaglandins, LTB_4, and cysteinyl-containing leukotriens. The IC 50 for inhibition was approximately 3.5 m*M*. Perhaps there is a species difference to the rat with respect to the efficacy of the drug.

SHARON

Perhaps; we checked it in man, and we used up to 5 m*M* of 5-aminosalicylic acid, and we could not get any inhibition of the lipoxygenase in the TLC system which we used.

PESKAR

Maybe we should compare the methodology used.

SHARON

Did you use also rats?

PESKAR

No, we did not use the rat.

SHARON

But it is known that this model is quite easy, and we were excited by the fact that basically the arachidonic-acid metabolism in man and acetic-acid model were similar.

DOMSCHKE

May I shall try to sum up briefly? When we were talking about the clinical importance of prostaglandins in the context of inflammatory bowel disease, we began with Dr. Rampton's presentation dealing with the effects of nonsteroidal antiinflammatory drugs in ulcerative colitis patients in the active as well as in the quiescent phase of that disease. He showed us that these compounds do more harm than good, and consequently one can speculate that this may be due to a consecutive prostaglandin deficiency or, in other word, that cytoprotective actions might be attributed to prostaglandins. This is why in the following paper Dr. Rachmilewitz spoke of the effects of exogenous prostaglandins on inflammatory bowel disease, presenting evidence mostly militating against an essential involvement of prostaglandins as a therapeutic means in this clinical condition. As an alternative explanation for the deleterious effects on nonsteroidal anti-inflammatory drugs, it can be hypothesized that the metabolic activity is shifted to the other arm of the eicosanoid metabolism, that is to say, to the formation of lipoxygenase-mediated products. This latter point has been emphasized and further supported by the last paper, that delivered by Dr. Sharon, firstly, by the fact that the inflamed colonic mucosa synthesized leukotrienes at a higher rate than it synthesizes prostaglandins, and, secondly, by the fact that the clinically active compounds in the context of inflammatory bowel disease, namely sulfasalazine as well as one of its breakdown products, 5-aminosalicylic acid, inhibits both enzyme activities, i.e,. lipoxygenase as well as cyclooxygenase, whereas the other breakdown product, sulfapyridine, only inhibits cyclooxygenase activity, and this latter breakdown product has been shown to be clinically inactive.

Prostaglandins: Their Potential Therapeutic Value in the Upper Gastrointestinal Tract

The Natural History of Ulcer Disease and its Impact upon Therapeutic Options and Assessment of Drug Safety

M. J. S. LANGMAN

Introduction

In deciding what influence upon outcome there might be from the introduction of effective medical treatment for ulcer, we are greatly hindered by the lack of a stable background of ulcer frequency. Figures coming from countries with Western cultural patterns suggest a general decline in ulcer mortality. These may form a poor proxy for occurrence rates, but other data, which include sickness absence rates in the United Kingdom [1] attributed to ulcer, and hospital admission rates for all varieties of ulcer disease both in the United Kingdom and the USA show pronounced falls [23]. Using these figures by themselves, it is not possible to distinguish the influence of changing fashions in management from a true decline in disease frequency.

Taking United Kingdom admission data for all duodenal ulcer in men by themselves, the pattern seems to have been that of a reasonably stable frequency rate until about 1970, followed by a precipitous fall. This fall antedates the introduction of effective medical treatment and presumably reflects changing fashions of management. However, the pattern is almost certainly more complex. When ulcer perforation is considered by itself there has been a steady decline in the number of cases. Clearly not all of these are new but cases of perforated ulcer probably give as close an approximation to the frequency of newly occuring disease as can be obtained.

The decline in perforated ulcer frequency has mainly occurred in younger men, whereas in older women the disease has become markedly more frequent associated with, but probably only partly due to, treatment with non-steroidal anti-inflammatory drugs [4]. The reasons for these general changes are largely obscure, but they present morals in considering choices of treatment. The frequency of associated disease of, for instance, the cardiovascular system is high in the elderly, and elderly patients withstand the stresses imposed by ulcer complications and by surgery, elective or emergency, poorly.

Table 1 shows the average mortality rate associated with gastric surgery in 1975 in Scotland [5]. The high mortality rated in part reflect the combined data obtained from considering emergency plus elective operations. However, they still supply a useful counter-weight to series of data obtained in patients operated upon in specialist centres. Surgeons are understandably reluctant to operate on older patients and ask that the elderly should be considered for operation many years earlier. However, this idealistic approach ignores the probability that much of the ulcer disease in the elderly is new and not of long standing and even in that of long standing it was not necessarily

Table 1. Mortality associated with gastric surgery in Scotland 1975 [5]

	Age in years		
	50–	60–	70–
Operation	% deaths		
Vagotomy + g. enterostomy	0.7	2.8	5.9
+ other products	2.4	2.6	12.7
All operations	3.7	8.1	16.5

apparent that the disease course would indeed prove to be unsatisfactory during conventional medical treatment.

Anti-ulcer Treatment-Datas

Some idea of what happens to ordinary patients receiving anti-ulcer treatment can be obtained by considering the surveillance study conducted in Nottingham, Oxford, Portsmouth and Glasgow where morbidity and mortality patterns were examined in random samples of some 10000 cimetidine recipients and age-sex-matched controls. The use of controls allowed comparisons with experience with the ordinary population in the United Kingdom, with, as an added check, a further comparison with age- and sex-specific mortality data published by the Office for Population Censuses and Surveys (OPCS).

Data obtained therefore reflected a combination of information about

a) ordinary disease patterns in the population
b) the disease experience of ulcer patients and of dyspeptics in general (since prescriptions were freely issued for any indication a practitioner considered appropriate)
c) the symptom and disease patterns present in those issued with prescriptions who could not be assumed to be a random sample of the symptomatic population
d) any illness associated with and caused by treatment.

Results obtained have been reported in detail elsewhere [6–9]. They indicate that the events recorded mainly arose in association with disease already present in the cimetidine takers prior to drug prescription or else in association with the social habits of those individuals, particularly smoking and alcohol consumption.

Hospital admission, or attendance as an outpatient, was more frequent in takers than in controls for a wide variety of non-dyspeptic complaints, these including, for instance, excesses of lung cancer, hepatic cirrhosis and accidental poisoning and violence, which emphasized the role of smoking and alcohol although a subsample survey suggested, somewhat oddly, that drug recipients smoking habits did not differ materially from those of the controls.

Table 2a. Observed and expected deaths in recipients of cimetidine [6–9]. Overall mortality during first study year

	Observed deaths		Expected deaths
	Takers	Matched controls	in takers
Men	246	122	129
Women	129	76	80

Table 2b. In the first and fourth years of study [6–7]

	Takers		Controls	Expectation
	Year 1	Year 4	Year 1	
Malignant neoplasm of stomach	45	8	3	3.5
Malignant neoplasm of trachea				
Malignant neoplasm of bronchus & lung	35	22	11	12.5
Diseases of circulatory system	131	79	94	90.8
Diseases of respiratory system	40	24	28	26.3
Diseases of digestive system	33	11	7	5.0

Mortality Rate

In keeping with those findings, mortality rates in the first year were almost twice those of the ordinary community, subsequently falling steadily towards population expectation (Table 2). In the face of these general changes it would be well-nigh impossible to detect drug-induced changes in disease experience if these were similar in type to ordinary illness.

However, the close approximation of mortality rates to population experience by the end of the fourth year following initial prescription, and the very low recorded mortality from ulcer and the low recorded rate of ulcer complications, with these occurring randomly without any particular relation to treatment timing or intensity, argued for the general safety of treatment.

The overwhelming likelihood would be that surveillance studies conducted following treatment with any other drug would give much the same answers. The findings suggest that what happens to dyspeptics is influenced in great part, not by any ulcer present but by their age and their general health.

Examination of operation rates for peptic ulcer is in broad conformity with this view, thus the general slow decline in the number of operations performed became rather greater at the time that cimetidine was marketed [10–12]. Subsequently, operation rates rose slightly, perhaps reflecting clinical realization that the treatment did not fundamentally change disease behaviour before the decline resumed. The overall fall is itself likely to be due to the general decline in the impact of ulcer disease especially in young people. If these overall trends continue the need to find reliable and effective means of deciding which patients will suffer life-threatening complications will become pressing. As matters stand, our information is limited. At least in patients with bleeding gastric ulcer who have been treated successfully in the short-term medically the number who suffer further life-threatening complications seems to be small. Unfortunately we are quite unable to predict which individuals will enter this high risk group.

Summary

The changing pattern of ulcer disease in the United Kingdom and possibly elsewhere, with decreasing impact in the young and rising frequency in the elderly, emphasizes the need for safe and effective medical treatments because the elderly tolerate surgery poorly. The high frequency of coincident disease of other systems in elderly people in general and in dyspeptics in particular makes it very difficult to confirm with confidence that treatment is as safe as clinicol trial results would lead us to believe.

References

1. Taylor P (1974) Sickness absence facts and misconceptions. J Roy Coll Physicns (Lond) 8: 315–319
2. Coggon D, Lambert P, Langman MJS (1981) 20 years of hospital admissions for peptic ulcer in England and Wales. Lancet i 1302–1304
3. Kurata JH, Honda GD, Frankl H (1982) Hospitalization and mortality rates for peptic ulcers: a comparison of a large health maintenance organisation and United States data. Gastroenterology 83: 1008–1015
4. Walt RP, Katschinski B, Logan R, Ashley J, Langman MJS (1986) Rising frequency of ulcer perforation in elderly people in the United Kingdom. Lancet i 489–492
5. Scottish Health Service. Common Services Agency (1979) What has been happening to peptic ulcer in Scotland? An analysis of hospital inpatient data. Scrips Review No. 2, Edingburgh
6. Colin Jones DG, Langman MJS, Lawson DH, Vessey MP (1982) Cimetidine and gastric cancer: preliminary report from post marketing surveillance study. Br Med J 285: 1311–1313
7. Colin Jones DG, Langman MJS, Lawson DH, Vessey MP (1985) Post marketing surveillance of the savety of cimetidine: 12 month morbidity report. Quart J Med 54: 253–268
8. Colin Jones DG, Langman MJS, Lawson DH, Vessey MP (1983) Post marketing surveillance of the safety of cimetidine: 12 month mortality report. Brit Med J 286: 1713
9. Colin Jones DG, Langman MJS, Lawson DH, Vessey MP (1987) Post marketing surveillance of the safety cimetidine: mortality during second, third, and fourth years of follow-up. Brit Med J 291: 1084–1088
10. Hospital Inpatient Enquiry. Main tables 1976, 1977, 1978 Department of Health & Social Security, Office of Population Censuses & Surveys 1980, 1980 and 1981 HMSO
11. Hospital Inpatient Enquiry. Summary tables 1979, 1980, 1981, 1982, 1983, 1984. Department of Health & Social Security, Office of Population Censuses & Surveys, 1982, 1983, 1984, 1985, 1986 HMSO
12. Wyllie JH, Clark CG, Williams JA, Bell PRF, Kennedy TL, Kirk RM, Mackay C (1981) Effect of cimetidine on surgery for duodenal ulcer. Lancet i 1307–1308

Benefits and Risks of Long-term Medical Therapy with Histamine H_2-receptor Antagonists in Ulcer Disease – A Physician's View

W. P. FRITSCH

Introduction

The aim of medical therapy in ulcer disease is to accelerate ulcer healing i. e., to remove pain and complaints and to prevent ulcer recurrence and, in so doing, ulcer complications. As the results of many controlled clinical trials in duodenal ulcer disease show, long-term medical therapy with histamine H_2-receptor antagonists is able to reduce ulcer recurrences from 50% to 90% per year to about 25% per year [9]. Regarding the efficacy of cimetidine and ranitidine, the difference between these two drugs is very slight, if at all demonstrable, significance is shown only in trials with study groups larger than 400. The percentage of asymptomatic ulcer recurrences in the cimetidine group is half that of the placebo group: 12% and 24%, respectively.

Asymptomatic ulcers are discovered endoscopically at intervals of 3 or 6 months; this means a diagnostic uncertainty. During long-term medical treatment with histamine H_2-receptor antagonists, complaints were reduced significantly, consumption of antacids was less, and some studies were able to show a reduced complication rate.

Side effects of the histamine H_2-receptor antagonists include endocrine effects, interactions with other drugs, mental disorders, and injury of some organs. The antiandrogenic effects are usually side effects of cimetidine given in high doses of more than 2 g per day. Impotence is seen rarely and is described during therapy with all H_2-receptor antagonists. Interactions with other drugs are caused by the inhibition of hepatic elimination or by the inhibition of real elimination. The possibility of clinical relevance is given in case of a therapy with lidocain, theophylline, phenytoin, and warfarin [16]. On the basis of evidence of the last decade, side effects are rarely observed; in nearly all cases they are fully reversible. Side effects were seldom observed during long-term medical treatment if the acute medication was tolerated well.

The placebo recurrence rate in Great Britain amounts to 75% per 6 months. Studies in Europe show comparable results during placebo maintenance per 12 months. There is a clear correlation between placebo healing rates and intervals free of recurrence [23] (Fig. 1). Therefore benefits of long-term medical treatment would be better for patients with a lower than for those with a higher placebo healing rate.

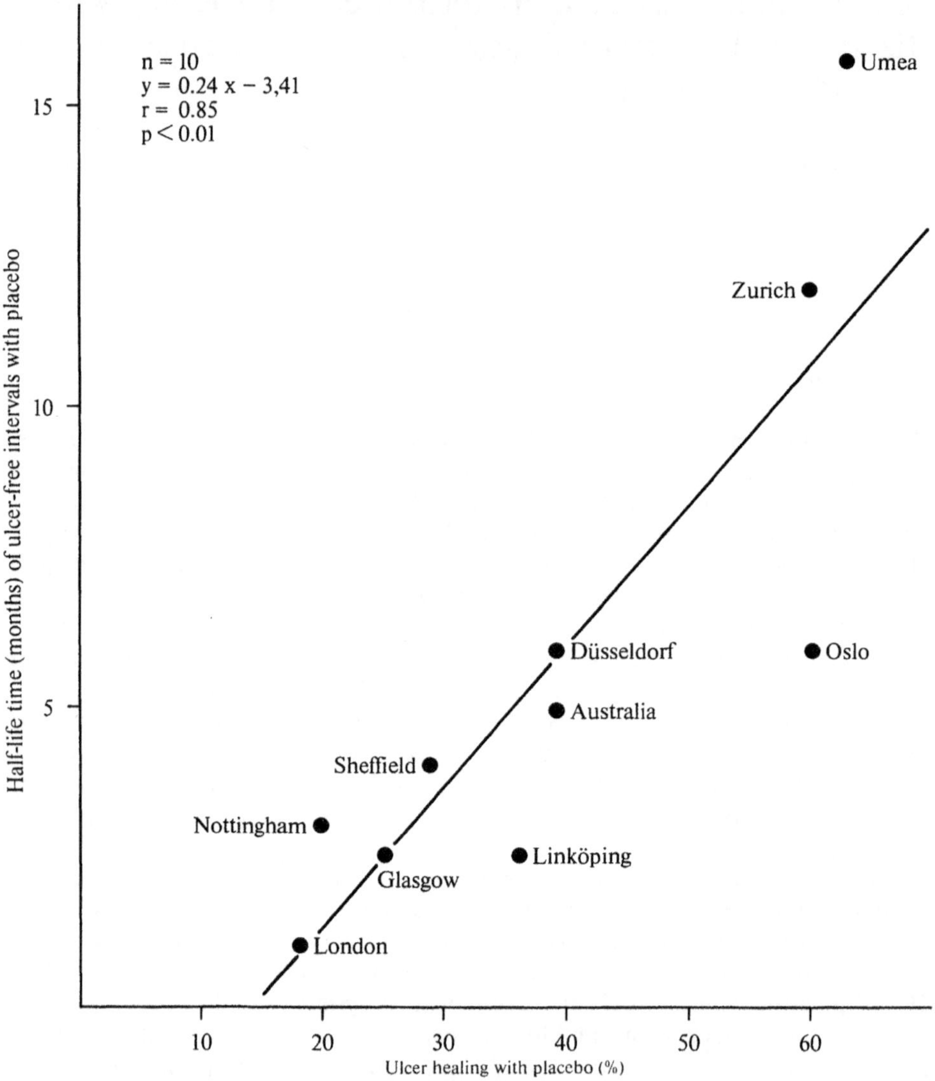

Fig. 1. Correlation between half-life time of ulcer-free intervals and ulcer healing (%) during placebo medication. Results of ten controlled clinical trials

Results

With acid inhibition we produce a reduction of the secretory status of the gastric mucosa, and we have to ask whether that means disposition for ulcer recurrence. The question whether the recurrence rate depends on the special drug used in acute ulcer therapy cannot be conclusively answered at this time [8]. Acid secretion is reduced by about 40%-60% in long-term medication with H_2-receptor antagonists. The stimulated gastrin is raised according to the inhibited acid secretion; the higher the medication, the longer it is administered. Basal serum gastrin levels do not change [12].

There are some studies comparing the efficacy of H_2-receptor antagonists with other ulcer drugs in acute ulcer episodes. These show what happens with ulcer recurrence after stopping the medication. There is only one study [6] comparing pirenzepine and H_2-receptor antagonists. In this study no difference between recurrence rates of the two groups was calculated. In two studies, sucralfate and H_2-receptor antagonists are compared. The study of Marks et al. [20] showed less recurrence in the sucralfate group; Hentschel et al. [13] did not find any difference.

In comparing bismuth with H_2-receptor antagonists, more studies show fewer recurrences [4, 11, 18, 19, 21, 25] after bismuthate therapy than after H_2-receptor antagonists [15, 22]. To our knowledge, there is no study comparing H_2-receptor antagonists with other ulcer drugs or with a placebo medication which is able to demonstrate a lower ulcer relapse rate in the H_2-receptor antagonist group.

Studies from Australia [14] and England [2] show the superiority of long-term treatment with cimetidine in ulcer recurrence and complaints compared with intermittent medication. Only half the ulcer patients were satisfied with intermittent therapy.

Discussion

Are there any criteria to help in the selection, between these two possibile forms of therapy? There is no relationship between the length of ulcer disease and frequency of ulcer recurrences [1]. No correlation exists between the last ulcer-free interval and the length of a future remission [2]. Therefore, no criteria are available for an individual recommendation either for long-term treatment or intermittent medication. If long-term treatment with H_2-receptor antagonists were accepted, each patient with duodenal ulcer disease would have to undergo treatment.

What happens in the natural history of ulcer recurrence disease if long-term treatment with H_2-receptor antagonists is stopped? The frequency of ulcer is the same whether long-term treatment ist stopped or whether placebo medication is administered after the ulcer has healed [10] (Fig. 2). Also, there is no difference between the runter of complaints and frequency of surgery [5].

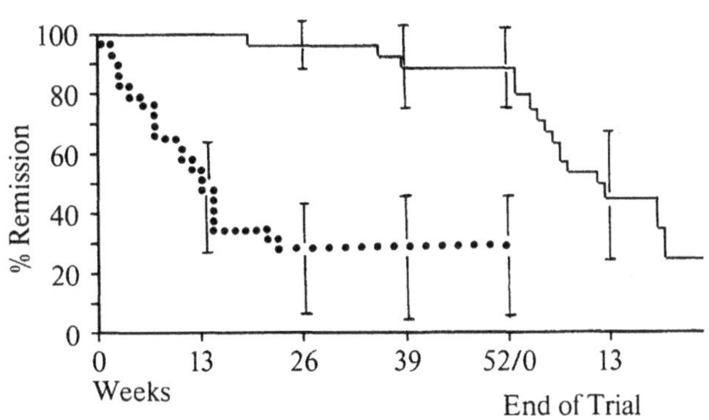

Fig. 2. Life-table analysis according to method of Peto et al. showing estimated percentage probability (±2 SE) of continued remission during and after cimetidine treatment for 1 year (*solid line*) and during placebo treatment for 1 year (*broken line*). (From [10])

When long-term therapy with H_2-receptor antagonists is ceased, placebo recurrence amounts to 77% per 6 months; on the other hand, further drug maintenance results in a continuous reduction of ulcer recurrence [17]. Therefore, it is obvious that the natural history of duodenal ulcer disease is not changed by long-term treatment with H_2-receptor antagonists.

Long-term treatment with cimetidine, 1 g per day, is not able to prevent ulcer recurrence. Frequency of ulcer recurrence is comparable to maintenance with 400 mg cimetidine daily. The longer H_2-receptor medication is administered, the quicker ulcer recurrence is demonstrable after the therapy is stopped [3, 7]. The recurrence rate amounts to 90% 2 years after medication.

Conclusion

In conclusion, arguments in favor of long-term therapy with H_2-receptor antagonists are:

- Decrease of ulcer recurrence
- Decrease of pain and complaints
- Decrease of ulcer complications and perhaps
- Decrease of surgical treatment

In spite of the favorable results of controlled clinical trials some aspects should be noted for critical evaluation:

- Benefits of this treatment in duodenal ulcer patients with relatively high placebo healing rates are not proven
- Up to now it is uncertain whether H_2-receptor antagonists predispose to higher ulcer recurrence rates
- Is long-term medical therapy indicated for each patient with ulcer disease or which are the criteria of choice
- H_2-receptor antagonists have no influence on the natural history of ulcer disease
- On the basis of epidemiological studies, there is no termination to the treatment
- Nonsmokers seem to have no benefit from long-term therapy with an H_2-receptor antagonist, as the results of a study by Sontag et al. [24] show.

On the basis of this critical evaluation, a physician, although aware of high placebo healing rates in duodenal ulcer patients, especially in the Federal Republic of Germany, has to conclude that today long-term medical treatment with H_2-receptor antagonists cannot be recommended for each duodenal patient. This therapy should be given to patients with high-risk factors, to patients who refuse surgical treatment, and to patients with Zollinger-Ellisonsyndrome only.

References

1. Bardhan KD, Saul DM, Edwards JL, Smith PM, Haggie SJ, Wyllie JH, Duthie HL, Fussey IV (1979) Double-blind comparison of cimetidine and placebo in the maintenance of healing of chronic duodenal ulceration Gut 20: 158–162
2. Bardhan KD (1980) Intermittent treatment of duodenal ulcer with cimetidine Brit Med J II: 20–22
3. Bardhan KD, Cole DS, Hawkins BW, Franks CR (1982) Does treatment with cimetidine extended beyond initial healing of duodenal ulcer reduce the subsequent relapse rate? Brit Med J 284: 621–623
4. Bianchi Porro G, Petrillo M (1982) An endoscopic controlled trial comparing De Nol tablets and cimetidine tablets in the treatment of duodenal ulcer Scand J Gastroenterol 17: Suppl. 78, 99
5. Bodemar G, Wallan A (1980) Two-year follow-up after one year's treatment with cimetidine or placebo Lancet I: 38–39
6. Brunner H (1982) Pirenzepine and cimetidine in the treatment of peptic ulcer Scand J Gastroenterol 17: Suppl 72: 207–210
7. Cargill JM, Peden N, Saunders JHB, Wormsley KG (1978) Very long-term treatment of peptic ulcer with cimetidine Lancet II: 1113–1115
8. WP Fritsch (1982) Medikamantöse Langzeittherapie des peptischen Ulkusleidens Dtsch med Wschr 107: 1681–1683
9. WP Fritsch (1986) Differentialtherapie bei Ulkuskrankheit Internistische Welt, in press
10. Gudmand-Høyer E, Birger Jensen K, Krag E, Rask-Madsen J, Rahbeck I, Rune SJ, Wulff HR (1978) Prophylactic effect of cimetidine in duodenal ulcer disease Brit med J I: 1095–1097
11. Hamilton I, O'Connor HJ, Axon ATR (1982) The treatment of duodenal ulcer with De Nol tablets or cimetidine Scand J Gastroenterol 17: Suppl. 78, 99
12. Hansky J, Stern AI, Korman MG, Waugh J (1979) Effects of long-term cimetidine on serum gastrin in duodenal ulcer Dig Dis Scien 24: 468–470
13. Hentschel E, Schütz K, Dufek W (1985) Rezidive des chronischen Ulcus duodeni nach initialer Therapie mit Pirenzepin oder Cimetidin Z Gastroenterologie 23: 14–17
14. Hetzel DJ, Hecker R, Shearman DJC (1980) Long-term treatment of duodenal ulcer with cimetidine – intermittent or continous therapy? Med J Aust 2: 612–614
15. Kang JY, Piper DW (1982) Cimetidine and colloidal bismuth in treatment of chronic duodenal ulcer Digestion 23: 73–79
16. Klotz U, Reimann IW (1986) Wechselwirkungen zwischen H_2-Blockern und anderen Pharmaka In: B Simon, Bianchi Porro G, Dammann HG (Hrsg.) Famotidin, ein Fortschritt in der Therapie säurebedingter Erkrankungen S. 22–48 Thieme, Stuttgart
17. Korman MG, Hetzel DJ, Hansky J, Shearman DJC, Don G (1980) Relapse rate of duodenal ulcer after cessation of long-term cimetidine treatment Dig Dis Scie 25: 88–91
18. Lee FI, Samloff IM, Hardman M (1985) Comparison of tripotassium dicitrato bismuthate tablets with ranitidine in healing and relapse of duodenal ulcers Lancet I 1299–1302
19. Lee SP, Nicholson GI (1977) Increased healing of gastric and duodenal ulcers in a controlled trial using tripotassium dicitrato bismuthate Med J Aust 1: 808–812
20. Marks IN, Wright JP, Luke W, Girdwood AH (1982) Relapse rates following initial ulcer healing with sucralfate and cimetidine Scand J Gastroenterol 17: 429–432
21. Martin DF, Hollanders D, May SJ, Ravenscroft MM, Tweedle DEF, Miller JP (1981) Difference in relapse rates of duodenal ulcer after healing with cimetidine or tripotassium dicitrato bismuthate Lancet I: 7–10
22. Shreeve DR (1975) A double-blind study of tripotassium dicitrato bismuthate in duodenal ulcer Postgrad Med J 51 Suppl. 5: 33–36
23. Sonnenberg A, Kiene K, Weber KB, Pelloni S, Peter P, Wienbeck M, Strohmeyer G, Blum AL (1979) Rezidivprophylaxe des Ulcus duodeni mit Cimetidin Dtsch med Wschr 104: 725–730
24. Sontag S, Graham DY, Belsito A (1984) Cimetidine, cigarette smoking, and recurrence of duodenal ulcer N Engl J Med 311: 689–693
25. Vantrappen G, Schuurmans P, Rutgeerts P, Janssens J (1982) A comparative study of colloidal bismuth subcitrate and cimetidine on the healing and recurrence of duodenal ulcer Scand J Gastroenterol 17 Suppl. 80: 23–30

Benefits and Risks of Long-term Medical Therapy with Histamine H_2-Receptor Antagonists in Ulcer Disease: A Surgeon's View

V. SCHUMPELICK, G. ARLT, and G. WINKELTAU

Introduction

Who could be satisfied with the therapy results of a disease which still kills more than 3000 patients per year in the Federal Republic of Germany? This is the situation in ulcer disease with 3200 casualities from hemorrhage or perforation during 1984 [8]. There is no question that H_2-receptor antagonist treatment is of great benefit for the ulcer patients, but it does not solve the problem completely. Gastric and duodenal ulcers are major killers in our society resulting in a death toll of as much as one-third of the number of fatal traffic accidents in the Federal Republic of Germany. Therefore, we cannot be complacent about peptic ulceration and its treatment. Without any doubt, the H_2-receptor antagonists resulted in a drastic reduction of elective ulcer surgery all over the world. According to many authors, the frequency of peptic surgery decreased by at least 50% [9, 28].

On the other hand, the rate of emergency ulcer surgery has not dropped over the years. In most clinics, for example in the McKay's clinic [18], or in my clinic at the University of Hamburg, or now also at the University of Aachen, the rate of emergency operations due to bleeding or perforation has not shown a decline to date [27]. If the age distribution of the patients is examined in detail, one notices a change: the average age of the patients has increased from 56.5 years in Hamburg 10 years ago to 64.8 years at the clinic of Aachen at present. We are no longer dealing with the same age group we are now operating mainly on the elderly population. Of those who have died of gastroduodenal ulcers since 1984, 66% of the women and 57% of the men were more than 75 years old.

This section of the population lives with a constant risk factor, and sometimes it seems that, by treating the young and middle-aged population conservatively, surgeons delay the bleeding episode until later when the patients are not able to withstand any complications. In our patients, we could demonstrate that the mortality rate of elective treatment compared to emergency treatment shows a widening gap with increasing age [27]. On the other hand, there is a tendency to withhold elective surgery because of intractability of ulcer disease in elderly patients. Between 1940 and 1955 Cutler still had a surgery rate of 44% due to intractability; this rate changed to 0% in the study of Permutt in 1982 [20]. Today the tendency is the same with nearly no patients above the age of 75 undergoing elective ulcer surgery.

What can we do, from the surgeon's point of view, to reduce the mortality rate, seeing that death is the ultimate result of inconsequent and ineffective ulcer treatment?

We have to consider four different factors influencing the success of our treatment:

1. The administration, modality, and effect of the drug treatment, which we call the "medical treatment factor"
2. The natural history of the ulcer disease, the patients' choice of treatment, and the compliance which we want to summarize as the "patient factor"
3. The results and risks of surgery summarized as the "surgical method factor"
4. The socio-economic impact of the different treatment methods summarized as the "social factor"

Let us start with the medical treatment factor. Everybody will agree that H_2-antagonists are very effective in the treatment of acute ulcer. But what about the maintenance treatment studies? A lot of clinical and empirical work has been done to evaluate the results of maintenance treatment with H_2-receptor antagonists. The results after 1 year of cimetidine treatment with recurrency rates from 17.3% to 39% did not convince the surgeon, who is used to having less than 3% recurrency rate in the 1 year after the selective proximal vagotomy [3, 7, 16]. Even the more sophisticated drugs such as famotidine and ranitidine, did not show any significant advance in comparison to the results with cimetidine [2, 19]. These are only 1-year results, representing only a very short period compared to the natural history of ulcers. But what about the true long-term recurrence prevention by H_2-receptor antagonists?

In a multicenter study of 44 centers in 12 countries published by Rohner, there was a 1-year recurrence rate with cimetidine treatment of 26%, a 2-year recurrence rate of 38%, and a 3-year recurrence rate of 48% [22]. Even if a lot of these patients could be treated by a higher dose of H_2-receptor antagonists, especially those who had an asymptomatic ulcer, these results, from the surgeon's point of view, are unacceptably poor. No surgical procedure would survive with such a high recurrence rate in duodenal ulcer. Furthermore, we know from the study of Gray et al. that of the 40% of patients who had to be operated on during the 5-year maintenance treatment with cimetidine, only 25% were operated on in an elective situation, whereas 75% had to be operated on because of pain or complications. Surgical procedures in these cases were truncal vagotomy combined with gastrojejunostomy or distal gastric resection [11]. As a result, these patients undergoing H_2-antagonist treatment had to undergo a more complicated procedure with higher risk of mortality and morbidity than the selective vagotomy originally planned.

This should suffice regarding the situation in duodenal ulcer therapy. What about the gastric ulcer? Here nearly identical recurrence rates are found as for duodenal ulcer. Drug prevention of recurrence failed in about 20%–35% of cases during the 1st year of cimetidine treatment [6, 17]. Beside this poor long-term result, the maintenance treatment of gastric ulcer carries the risk that a gastric cancer might be missed, as shown by Poegel in 1985 [21]. Therefore, with maintenance treatment repeated endoscopies and biopsies are necessary. As a consequence, the quality of life is definitely reduced by never-ending diagnostic procedures.

We now proceed to the patient factor. We can conclude that about 50%–70% of the patients with uncomplicated ulcer disease can be kept free of symptoms by maintenance treatment with H_2-antagonists. But this is true only with good patient compliance. Can we trust the patient and his compliance even if he is free of symptoms?

We know that H_2-blockers do not influence the natural history of peptic ulcer disease. Once the drug therapy is discontinued the percentage of relapses during the following year is nearly 100%, as shown by Porro and coworkers in 1986 [5]. This means that cimetidine-treated patients have the same recurrence rate within 6 months as a randomized placebo group regardless of how long they had been treated before. Patients undergoing maintenance drug treatment are therefore forced to take the drug for at least 10 years or possibly for the rest of their lives. We know from other drugs that in ambulatory long-term treatment less than 50% of the drugs were taken and patients' compliance may decrease within 5 years to a poor 17% rate.

Another aspect is the patient's choice. The gastroenterological departments of Aarhus and Odense studied this aspect in a joint project [1]. Patients had been informed about all the available methods and were allowed to choose their personal therapy in a rather liberal way. Patients tending toward early surgery were operated on within 3 years in 74% of the cases. About 60% of the patients allocated to long-term H_2-blocker treatment were operated on within the same period. The study shows that patients with severe symptoms are inclined to surgery after they have tried all types of drug treatment. The following points may indicate reasons for this tendency:

1. The failure to feel cured because of frequent recurrences under drug treatment
2. Doubts about the long-term safety of the drug
3. Concern about the short-term side effects of the drug
4. The hope of definite treatment by surgery

This choice reflect the surgical factor: we have to consider the surgical results when we compare benefits and risks of long-term H_2-antagonist treatment. There are at least two methods of gastric operation in ulcer surgery: gastrectomy or gastric resection in gastric ulcers and vagotomy in duodenal ulcers [23]. Generally speaking, there seems to be an inverse correlation between recurrence rate and postoperative mortality and morbidity. The lowest mortality and morbidity rates occur after selective proximal vagotomy with 0.3% lethality and less than 10% morbidity [14]. But the relapse rate in duodenal ulcer reaches 10%–15% after 5 years [14]. Selective proximal vagotomy is the first choice of surgical treatment in duodenal ulcer.

In randomized trials of selective vagotomy versus cimetidine treatment, the recurrence rate under cimetidine treatment was two to three times higher than after vagotomy [10, 12]. In the study of Harling and coworkers in 1985 [12], 35% of the cimetidine group had to undergo subsequent surgery. In 26% of these patients additional drainage had to be performed because of a complicating pyloric stenosis which developed under cimetidine treatment.

Gastric ulcer is best treated by distal resection and Billroth I anastomosis. This procedure has a mortality rate of lower than 2%. The recurrence rate and the rate of postgastrectomy syndromes after the Billroth I procedure is less than 5% [4, 25]. Recurrence rates under long-term H_2-antagonist treatment in gastric ulcer are, as we demonstrated earlier, four to ten times as high. Furthermore, gastrectomy makes the repeated endoscopies and biopsies to detect any malignant transformation unnecessary.

Finally I would like to say something about the socioeconomic impact of medical or surgical treatment. The costs of a disease include direct and indirect costs. The direct costs are the costs of diagnosis, treatment, and prevention of the disease. In the evaluation of maintenance treatment versus surgery, these costs are different in different countries depending on the costs of surgery and drugs. But even in countries with lower drug costs and higher surgery costs, the expenses for maintenance treatment will exceed the costs of selective proximal vagotomy after some years [13, 15]. The indirect costs of a disease are the costs of loss of productivity, disability, and premature death. These costs usually reach 70% of the total costs of a disease. Indirect costs, as far as working disability is concerned, have been studied by Walan and Ström 1985 in Sweden [26]. They could not find any difference in the working disability in patients in the 1st or 2nd years of H_2-blocker treatment or after selective proximal vagotomy. This held true for complaints related to peptic ulcer disease as well as other complaints.

In conclusion, we can summarize the benefits and risks of long-term H_2-antagonist treatment: there is no question that 50%–70% of patients with uncomplicated ulcer disease can be kept free of symptoms for a long period. About 40%–60% of these patients will not have to be operated on as long as they take their drugs. This may be of particular benefit in patients with additional diseases which would increase the risk of surgery. Another group of patients with unresectable gastrinoma should be treated by long-term H_2-antagonists as a treatment of first choice.

On the other hand, there are still many patients who must be operated on in spite of maintenance H_2-antagonist treatment. For these patients it is important to perform surgery before complications take place. These patients should preferably be operated on as an elective treatment at an uncomplicated stage. This fact was recently demonstrated by Taylor [24]: with respect to 24000 patients who develop peptic ulcer disease per year in the United Kingdom, one could presume that 6000 ulcer bleedings and 2400 perforations would occur in those aged 50–60. Out of these about 600 would die from the first bleeding and 240 would die from the first perforation. If we calculate a rebleeding rate of 60% and a reperforation rate of 10%, there would be 400 more deaths from rebleeding and 24 more deaths from reperforation. This means a total death toll of 1264 patients per year from ulcer complications. If the same group had been operated on by selective proximal vagotomy, only 48 patients would have died because of the operation. If we calculate 2400 recurrences and perform a truncular vagotomy in about 50% of the recurrences, 24 additional patients would die. This means that in the case of an early elective vagotomy in all 24000 patients, only 72 patients would die from the peptic ulcer disease.

These data should illuminate the role of elective surgery in peptic ulcer. In future, we have to separate carefully those patients who may respond to long-term medical treatment without complications from those who should undergo elective surgery at an early stage. Otherwise the death rate from ulcer disease will not be reduced because we will have to operate on more and more elderly patients with complications, giving poor results in many cases. Therefore, from the surgeons's point of view, we would recommend the operation:

1. If three or more relapses occur over a period of 2 years of maintenance treatment
2. If there are the typical "break-through ulcers" during maintenance treatment
3. If there is no sign of healing after 6–12 weeks
4. If there is bad compliance

References

1. Andersen A (1985) Prevention of ulcer recurrence – Medical vs. surgical treatment. The surgeons view. Scand J Gastroenterol 110 (Supp 20): 89–92
2. Baglioni A, Barbara L, Bianchi-Porro G, et al (1985) Famotidine versus Plazebo in der Rezidivprophylaxe der Ulcus-duodeni-Erkrankung. Z Gastroenterologie 23: 665–669
3. Battaglia G, Farini R, Di Mario F, Piccoli A, Plebani M, Vianello F, Burlina A, Naccarato, R (1984) Reccurence of duodenal ulcer under continuous antisecretory treatment: An approach to the detection of predictive markers. Am J Gastroenterol 79 (11): 831–834
4. Becker HD, Lehmann L, Löhlein D, Schumpelick V, Troidl H (1982) Selektiv-proximale Vagotomie mit Ulcusexcesion oder Billroth I-Resektion beim chronischen Ulcus ventriculi. Chirurg 53: 773–777
5. Bianchi-Porro G, Petrillo M (1986) The natural history of peptic ulcer disease: The influence of H2-antagonist treatment. Scand J Gastroenterol 21 (Supp 121): 46–52
6. Bianchi-Porro G, Petrillo M (1979) A controlled trial comparing cimetidine with carbenoxolon sodium in gastric ulcer. Drugs Exp Clin Res 5: 173–176
7. Burland WL, Hawkins BW, Beresford J (1980) Cimetidine treatment for the prevention of recurrence of duodenal ulcer: An international collaborative study. Postgrad Med J 56: 173–176
8. Effenberger Th, Schumpelick V (1984) Magenchirurgie im Alter. Zbl Chir 109: 338–346
9. Fineberg HV, Pearlman LA (1981) Surgical treatment of peptic ulcer in the United States. Lancet I: 1305–1307
10. Gear MWL (1983) Proximal gastric vagotomy versus long-term maintenance treatment with cimetidine for chronic duodenal ulcer: A prospective randomised trial. Brit Med J 286: 98–99
11. Gray GR, McWhinnie D, Smith IS, Gillespie G (1982) Five-year study of cimetidine or surgery for severe duodenal ulcer dyspepsia. Lancet I: 787–788
12. Harling H, Balslev I, Bentzen E (1985) Parietal cell vagotomy or cimetidine maintenance therapy for duodenal ulcer? Scand J Gastroenterol 20: 747–750
13. Hotz J (1982) Konservative Therapie des Magen- und Duodenalulkus. Indikation zur Operation. In: Bünte H, Langhans P (ed): 100 Jahre Ulkuschirurgie. Urban & Schwarzenberg, München–Wien–Baltimore
14. Jordan PH, Thornby J (1987) Should it be parietal cell vagotomy or selective vagotomy-antrectomy for treatment of duodenal ulcer? Ann Surg 205: 572–590
15. Largiader F (1985) Failures of drug therapy in ulcer patients – What should we do? Langenbecks Arch Chir 366 (Kongreßber): 127–129
16. Massarrat S, Heuser E, Hausmann L, Schubotz R (1982) Long-term prevention of duodenal ulcer with cimetidine. Dtsch Med Wschr 107: 1085
17. McAdam WAF, Pacsoo C, Morgan AG (1980) A comparsion between Caved-S and cimetidine in gastric ulcer treatment and subsequent maintenance therapy. Acta Hepato Gastroenterol (Stutt), (Abs 205)
18. McKay AJ, McArdle CS (1982) Cimetidine and perforated peptic ulcer. Br J Surg 69: 319–320
19. Paul F, Neuhaus H, Homann J, Kamenisch W, Eimüller A (1986) Dosisvergleichsstudie mit Ranitidin zur Therapie und Prophylaxe des Ulcus duodeni. Z Gastroenterologie 24: 141–148
20. Permutt RP, Cello JP (1982) Duodenal ulcer disease in the hospitalized elderly patient. Dig Dis Sci 27: 1–6
21. Poegel K, Riedel H, Friedrich P, Wolf K (1985) Rate of malignization of peptic gastric ulcers. Z Klin Med 40: 1661–4
22. Rohner H-G (1985) Long term cimetidine therapy for the prevention of recurring peptic ulcer: A multicenter study. Z Gastroenterologie 23: 403–411
23. Schumpelick V, Arlt G, Winkeltau G, Klinge G (1987) Gastroduodenal recurrent ulcer: Controversies in primary and reconstructive surgery. Langenbecks Arch Chir 372 (Kongreßber): 189–198
24. Taylor TV (1985) Deaths from peptic ulceration. Brit Med J 291: 653–654
25. Thomas WEG, Thompson MH, Williamson RCN (1982) The long-term outcome of Billroth I partial gastrectomy for benign gastric ulcer. Ann Surg 195: 189–195
26. Walan A, Ström M (1985) Prevention of ulcer recurrence – Medical vs surgical treatment. The physician's view. Scand J Gastroenterol 110 (Supp 20), 83–88

27. Winkeltau G, Arlt G, Truong S, Schumpelick V (1986) Indikation und chirurgische Verfahrenswahl beim blutenden gastroduodenalen Ulkus. Zbl Chir 111: 1441–1449
28. Wyllie JH, Clark CG, Alexander-Williams J, Bell PRF, Kennedy TL, Kirk RM, MacKay C (1981) Effect of cimetidine on surgery for duodenal ulcer. Lancet I: 1307–1308

The Surgical Approach to Ulcer Disease and its Complications – Has there been a Change in the Last Decade?

E. H. FARTHMANN, P. BUSS, St. EGGSTEIN, and A. IMDAHL

Introduction

The aim of this presentation is to review briefly the development during the last decade and the present spectrum of surgical treatment for peptic ulceration in the duodenum and stomach. Since elective surgery as well as surgical treatment of ulcer bleeding, ulcer perforation, and pyloric stenosis shall be covered, only a broad overview can be given.

Elective Ulcer Surgery

It has been well recognized that the incidence as well as the prevalence of peptic ulceration has shown a general decline during the last 20–30 years [1]. This reduction pertains especially to males and to gastric ulcer and it has been observed in different regions worldwide. The causes remain speculative. There is no doubt, however, that the decline antedates and is thus superimposed on the effect of the introduction of H_2-receptor antagonists in 1976.

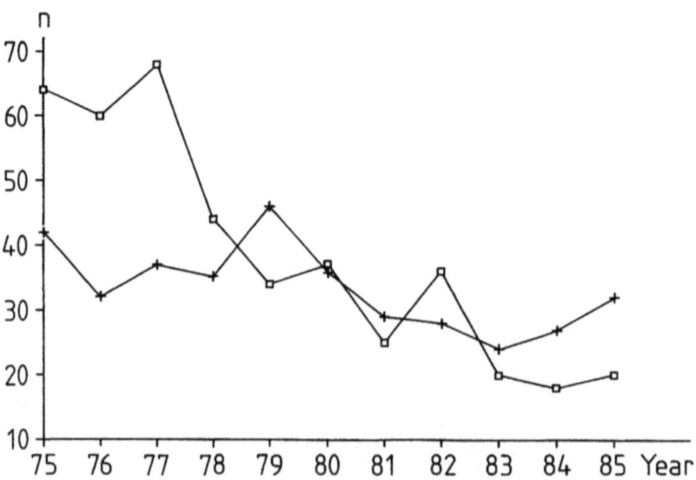

Fig. 1. Number of operations for peptic ulcer disease per year from 1975 to 1985 (total = 794). The decrease is more pronounced for duodenal ulcer. *Crosses*, gastric ulcer, n = 368; *squares*, duodenal ulcer, n = 426

The general experience in surgical units is reflected in the figures from our institution (Fig. 1). During the last decade there has been a general drop in the total number of operations both for gastric and duodenal ulcer, which appears to be more pronounced for duodenal ulcer. At the same time the spectrum of the disease as seen by surgeons has changed, too (Figs. 2, 3). While the number of uncomplicated duodenal ulcers, i. e., of those operated upon because of medical intractability, has declined sharply to almost zero, the complications necessitating surgery have risen without exception, the

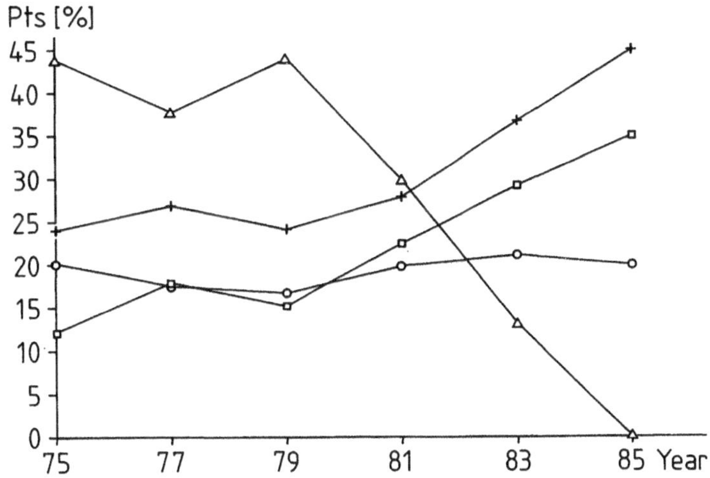

Fig. 2. Rate of duodenal ulcer complications requiring surgery from 1975 to 1985. Complications increased on the whole with bleeding being most frequent. The yearly rate of uncomplicated ulcers, i. e., operated upon for intractability, has recently approached zero. n = 426.*quares*, perforation and penetration; *crosses*, bleeding; *circles*, stenosis; *triangles*, no complications

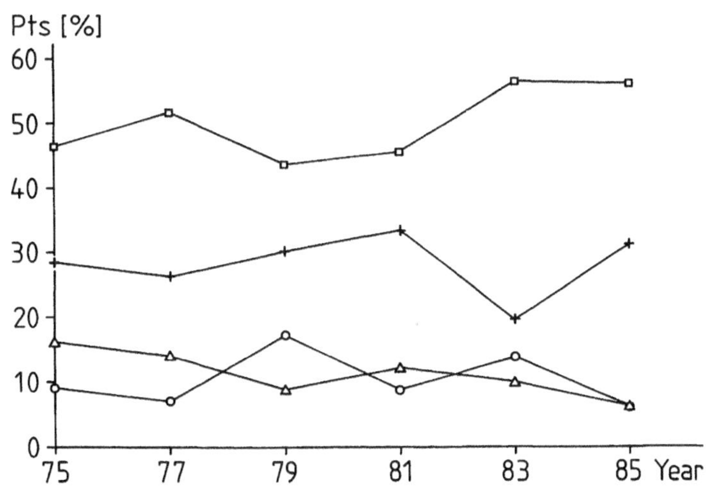

Fig. 3. Rate of gastric ulcer complications requiring surgery from 1975 to 1985. The ratio of complicated versus uncomplicated gastric ulcer has remained stable over the 10-year period. n = 368.*Squares*, perforation and penetration; *crosses*, bleeding; *circles*, sten; *triangles*, no complications

increase being most pronounced for bleeding. Gastric ulcer, on the other hand, has remained rather stable as far as its manifestations are concerned.

This observation has been made by others as well [2, 3]. It is generally interpreted as being the combined effect of the general decline in ulcer disease and the introduction of potent antiulcer drugs. The disturbing consequence is a shift in ulcer surgery toward more complication-prone operations with subsequently increasing risks and corresponding results which might augment even further the tendency to rely on nonoperative means of treatment. In short, a negative selection of patients coming to surgery is taking place.

Ulcer Bleeding

The general problems of ulcer bleeding remain unchanged:
a) to estimate the individual risk of bleeding;
b) to quantitate bleeding intensity;
c) to determine the optimal time of intervention;
d) to choose the appropriate surgical method.

Retrospective analyses of the literature are of little help. Reported mortality rates and rebleeding rates for duodenal and gastric ulcer and the methods employed vary widely. It can be generally stated that the reported total mortality of conservative and surgical treatment range between 5% and 25% [4].

We studied 453 patients with ulcer bleeding treated from 1975 to 1985. Of the total number, 202 had to be operated upon immediately because of persistent bleeding, 122 from duodenal, 80 from gastric ulcers. The median age was 54.4 and 58.5 years, respectively, and the male : female ratio 3 : 1 and 2 : 1. There was a high incidence of coexisting diseases (Fig. 4) and of additional ulcer complications (Fig. 5). Global treatment results did not differ from those reported in the literature and were mainly independent of the method employed except for simple suture in high-risk patients, who had a high mortality and rebleeding rate.

When mortality was correlated with bleeding intensity, it became obvious that it rose sharply when signs of shock were present at admission. Even more pronounced was the correlation of mortality with the presence of high-risk factors: mortality was in the range of elective surgery in the absence of those factors, while it exceeded 50% with three such factors (Fig. 6). The risk of bleeding from both duodenal and gastric ulcer rose sharply with increasing age and the amount of blood transfused (Figs. 7, 8). These risk factors were validated statistically by employing the χ^2-test and logistic regression analysis.

It became obvious from our analysis that early occurrence of rebleeding after initial cessation of hemorrhage constitutes an extremely dangerous situation as has been pointed out by others [5]. Read et al. [6] had demonstrated previously that mortality could be reduced to the elective range by identifying and operating on those 30% of patients who were thought most likely to rebleed within 48 h following the cessation of the initial bleeding episode. This strategy of early elective surgery has become our standard procedure. We hope that besides clinical and endoscopic criteria the use of doppler ultrasound to determine patency of a visible vessel will be helpful in further clarifying this issue [7].

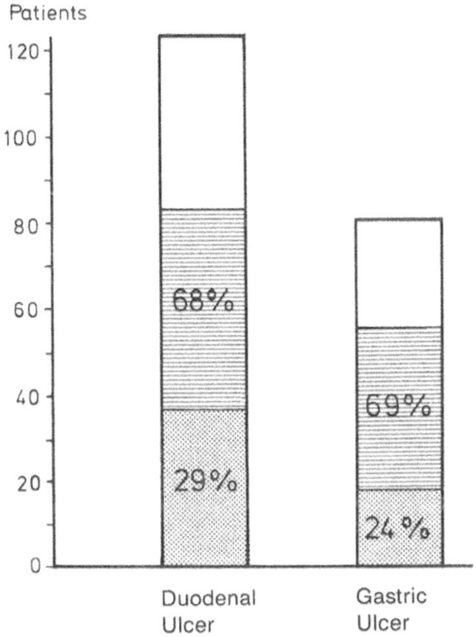

Fig. 4. Frequency of coexisting diseases among 202 patients operated upon as an emergency for bleeding peptic ulcer. Less than one-third of both groups was free from at least one severe coexisting disease. *Hatched area*, one severe coexisting disease; *dotted area*, more than one severe coexisting disease

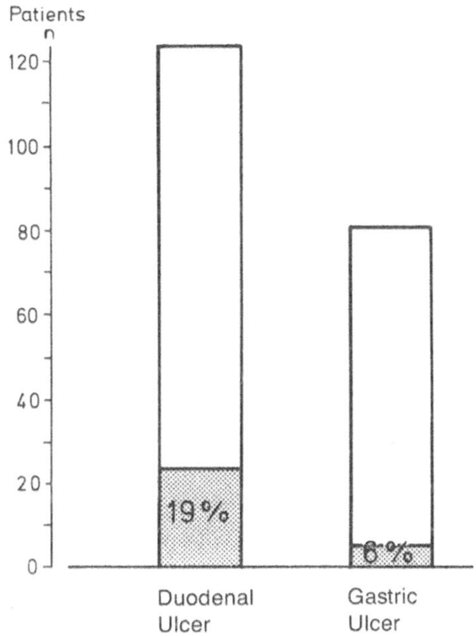

Fig. 5. Rate of additional ulcer complications *(dotted area)* among 202 patients operated upon as an emergency for bleeding peptic ulcer. Penetration, perforation, and stenosis were three times as frequent among duodenal ulcer patients

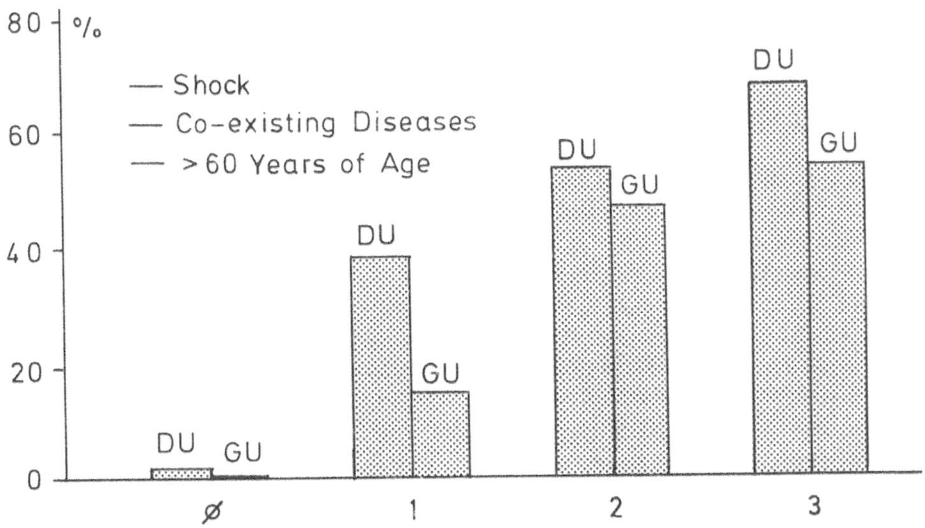

Fig. 6. Mortality related to number of high-risk factors in 202 patients operated on as an emergency for bleeding peptic ulcer. In the absence of shock at admission, coexisting diseases, and age beyond 60 years, operative risk was in the range of elective ulcer surgery. In the presence of all three risk factors more than half of the patients died irrespective of the location of the bleeding ulcer. *DU*, duodenal ulcer; GU, gastric ulcer

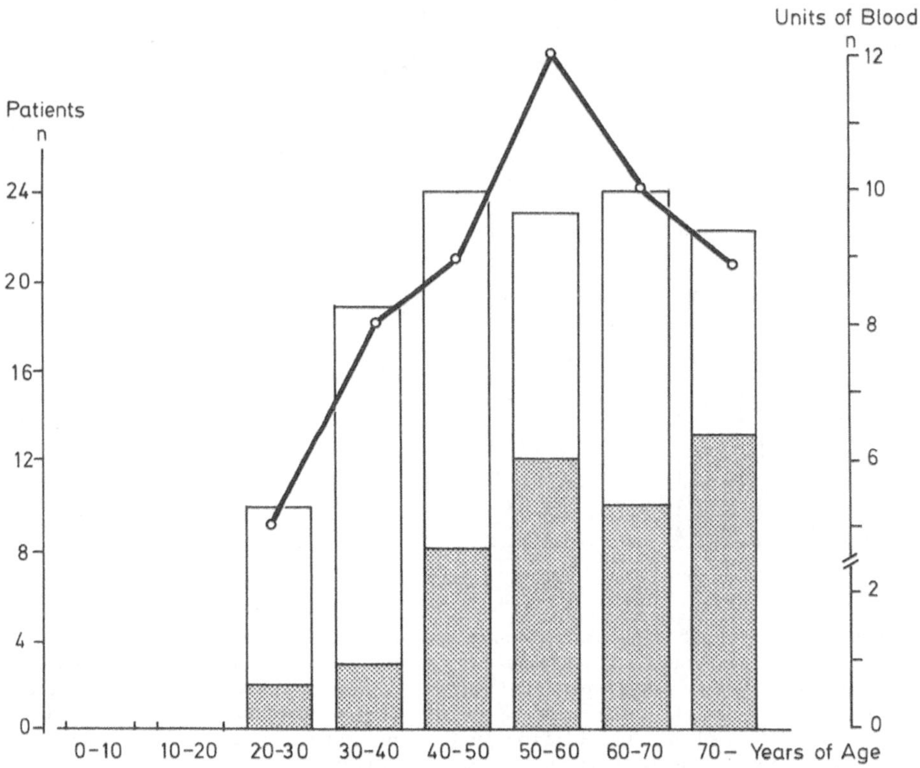

Fig. 7. Mortality *(dotted area)* from bleeding duodenal ulcer related to age and units of blood transfused *(line)*. There is an almost linear correlation up to the age of 60 years

Ulcer Perforation

The general incidence of perforation does not seem to have changed in the last decade. Figures from the Oxford Record Linkage Study indicate the incidence to be between 8.7 and 6.9 in recent years [8]. There seems to be an increase in the proportion of female patients with the male: female ratio declining from 4.9: 1 to 1.9: 1. It is unproven but not unlikely that the increasing use of nonsteroidal anti-inflammatory drugs (NSAIDs) is involved in the pathogenesis of a major part of ulcer perforations. Especially if looked for in a prospective manner, the proportion of patients on this type of medication may surpass 80% [9].

The choice of method for surgical treatment of perforated ulcer is characterized by a lack of controlled data. Criteria for this decision could be theoretically derived from patient data, ulcer location, ulcer history, additional ulcer complications, and the time interval between perforation and surgical treatment. The latter is obvious because frank peritonitis would exclude any major procedure directed at the elimination of ulcer disease. In this context, there is some indication that peritonitis following perforation might be more serious in patients taking H_2-receptor antagonists because of bacterial overgrowth in their stomachs [10].

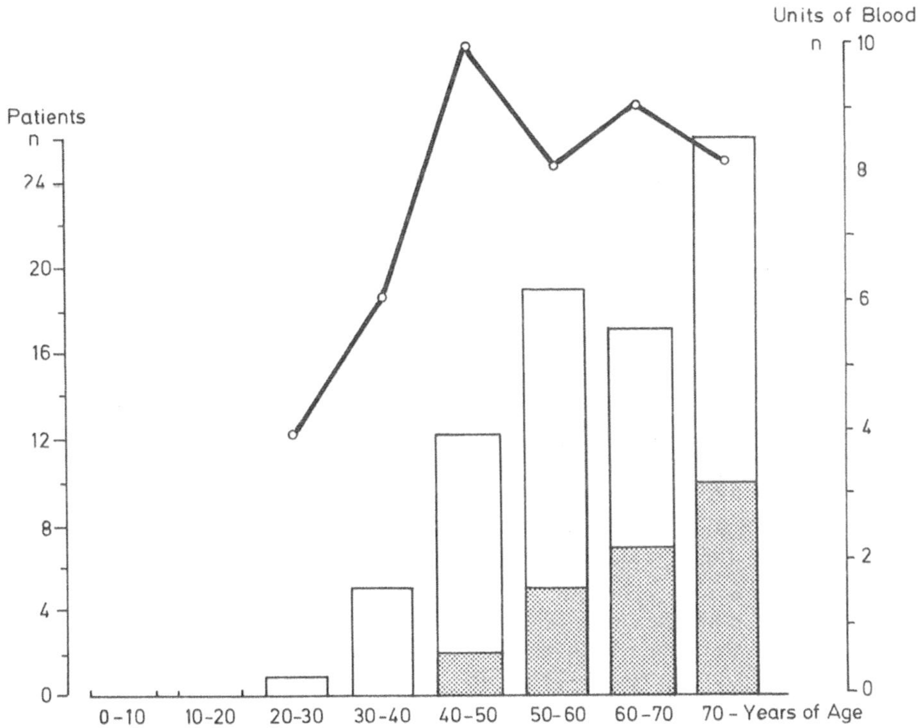

Fig. 8. Mortality *(dotted area)* from bleeding gastric ulcer related to age and units of blood transfused *(line)*. A trend identical to Fig. 7 is seen. Number of units of blood includes the transfusion requirements for cardiovascular stabilization in patients admitted with hemorrhagic shock

There is general agreement that among the criteria listed above the presence or absence of previous ulcer history is most likely to influence the choice of operative treatment. It has been shown that following simple suture of the perforation in all patients, there will be one-third who will need further surgical treatment, one third who will continue to have medically controlled ulcer symptoms, and one-third who will remain symptom free [11]. If only patients with no prior history are evaluated, almost three-quarters will remain symptom free following simple suture. On the other hand, this proportion decreases to about one-quarter in patients with prior symptoms of more than 3 months' duration with a corresponding increase of those needing further surgery to almost one-half.

These results were corroborated by a prospective study comparing simple suture and immediate definitive surgery by proximal gastric vagotomy or truncal vagotomy plus drainage [12]. Although more than half of the patients entered into the study had to be excluded, and the proportion of males was unusually high, it became apparent that the long-term results of vagotomy and drainage as well as of proximal gastric vagotomy were superior to simple closure of the perforation. It is generally accepted, therefore, that patients with a previous ulcer history should receive some form of definitive surgical treatment at the time of perforation if the general condition and local situation permits. The problem remains that not all chronic ulcers will relapse following perforation and, on the other hand, not all acute ulcers will heal following closure. Therefore, more prospective controlled studies are needed. Few data are available on the problem of ulcer perforation in patients who are being treated with H_2-receptor antagonists. There is no doubt that this may occur. A recent study seems to indicate that this subgroup of patients will, without exception, eventually need definitive surgery [13].

Pyloric Stenosis

There is a general feeling that gastric outlet obstruction due to scarring from recurrent duodenal ulceration seems to be on the increase, although the published evidence is conflicting [2, 14, 15]. This phenomenon would not be at all unlikely in view of the increasing number of duodenal ulcer patients being medically treated for recurrent ulcer episodes on a long-term basis. It has been shown that surgical treatment becomes virtually unavoidable once organic pyloric stenosis has been established. Even following initial resolution of gastric outlet obstruction by conservative treatment symptoms will recur in most patients, making surgery necessary in more than 80% of those developing stenoses [14].

In this situation some form of drainage procedure is called for. Short of partial gastrectomy, followed by gastroduodenostomy or gastrojejunostomy, pyloroplasty seems to be the favored procedure with gastroenterostomy being less frequently employed. The combination of proximal gastric vagotomy and pyloroplasty in this setting has been shown to be as effective and successful as proximal gastric vagotomy in the absence of pyloric stenosis if the long-term results are evaluated according to Visick grading [15]. Interestingly enough, the rate of recurrent ulceration was shown to be strikingly different following these two procedures: 1.3% for proximal gastric vagotomy plus pyloroplasty and 11.4% for proximal gastric vagotomy in the absence of pyloric stenosis. This finding further supports the notion that once gastric outlet obstruction is present, some form of drainage becomes necessary. It can be safely assumed that this problem will become increasingly frequent in the future. This, in turn, will hopefully furnish more data as a basis for decision-making.

Conclusions

There is no doubt that surgery has a place in the elective treatment of peptic disease and of its complications. The data available are sufficiently stable to allow for rational indication and prediction of results. This applies more to the elective setting than to emergency treatment of complications where patient variation and empirical decision-making prevail. It has to be stated, too, that present-day ulcer surgery is mainly the surgical treatment of ulcer complications. This fact poses problems regarding both the development of reproducible data as a basis for decision and the availability of expertise.

If other and more potent drugs became available for the control of ulcer disease it would seem possible that the extent of surgery for ulcer complications could be reduced to treating the complication as such, leaving the control of ulcer disease to subsequent medical treatment and/or elective surgery at a later date. On the other hand, the place and the effectiveness of elective ulcer surgery should not be forgotten today, because this trend seems to postpone necessary surgery to a situation where the risk becomes prohibitive. After all, the aim of treating peptic ulcer disease should not be to avoid an operation but rather to heal the patient.

References

1. Elashoff JD, Grossmann MJ (1980) Trends in hospital admissions and death rates for peptic ulcer in the United States from 1970-1978. Gastroenterology 78: 280-285
2. Rohner HG, Bloemer A, Echterhoff HM, Gugler R (1983) Chirurgische Behandlung der Ulcuskrankheit 5 Jahre vor und nach Einführung des Cimetidins. Z Gastroenterol 21: 585-592
3. Linder MM, Petermann Ch, Arens B (1985) Standardisierte Ulcuschirurgie. Ergebnisse zehnjähriger Erfahrung. Dtsch med Wschr. 110: 719-720
4. Gyr K, Kayasseh L (1982) Gastrointestinale Blutung: Ulcus ventriculi et duodeni. Indikation und Verfahrenswahl; in Siewert JR, Blum AL, Farthmann EH, Lankisch PG: Notfalltherapie. Berlin – Heidelberg – New York: Springer: 233-245
5. Morris DL, Hawker PC, Brearley S, Simms M, Dykes PW, Keighley MRB (1984) Optimal timing of operation for bleeding peptic ulcer: prospective randomized trial. Br Med J: 288: 1277-1280
6. Read RC, Huebl HD, Thal AP (1970) Randomized study of massive bleeding from peptic ulceration. Ann Surg 162: 561
7. Beckly DE, Casebow MP (1986) Prediction of rebleeding from peptic ulcer. Experience with an endoscopic doppler device. Gut 27: 96-99
8. Watkins RM, Dennison AR, Collin J (1984) What has happened to perforated peptic ulcer? Br J Surg 71: 586
9. Jørgensen TG (1977) Drug consumption before perforation of peptic ulcer. Br J Surg 64: 247
10. Muscroft TJ, Deane SA (1982) Prevention of sepsis in gastroesophageal surgery. World J Surg 6: 293-300
11. Sawyers JL, Herrington J, Mulheim JL, Whitehead WA, Mody B, Marsh J (1975) Acute perforated duodenal ulcer. Arch Surg 110: 527
12. Boey J, Lee NW, Koo J, Lam PHM, Wong J, Ong GB (1982) Immediate definitive surgery for perforated duodenal ulcer. Ann Surg 196: 338-344
13. Sherlock DJ, Holl-Allen RT (1982) Duodenal ulcer perforation whilst on cimetidine therapy. Br J Surg 143: 90-93
14. Weiland D, Dunn D, Humphrey E, Schwarz M (1982) Gastric outlet obstruction in peptic ulcer disease. Am J Surg 143: 90-93
15. Lunde OC, Liavag I, Roland M (1985) Proximal gastric vagotomy and pyloroplasty for duodenal ulcer with pyloric stenosis: A thirteen-year experience. World J Surg 9: 165-170

The Efficacy of Prostaglandins in the Prevention of Stress Lesions in the Critically Ill Patient

R. SCHIESSEL

Introduction

Acute stress lesions of the stomach and duodenum are epithelial defects of the mucosa reaching to the lamina propria or submucosa. The mucosal defects can either appear as multiple small erosions or single large ulcerations. The development of such lesions usually occurs within a few hours after severe burns, polytrauma, major operations, apoplexia, and sepsis. We know from prospective studies with routine endoscopy that the incidence of stress lesions ranges between 80% and 100% in burns, polytrauma, major operations, apoplexia and sepsis (Table 1) [3, 9, 10, 19, 21]. Acute stress lesions are still a serious threat to a severely ill patient because complications such as bleeding and perforation are common. The mortality from the established complication is very high when the severely ill patient suffers from an additional problem.

Table 1. Incidence of stress lesions: prospective studies with routine endoscopy

Author		Patients	*(n)*	Mucosal lesion (%)	Bleeding (%)
Czaja et al.	[3]	Burns	32	86	22
Schiessel et al.	[19]	Polytrauma	38	97	42
Le Gall et al.	[10]	Sepsis	14	100	68
Kitamura and Ho	[9]	Apoplexia	177	52	19
Schiessel et al.	[21]	Renal transplant	28	28	7

The pathophysiology of these lesions has been investigated intensively in recent years. The definition of the protective mechanisms of the gastric and duodenal mucosa has shown that a major cause of the development of stress lesions is the impairment of the protective mechanisms; it is not an overproduction of acid. Since treatment of bleeding lesions is difficult and often unsuccessful, the prophylaxis in high – risk patients has been established for many years. Theoretically, there are two possibilities by which to perform stress ulcer prophylaxis:

a) to reduce acid with H_2 blockers or antacids;

b) to stimulate the protective mechanisms with prostaglandins and related compounds.

Clinical Trials

There have been several clinical trials in the development of an effective stress ulcer prophylaxis. The first series of trials compared the effect of antacids versus placebo (Table 2). In 1976 McAlhany [13] and in 1978 Hastings [8] showed a significant reduction in the frequency of stress ulcer bleeding in burn patients and intensive care patients, respectively. In another series of trials cimetidine was tested versus placebo (Table 3). McDougall [15] showed a significant reduction in the bleeding frequency of patients with liver failure, Halloran [7] a reduction of bleeding frequency in brain trauma, Lorenz [12] in polytrauma. A trial by my group in renal transplantations showed no effect [20]. A further series of trials compared cimetidine versus antacids (Table 4). McElwee [14], Stothert [24], and Martin [16] showed no difference between cimetidine and antacids in the frequency of bleeding. Only a study by Priebe [18] has shown a significantly lower bleeding frequency in the antacid group. A trial by Zinner [26] on intensive care patients also showed a better result with antacids than with cimetidine or placebo (Table 5). In a similar trial by Basso [1] cimetidine and antacids showed no difference, but were much better than placebo.

Table 2. Antacids vs. placebo

Author	Patients	*(n)*	Bleeding
McAlhany et al. [13]	Burns	A 24	1*
		P 24	6*
Hastings et al. [8]	ICU	A 51	2*
		P 49	12*

* $P < 0.05$; A antacids; P placebo

Table 3. Cimetidine vs. placebo

Author	Patients	*(n)*	Bleeding	ML (%)	Dose (g)
McDougall et al. [15]	Liver failure	C 26	1	–	2.4
		P 24	13*		
Halloran et al. [22]	Brain injury	C 26	5	18	1.8
		P 24	18*	21	
Silvestri et al. [22]	Brain injury	C 10	0	0	1.0
		P 10	0	70*	
Lorenz et al. [12]	Polytrauma	C 14	0	–	1.2
		P 14	5*	–	–
Schiessel et al. [21]	Renal transplant	C 27	3	27	1.6
		P 28	2	28	

* $P < 0,05$; C, cimetidine; P, placebo; ML, mucosal lesions

Table 4. Cimetidine vs. antacids

Author		Patients	(n)	Bleeding	ML (%)	Dose
McElwee et al.	[14]	Burns	C 13	0 *	30	1.6 g
			A 14	0	79**	15 ml/h
Stothert et al.	[24]	ICU	C 65	1 *	–	1.2 g
			A 58	0	–	30–60 ml/h
Martin et al.	[16]	ICU	C 40	3 *	–	1.8 g
			A 37	2	–	60 ml/h
Priebe et al.	[18]	ICU	C 38	7	–	1.2–2.4 g
			A 37	0**	–	30–120 ml/h

* NS; ** $P < 0.05$; C cimetidine; A antacids; ML mucosal lesions

Table 5. Cimetidine vs. antacid vs. placebo

Author		Patients	(n)	Bleeding	Dose
Basso et al.	[1]	ICU	C 44	0*	0.8 g
			A 44	1*	10 ml/h
			P 49	8	–
Zinner et al.	[26]	ICU	C 100	14	1.2 g
			A 100	5*	10–40 ml/h
			P 100	20	–

* $P < 0.05$; C cimetide; A antacid; P placebo

From these studies we learned that antacids, and also cimetidine and ranitidine, reduced the incidence of stress ulcer bleeding in comparison to placebo. However, several problems have been found to be associated with increasing the pH of the gastric contents. It has been shown that the reduction of H ions in gastric juice leads to bacterial contamination of the gastric juice which is in a linear correlation with the pH [17]. This means that the higher the pH, the higher is the bacterial count in the stomach. In addition, it has been shown that bacteria found in the stomach can also be cultivated from the tracheal-bronchial tree. From this it has been implicated that a gastrobronchial reflux in intensivercare patients may lead to severe pulmonary infections. Another problem associated with cimetidine was the finding that the mental status of intensive care patients was worse in cimetidine-treated patients than in patients not treated with cimetidine. It was hypothesized that this occurs because cimetidine crosses the blood brain barrier.

Results

Since the principle of reducing gastric acidity has its potential hazards, it seemed likely that prostaglandins in a dose which does not reduce gastric acidity might be more useful for stress ulcer prophylaxis. The theoretical advantages of prostaglandins are:

1. Gastric pH unchanged, therefore no bacterial contamination
2. Stimulating protective mechanisms
3. Experimental data showing protection of gastric mucosa against various damaging agents (cytoprotection)

There numerous experimental data available showing that prostaglandins stimulate alkaline secretion of the stomach and duodenum, stimulate mucus secretion, and increase the pH gradient between the gastric lumen and the mucosal surface [5. 6]. In addition, prostaglandins probably have an effect in stabilizing intracellular pH [20]. It has also been shown that prostaglandins protect the gastric mucosa against injury by alcohol and high acid concentrations, etc., when given shortly before the damaging agent was applied. Although there were some doubts about the extent of mucosal protection, the phenomenon of cytoprotection has been observed by many authors in different species.

It seemed that prostaglandins applied topically should be the ideal agent for stress ulcer prophylaxis. At present there are data available from several studies. In 1984 Skillman [23] published a study on intensive care patients comparing 15,15-PM-PGE_2 with antacid (Table 6). The result was disappointing, showing that antacid was much better than prostaglandins. In 1985 appeared two studies comparing PGE_2 versus placebo (Table 7). Van Essen [4] showed no difference in the incidence of bleeding between PGE_2 and placebo. Levine [11] used prostaglandins in gastric bleeding mainly from erosions. There was no difference between placebo and 15,15-DM-PGE_2. Thus,

Table 6. PGE_2 vs. antacid

Author	Patients	(n)	Bleeding	Dose/24 h
Skillman et al. [23]	ICU	PGE_2 24	12*	15, 15-DM-PGE_2 100 μg i.g. 6 ×
		A 22	3*	Mylanta II 30 ml/h

* $P < 0.0008$; ** pH > 3.5; A antacid

Table 7. PGE_2 vs. placebo

Author		Patients	(n)	Bleeding	Dose/24 h
Van Essen et al.	[4]	ICU	PGE_2 29 P 28	9* 13*	PGE_2 0.5 mg i.g. 6 ×
Levine et al.	[11]	Gastric Bleeding	PGE_2 32 stop P 28	11* 13*	15, 15-DM-PGE_2 50 μg i.g. 4 ×

* NS

Table 8. Sucralfate vs. antacid, cimetidine

Author		Patients	*(n)*	Bleeding	Dose/24 h
Borrero et al.	[2]	ICU	S 80	3 *	1 g 4×
			A 75	2	30–60 ml/h
					pH > 3.5
Tryba et al.	[25]	ICU	S 34	0	1 g 6×
			A 33	2 **	50 g Pirenzepine
			C 33	2	2 g

* NS; ** NS; S sucralfate; A antacid; C cimetidine

until now there has been no study showing that PGE is effective in stress ulcer prophylaxis. Recently trials were conducted with sucralfate, a substance that stimulates prostaglandin biosynthesis (Table 8). In 1985 Borrero [2] published a study comparing antacid with sucralfate showing no difference between sucralfate and antacid. Tryba [25] compared sucralfate, antacid, and cimetidine which showed no difference between the three groups undergoing a basic therapy with pirenzepine.

Summary

In summary, at the present time there are no data showing an effect of prostaglandins in stress ulcer prophylaxis. Sucralfate seems to be as effective as antacid or cimetidine in preventing bleeding from stress ulceration. Whether this is due to prostaglandin biosynthesis or another effect of the drug is uncertain. We might hypothesize why prostaglandins do not work in stress ulcer prophylaxis:

1. The right compound has not been found
2. The prostaglandin is only cytoprotective when given before the lesion is established; in intensive care patients the compound is given too late
3. For stress ulcer prophylaxis a drug has to favor rapid epithelial repair. This is achieved by increasing the luminal pH rather than by prostaglandins.

References

1. Basso N, Bagarani M, Materia A, Fiorani S, Lunardi P, Speranza V (1981) Cimetidine and antacid prophylaxis of acute upper gastrointestinal bleeding in high risk patients. Am J Surg 141 : 339–341
2. Borrero E, Bank S, Margolis I, Schulman ND, Chardavoyne R (1986) Comparison of antacid and sucralfate in the prevention of gastrointestinal bleeding in patients who are critically ill. Am J Medicine 7 (suppl 2C): 62–64
3. Czaja AJ, McAlhany JC, Pruitt BA (1974) Acute gastroduodenal disease after thermal injury. An endoscopic evaluation of incidence and natural history. N Engl J Med 291 : 925–929
4. van Essen HA, van Blankenstein M, Wilson JHP, van den Berg B, Bruining HA (1985) Intragastric prostaglandin E_2 and the prevention of gastrointestinal hemorrhage in ICU patients. Critical Care Medicine 13 : 957–960
5. Flemström G, Garner A (1982) Gastroduodenal HCO_3-transport: characteristics and proposed role in acidity regulation and mucosal protection. Am J Physiol 242: G183–193

6. Flemström G, Kivilaakso E (1983) Demonstration of a pH gradient at the luminal surface of rat duodenum in vivo and its dependence on mucosal alkaline secretion. Gastroenterology 84: 787–794
7. Halloran LG, Zfass AM, Gayle WE, Wheeler CB, Miller JD (1980) Prevention of acute gastrointestinal complications after severe head injury: A controlled trial of cimetidine prophylaxis. Am J Surg 139: 44–48
8. Hastings PR, Skillmann JJ, Bushnell LS, Silen W (1978) Antacid titration in the prevention of acute gastrointestinal bleeding. A controlled randomized trial in 100 critically ill patients. N Engl J Med 298: 1041–1045
9. Kitamura T, Ho K (1976) Acute gastric changes in patients with acute stroke. Part 1: With reference to gastroendoscopic findings. Stroke 7: 460–463
10. Le Gall JR, Mignon FC, Rapin M, Radjeni M, Harasi A, Bader JP, Soussy CJ (1976) Acute gastroduodenal lesion related to severe sepsis. Surg Gynecol Obstet 142: 377–380
11. Levine BA, Sirinek KR, Gaskill HV (1985) Topical prostaglandin E_2 in the treatment of acute upper gastrointestinal tract hemorrhage. A prospective, randomized, double-blind study. Arch Surg 120: 600–604
12. Lorenz W, Fischer M, Rhode H, Troidl H, Reimann HJ, Obmann C (1980) Histamine and stress ulcer: New components in organizing a sequential trial on cimetidine prophylaxis in seriously ill patients and definition of a special group at risk (severe polytrauma). Klin Wochenschr 58: 653–665
13. McAlhany JC, Jr, Czaja AJ, Pruitt BA (1976) Antacid control of complications from acute gastroduodenal disease after burns. J Trauma 16: 645–649
14. McElwee HP, Sirinek KR, Levine BA (1979) Cimetidine affords protection equal to antacids in prevention of stress ulceration following thermal injury. Surgery 86: 620–625
15. McDougall BRD, Bailey RJ, Williams R (1977) H_2-receptor antagonists and antacids in the prevention of acute gastrointestinal hemorrhage in fulminant hepatic failure. Two controlled trials. Lancet 1: 617–619
16. Martin LF, Max MH, Polk HC,Jr (1980) Failure of gastric pH control by antacids or cimetidine in the critically ill: a valid sign of sepsis. Surgery 88: 59–66
17. Moulin GC,du, Patenson DG, Hedley-White J, Lisbon A (1982) Aspiration of gastric bacteria in antacid-treated patients: a frequent cause of postoperative colonisation of the airway. Lancet I: 242–245
18. Priebe HJ, Skillmann JJ, Bushnell LS, Lang PC, Silen W (1980) Antacid versus cimetidine in preventing acute gastrointestinal bleeding. A randomized trial in 75 critically ill patients. N Engl J Med 302: 426–430
19. Schiessel R, Deisenhammer N, Opitz A, Dinstl K, Poigenfürst J, Voill M, Sporn P (1978) Stressveränderungen des Magens und Duodenums bei Mehrfachverletzten. Ergebnis einer prospektiven Studie. Kongressbericht der Österr.Ges.f.Chirurgie, Wayand E and Brücke P eds, Egermann Verlag Wien, pp 53–56
20. Schiessel R, Matthews J, Barzilai A, Merhav A, Silen W (1980) PGE stimulates gastric chloride transport: Possible key to cytoprotection. Nature 283: 671–673
21. Schiessel R, Starlinger M, et al (1981) Failure of cimetidine to prevent gastroduodenal ulceration and bleeding after renal transplantation. Surgery 90: 456–458
22. Silvestri N, Curzio M, Motta M, Pletrio P,de, Bonanzina F, Minoja G (1980) Cimetidine to prevent stress ulcers. Lancet I: 885
23. Skillmann JJ, Lisbon A, Long PC, Silen W (1984) 15(R)-25-Methyl-prostaglandin E_2 does not prevent gastrointestinal bleeding in seriously ill patients. Am J Surg 147: 451–455
24. Stothert JC, Simonowitz DA, Dellinger EP, et al (1980) Randomized prospective evaluation of cimetidine and antacid control of gastric pH in the critically ill. Ann Surg 192: 169–174
25. Tryba M, Zervounov F, Torok M, Zenz M (1986) Prevention of acute stress bleeding with sucralfate, antacids, or cimetidine. Am J Med 79 (suppl 26): 55–61
26. Zinner MJ, Zuidema GD, Smith PL, Mignosa M (1981) The prevention of upper gastrointestinal tract bleeding in patients in an intensive care unit. Surg Gyn Obstet 153: 214–220

Discussion Following this Section

K. H. HOLTERMÜLLER

HOLTERMÜLLER

Dr. Langman, in view of your results, is there a need for similiar surveillance studies with other drugs?

LANGMAN

The answer is yes and no. Regulatory authorities will ask for this type of studies but it might be difficult in the long run to interpret whether an illness is caused by a drug or not.

TOME

What is the clinical course of duodenal ulcer disease treated in the acute phase with bismuth?

LANGMAN

The relapse pattern is slower. The explanation for this is not clear; it could be related to a bismuth-induced clearance of *Campylobacter*. It may then take some time for the Bacteria to come back.

HOLTERMÜLLER

What is the indication for maintenance therapy in ulcer disease?

LANGMAN

In general it is not done in the four centers mentioned (Nottingham, Oxford, Portsmouth and Glasgow). You can produce respectable arguments for maintenance therapy in people who are over 60 years old and have had episodes of bleeding. The important question in deciding about surgery in ulcer disease is, can we define a group of patients early on who we do or don't wish to operate on after 60 years of age? It looks to me from the pattern of appearance of ulcer disease in the UK that a high proportion of patients who are turning up at the age of 70 have new ulcers.

SCHUMPELICK

If we do not perform elective surgery in ulcer disease we may be postponing surgery in some patients until a later time in life – when they possibly run a higher risk in undergoing surgery. Some ulcers seen in older persons may be truly new ulcers, but there is a distinct group of patients who will still be developing ulcers in old age after 30 years of ulcer disease.

SCHIESSEL

In our unit we too operate on an increasing number of complications of longstanding ulcer disease like gastric outlet obstruction. These observations make it necessary to evaluate the longterm efficacy of maintenance therapy in ulcer disease. Especially in patients with complications of ulcer disease, like bleeding, which are the criteria for surgery?

FARTHMANN

For example, in ulcer bleeding, one of the important factors in deciding about surgery is the intensity of bleeding, as measured by the number of units of blood needed to compensate for the loss. Furthermore, there is a high risk of early rebleeding (30%) in these patients. To achieve good surgical results it is necessary to operate on these patients prior to their second bleeding episode.

SCHUMPELICK

In regard to maintenance therapy, it seems to me that there is no consensus among physicians when and how to do it.

FARTHMANN

But this is a general problem relating to what is called the process of medical decision making. We have to establish clearly outlined rules for the management of our patients, realizing that with new data being available we might have to modify our rules.

COHEN

Most surgeons operate now on elderly patients because of complications of ulcer disease. In these cases in my opinion parietal cell vagotomy (PGV) cannot be the operation of choice any more.

SCHUMPELICK

The goal of surgery is the reduction of acid secretion, and this can be achieved in the majority of patients by PGV.

FARTHMANN

PVG will reduce acid secretion, and is an effective surgical therapy for duodenal ulcer disease. However, since not many patients are referred to surgery we have a situation where we have a solution for a problem but we have to search for the problem.

WALAN

Surgery will not cure ulcer disease and, just like the disease itself, all surgical procedure will have some mortality. Considering this, I have chosen the approach of first treating patients with ulcer disease medically.

FRITSCH

Do we have sufficient epidemiological data to support this conclusion even in young patients with duodenal ulcer disease?

WALAN

We have only few studies examinig the natural course of ulcer disease. In the longterm trial over 3 years with 1800 patients there was a very low complication rate with regard to bleeding: one in 173 years of treatment.

HOLTERMÜLLER

The question to be answered is not "Maintenance therapy or surgery?" But can we define subgroups of patients with ulcer disease who might benefit more from early surgery than from longterm medical therapy?

FARTHMANN

I agree that ulcer disease is a heterogeneous disease and we have to find ways to analyse this heteogeneity in view of the therapeutic needs.

HALTER

It has been claimed that antacid titration is the treatment of choice in preventing stress ulcer formation and bleeding from these lesions. In a preliminary study we assessed a low-dose antacid regimen and ranitidine in the prophylaxis of stress bleeding and found no difference between the regimens.

SCHIESSEL

If an intragastric pH of 3.5 is reached with a low-dose antacid regimen, this may be sufficient, since the gastric acid secretion of the severely ill patient is not very high.

SZABO

To evaluate the efficacy of prostaglandins, I think that prostaglandins should be given prior to the development of stress lesions. Such a study might be possible in renal transplant patients, for instance.

COHEN

Stress ulcer is nowadays a rare lesion and the mucosal injury is by and large of little clinical significance. So far prostaglandins have not been shown to be very effective in preventing stress lesions.

WEIHRAUCH

Strengthening the defense mechanism may be one approach to reduce gastric mucosal lesions when aspirin is being taken. One other way might be to give buffered aspirin compounds or enteric coated preparations.

WALAN

I agree with your point completely.

HALTER

You suggested that complete inhibition of acid secretion will reduce gastric mudosal lesions induced by non-steroidal anti-inflammatory drugs (NSAID).

WALAN

I do not as yet have any data on the effect of omeprazole in regard to prophylaxis against gastrointestinal damage by NSAID. I guess omeprazole will decrease the mucosal damage as well as the bleeding.

HOLTERMÜLLER

Thank you, Dr. Walan.

Subject Index

GPSR Compliance

The European Union's (EU) General Product Safety Regulation (GPSR) is a set of rules that requires consumer products to be safe and our obligations to ensure this.

If you have any concerns about our products, you can contact us on ProductSafety@springernature.com

In case Publisher is established outside the EU, the EU authorized representative is:

Springer Nature Customer Service Center GmbH
Europaplatz 3
69115 Heidelberg, Germany

Batch number: 10704771

Printed by Printforce, the Netherlands